Rewarding Specialties
for Mental Health Clinicians

THE CLINICIAN'S TOOLBOX
A Guilford Series

Edward L. Zuckerman, *Series Editor*

Breaking Free of Managed Care: A Step-by-Step Guide to Regaining Control of Your Practice
Dana C. Ackley

The Essential Guide to Group Practice in Mental Health:
Clinical, Legal, and Financial Fundamentals
Simon H. Budman and Brett N. Steenbarger

Outcomes and Incomes: How to Evaluate, Improve, and Market Your Psychotherapy Practice
by Measuring Outcomes
Paul W. Clement

Treatment Plans and Interventions for Depression and Anxiety Disorders
Robert L. Leahy and Stephen J. Holland

Clinician's Thesaurus, 5th Edition: The Guidebook for Writing Psychological Reports
Edward L. Zuckerman

Clinician's Electronic Thesaurus, Version 5.0:
Software to Streamline Psychological Report Writing
Edward L. Zuckerman

The Paper Office, 3rd Edition: Forms, Guidelines, and Resources to Make Your Practice Work
Ethically, Legally, and Profitably
Edward L. Zuckerman

Rewarding Specialties for Mental Health Clinicians: Developing Your Practice Niche
Rona L. LoPresti and Edward L. Zuckerman

The Insider's Guide to Mental Health Resources Online: 2004/2005 Edition
John M. Grohol

Rewarding Specialties for Mental Health Clinicians

DEVELOPING YOUR PRACTICE NICHE

Rona L. LoPresti, PhD
Edward L. Zuckerman, PhD

THE GUILFORD PRESS
New York   London

© 2004 The Guilford Press
A Division of Guilford Publications, Inc.
72 Spring Street, New York, NY 10012
www.guilford.com

Printed in the United States of America

This book is printed on acid-free paper.

Last digit is print number: 9 8 7 6 5 4 3 2 1

Library of Congress Cataloging-in-Publication Data

LoPresti, Rona L.
    Rewarding specialties for mental health clinicians: developing your practice
niche / Rona L. LoPresti, Edward L. Zuckerman.
        p.   cm. — (The clinician's toolbox)
    Includes bibliographical references and index.
    ISBN 1-57230-934-2
    1. Mental health personnel—Vocational guidance.   I. Zuckerman, Edward L.
II. Title.   III. Series.
    RC440.8.L57 2004
    616.89′023—dc21
                                                                    2003010340

To Mario
with a grateful heart
—RLL

To Joan
for her endless support through all my career changing
—ELZ

About the Authors

Rona L. LoPresti earned a master's in clinical psychology from Fairleigh Dickinson University and a PhD from New York University in community psychology. In addition to 25 years in private practice, she has learned about practice opportunities through working with businesses, law enforcement agencies, partial hospitalization programs, and community mental health agencies.

Edward L. Zuckerman earned his PhD in clinical psychology from the University of Pittsburgh. He has experience in many work settings, including community mental health centers, psychiatric hospitals, and consultation to general hospitals; state institutions for adults with mental retardation; and (for many years) the independent practice of general clinical psychology and the teaching of college psychology classes.

Contents

Introduction

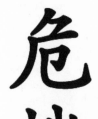 Together the two Chinese characters to the left represent "crisis." Individually, the top character means "danger," and (this is the point) the bottom one means "opportunity." We believe that "crisis" accurately represents the present state of professional psychology in the United States. There is no clinician who cannot name half a dozen major threats facing our profession. But seeing the opportunities is harder. Helping you see them is what this book is about. We offer the information you need to evaluate dozens of opportunities for you to put psychology to work helping people. These opportunities are supported by research and clinical literature; they do not require major reeducation; and they will enable you to utilize your skills and experience, do worthwhile work, and make a living.

The U.S. federal government is enthusiastic about the future of psychologists. The Occupational Outlook Handbook (2000–2001 online edition) says this about the "Job Outlook for Psychologists":

> Employment of psychologists is expected to grow faster than the average for all occupations through the year 2005. The need to combat alcohol and drug abuse, marital strife, family violence, crime, and other problems plaguing society should stimulate employment growth. Other factors spurring demand for psychologists include increased emphasis on mental health maintenance in conjunction with the treatment of physical illness and public concern for the development of human resources, including the growing elderly population and children in school. (Bureau of Labor Statistics, 2000)

The American Psychological Association (APA) convened a task force on future roles for psychological practitioners, and reached similar conclusions (Levant et al., 2001). We believe that the future is not dim. It is not one of

1

shrinking opportunities, of cutthroat competition between therapists, of retreat to a few safe places to survive for a few years. It is absolutely filled with opportunities.

You might ask, "If they are so wonderful, why haven't my colleagues and I heard about them?" Well, you probably have heard of some. For these, we offer specifics to help you explore them and decide whether you want to pursue them. But the better answer to your not knowing of them lies in a fuller understanding of ecology. We don't mean recycling paper or saving the whales (both noble efforts), but a different concept—that of "niches."

Let me (ELZ) tell you a story. I moved to a rural area 8 years ago and thought a pond would look nice, so I had a dank hole dug out, and soon I had my "pond." It was just a big, lifeless, clay-lined puddle at first. Some passing ducks came down, cruised around, dug up the sides, and left. As I looked out, I didn't like the view of the large black overflow pipes sticking out of the bank, and I decided to use several hundred medium-sized round rocks I had acquired (interesting story, but no space for it here) to conceal them. In a few hours I had placed them along on the bank and in the water, extending 10 feet on either side of the pipes. I liked the "natural" look and thought no more about them. A month later, while walking along, I saw motion on these rocks. Kneeling down, I saw a hundred little fish. New life had come to my pond! Later I learned that the ducks had brought eggs of many creatures on their feet and feathers. But these eggs and the small fish that hatched from them would quickly have been eaten if the larger space in the pond had not been subdivided by my rocks. The rocks created a special place in which they could survive—an ecological niche. Now there are many fish. My daughter feeds them each night; they follow in the water as she walks around the shore; and a great blue heron has made its home here because of the fish supply.

The same process is occurring in our professional world and has been going on for a long time. As each professional task or skill becomes more widely available, better understood, or more greatly valued, it grows and allows specializations—niches—to occur. Five hundred years ago there were only midwives, barber-surgeons, and bone setters; then there were physicians and dentists; the body hasn't changed, but now we have a hundred kinds of health care specialists. Why? Because knowledge and skills increased so greatly that no one could know it all, and specialists and specializations did a better job of meeting human needs.

We psychologists learn skills that have universal applicability. Does any human activity not have psychological aspects? Applied clinical psychology is barely 50 years old, and the time of the psychological generalist has passed. We must specialize to continue our mission of helping people and to survive as a profession. This book is simply about some of those specializations.

SPECIALIZATION AS EVOLUTION

The report of my death was an exaggeration.
—Psychology[1]

Advances in our scientific knowledge base occur in numerous but circum-scribed areas. The old witticism is accurate: We know more and more about less and less. This expansion of knowledge has resulted in improved out-comes with specific disorders treated with well-defined methods in specific populations. In addition, social, cultural, and demographic changes are con-tinually creating new needs, new demands, and thus new opportunities to improve our services and help us stand out from the crowd of generalist practitioners. Among the important changes that have influenced practice in recent times are these:

- The aging of the population.
- Greater numbers of women in the workplace.
- Delayed childbearing.
- An increase in the nondisabled lifespan.
- An orientation toward health, wellness, and prevention.
- A greater appreciation of the effects of stress on health and quality of life.

The combined forces of social change and refinement of our knowledge base have already had an impact upon the practice of psychotherapy. Improved understanding of disorders, the development of targeted treatments, greater sophistication among client populations, their demands for tailored services, and the industrialization of health care are exerting powerful pressures that are leading to the gradual extinction of the generalist therapist.[2] Some popu-lar but now generic specializations, such as testing and assessment or family therapy, have lost their perceived value and have produced a progeny of subspecialty areas. In the area of testing/assessment, just a few subspecial-ties include neuropsychological assessment; fitness-for-duty assessment; culture-fair assessment; presurgical evaluations for cosmetic or transgen-der surgeries; various forensic assessments; and assessments for children thought to have special gifts, learning disabilities, autistic-spectrum disor-ders, or attention-deficit/hyperactivity disorder (ADHD). In the family ther-apy realm, there are interventions for stepfamilies; interracial and interreli-gious families; families of children with disabilities; families of various ethnicities; gay and lesbian families; families of conduct-disordered, violent,

---

[1]With thanks to Mark Twain, who made the remark originally.
[2]The only remaining exceptions to this are in geographical areas with very few service provid-ers or some other unusual situation.

and/or suicidal youth; caregivers; siblings; families including a member with substance abuse or severe and persistent mental illness; families of divorce; families seeking enrichment; survivors of suicide; and many more.

Indeed, it is clear that the age of specialist practice is already upon us. Until recently, it was a rarity to encounter a practitioner of pediatric neuropsychology; infant or adolescent mental health work; psycho-oncology; exercise and sport psychology; geropsychology; ethnic minority interventions; psychological autopsy; organ transplantation, infertility, or genetic counseling; presurgical pain management training; treatment for motor-vehicle-accident-related posttraumatic stress disorder (PTSD); executive coaching; or even the now ubiquitous treatment for ADHD. Today specialists are sought out by clients who perceive value in the targeted interventions they can offer.

Because of these developments, Perrott (1998) advises psychologists to move in the direction of effective services for narrower niche markets and newly defined market segments: " . . . psychologists must now excel at marketing, creating, and delivering outstanding new services that bring demonstrable value to their consumers. Innovating psychotherapy-derived approaches that create the best total solutions for resolving client issues will be psychology's preferred positioning choices. Shifting paradigms to become a more customer-based, market-driven profession is the best means of repositioning applied psychology" (p. 173).

Likewise, Heller (1997) recommends specializing, particularly for the solo practitioner for very practical reasons: "The rule of thumb is that the smaller you are, the more you need to specialize. In a small business you don't need so many referrals, promotion is more efficient . . . and, once established, you can often charge premium prices because you have established yourself as an expert" (p. 52).

Whether you are just starting out or have been in general practice for some time, the strategy of focusing your energies on specializing in underserved or new practice arenas will help you to adapt to the trends that are eroding the foothold of the generalist practitioner. Just to survive and certainly to flourish, you need to add specialized practice areas to your repertoire of offerings—and these should be in areas such as the ones described in this book, where there is demand but not yet an oversupply of practitioners.

You don't need to abandon your current practice entirely. In addition to specializing within traditional clinical psychology, consider diversifying your practice outside the areas defined by this tradition (i.e., the "treatment" of "patients" or "clients" in line with a medical model). Such areas could be consulting with businesses, wellness applications, or forensics. According to Zur (2000), we can learn from dentists and auto mechanics:

> We need to educate people and ourselves that they do not need to be sick or broken in order to seek our services. Frequently, this is surprising news to consumers and therapists alike. . . . Dentists have their cleaning and check-up reminder postcards, and car mechanics have their oil change and tune-up routine. They should be our guides in helping people view our professional services as on-going and preventative, rather than exclusively reactive and crisis oriented. (p. 30)

That is what this book is about: where and how you can refocus your efforts by carefully choosing a few promising specialty areas where you can use your talents, do good work, benefit your clients, and make a decent living.

Where We Looked for Specializations

The specialized niches presented in this book were drawn from many types of research and observations. For the last 8 years, we have read the following professional literature:

- APA and non-APA psychology journals, and the abstracts in MEDLINE and PsycINFO.
- Practitioner-oriented newsletters and newspapers in the fields of psychology, couple and family therapy, counseling, and psychiatry.
- Professional newsletters, articles, and journals from areas outside our field (such as medicine, business, dentistry, law, social work, nursing, education, and even veterinary science), to discover potential linkages.

To get the varied perspectives of individual practitioners, we did these things:

- Actively participated in a variety of professional Internet lists.
- Attended professional conferences, continuing education workshops, and seminars on current and future practice possibilities.
- Participated in and contributed to APA practice-related divisions and our state psychological associations.
- Interviewed professionals involved in a variety of specialty areas.
- Searched the Internet for psychology-related Web sites, particularly those of practitioners working in niche areas.
- Read books written by people in niche practices.
- Talked to our peers.

To get a sense of professional associations, we did the following:

- Spoke with leaders in the field of psychology, such as presidents and past presidents of APA and of divisions of APA, and of our state psychological associations.
- Participated on boards and committees of divisions of APA and of our state psychological associations.

To sample the larger climate outside of our field, we took these approaches:

- Read the popular press, magazines, and other media both inside and outside our profession on business-related topics, managed care, health care, politics, and so on.
- Systematically surveyed trends in popular self-help topics in magazines and at Amazon.com.
- Subscribed to Internet discussion groups consisting of client groups, such as e-mail lists concerned with learning disabilities, midlife issues, and issues for gifted and talented individuals.
- Subscribed to Internet discussion groups on niche topics, such as creativity, training and development, virtual reality in mental health, technology, and coaching.

After having completed the observations and research described above, and having generated our own list of promising niches (originally 52 niche areas, many with subniches), we learned of a survey of psychologists in independent practice outside managed care (Walfish, 2001). Survey respondents identified 180 activities in which they engaged to diversify their psychotherapy practices. Although this study was restricted to independent non-managed care practice, its results corresponded well with our list of niche and subniche opportunities. We then pared down our list of niches, utilizing the criteria discussed next.

The Criteria We Used to Select Niches

As we came across a specialized kind of professional activity, we evaluated it with the following questions.

Is There a Knowledge Base for This Specialty Area?

As scientifically trained professionals, we want our work to have research support. However, this presents some problems:

- Empirical support varies among the specializations; some interventions have broad-based support, and some have never been evaluated.

- Few of these interventions have been in use long enough to have been thoroughly evaluated.
- Many of the interventions involved in a specialization have never been combined in this fashion before.
- Outcome evaluations for some specializations require methods and resources that are simply unavailable and so have not been performed.
- Researchers are not always interested in conducting research on clinical topics. For example, giftedness, wellness, and positive psychology have been neglected areas of research.
- Certain populations are not adequately represented among research subjects, particularly those we refer to as "underserved" and/or as members of minority groups.
- Even when there is empirical support, effectiveness is not the same as efficacy. What works in the lab may not in the field, and vice versa.
- The practices of individual clinicians may vary, despite their claims to use the same methods with the same population. Even among those using manualized treatment, there is significant variation.

Because of these considerations, we have chosen the following criteria for including niches in this book:

- We have given preference to areas with solid empirical validation of their methods.
- Although a particular intervention may not have been tested empirically, when highly similar or more basic interventions have been shown to be effective, we have assumed that this particular one will be as well. For example:

  —When an intervention is an extension of a supported method to a new population, we have assumed that it will be effective there as well.
  —Where a combination of supported interventions are used in a specialization, we have assumed that the combination will also be as effective as its components.
  —There should not be great controversy about the efficacy or validity of this type of intervention.
  —For some cutting-edge specializations with great need, we have accepted supporting rationales that were simply consistent with clinical experiences.
  —When a body of professionals recognizes the procedures as standard for a specialty, we have adopted those methods as very likely to be later proven valuable.

Are Learning Opportunities, Training, and Supervision Obtainable?

Although thus point may seem obvious, for some areas there are simply no learning opportunities aside from a few practitioners. We haven't required that graduate courses be available for each niche, but we chose niches where clinicians could acquire understanding and skills through the usual channels and could also arrange some kinds of personal training, supervision, or mentoring.

Does the Specialization Provide Autonomy?

We gave extra weighting to any practice area with good possibilities for self-pay clients; with, preferably, low or no managed care penetration or even interest; with few or no bureaucratic controls; and with a good possibility of a decent income. Independence of current or standard referral patterns would be best, but a reliance on other professionals for referral was quite acceptable.

Does the Specialization Provide Satisfactions for Clinicians?

Doing a particular type of work should produce a strong sense of having helped the most needy individuals or having made worthwhile changes in clients' lives. The work may not always be pleasant or exciting, but it should regularly satisfy typical clinicians' most important personal reasons for becoming clinicians.

Does the Specialization Offer a Real Opportunity?

Does a niche serve an undeveloped or underdeveloped market? Are there few competitors; a high demand for services or a large population; and a high awareness of a problem on the part of potential clients, referrers, or other payers?

When we had narrowed the list using these criteria we looked more deeply into each practice specialty. We organized the information we found under headings (see below) that we think are quite comprehensive ways of presenting the information and will make your comparing of different practice specializations much easier.

HOW WE PRESENT INFORMATION ABOUT EACH SPECIALIZATION

This book is intended to help you select and move into one or more specialized areas of practice. To select such an area, you need good-quality information.

We have clustered the specializations within these five broad sections:

Section 1. The Psychological Sides of Medical Illness
Section 2. Couples, Families, Children, and Schools
Section 3. The World of Work
Section 4. Forensics
Section 5. Underserved Populations and Developing Needs

We have placed each specialization in the section where we think most readers would expect to find it. However, because we all have different perspectives and backgrounds, most specializations have cross-references to related ones elsewhere in the book.

We have tried to use a consistent format for each niche. This provides equivalent information in each specialization to assist you in understanding the area's requirements and the nature of the work you would be doing. However, the specializations differ, and so there are cases where the information is organized a little differently. We start each section with an introduction intended to give a broad orientation to the specialized niche that follows. You will find information within each niche organized under the following headings.

Overview and Opportunities

We begin each niche with "Overview and Opportunities," an introduction to the clinical practice. This usually includes background, the activities psychologists currently perform, and some of the goals and value of this work.

Your Potential Satisfactions

There is no benefit in switching to a new practice area if you can only barely survive there, so under "Your Potential Satisfactions" we list the pleasures, excitements, and benefits that we believe you can receive from this kind of work. Since we cannot know your values and preferences, feel free to consider how each specialty might meet other needs of yours and offer additional personal benefits.

Your Skill Set

As we discuss later in this Introduction to the Book, we have assumed that you, our readers, are already competent and well-trained clinicians with many skills that can be of use. We have also assumed that our readers are seeking specializations that do not require major reeducation ("Retooling"), such as taking a postdoctoral internship. Under this heading, we try to answer this question: What skills and knowledge already in your possession can be immediately applied ("Recycling Your Current Competencies") for this specialization? Where more than these skills are needed, we indicate what training, experience, or other resources we believe are needed to practice under this heading and call this "Retreading for Added Skills."

Nature of the Work

For some specializations, we divide the "Nature of the Work" material into the phases of clinical work, "Assessment" and "Treatment." For other specialties, other descriptions (e.g., "Approaches and Techniques") are more appropriate. When there is a wide range of clinical work associated with a specialization, we have organized the work under "Areas of Practice." For example, interventions may vary with different medical diseases or different client types. We also offer "Cross-References to Related Specializations." Full citations for references made in the text can be found at the end of the book. In addition, where niches have "Subspecializations" we describe them as such, since they may be better suited to you or your setting than the more general niche.

Practice Models

In some specializations, clinicians may operate differently than in the usual outpatient practice. Such variations are described under "Practice Models."

Financial Considerations

Under "Financial Considerations," you will find answers to such questions as these: What kinds of financial arrangements are common in this specialization? Who will pay for your services? What are the costs involved in offering these services? We also address managed care's financial (not clinical or procedural) issues here.

Cautions, Ethical Dilemmas, Culture Clashes, and/or Managed Care Issues

Where appropriate, we include a "Cautions . . ." heading to raise issues you should be aware of involving ethics, managed care, interprofessional relations, or other concerns.

Prospects and Prospecting

Under "Prospects and Prospecting," we address four related issues.

Where Is the Need?

Before you devote the time and effort required to enter a field of specialization, you must know whether there is a sufficient need in your community to support your offering such a service. We offer all the information on needs we could obtain from government sources, authorities in the field, and research. Also, where possible, we offer suggestions for how to evaluate the need in your community.

Bear in mind that "need" is not identical with "demand." Therefore, we also consider demand—the ability of various clients to seek out and pay for the services involved—and we present this information when available. We have selected specializations for this book where we believe there will be openings and opportunities for significant numbers of new practitioners.

Competition

If there are need, demand, and opportunity, there also may be many providers—your potential competitors. Here we look at who would be your competitors (if any) and what their credentials and capabilities would be. We have chosen niches either where there is little or no competition, or where we believe psychologists bring unique skills and approaches to the specialization.

Reaching Clients

Here we describe and discuss the means of informing clients of the availability of your services, so that they will self-refer and seek your services. Clinicians often dislike the terms "advertising" and "marketing," but making efforts to be known in a community is essential to independent practice. The challenge is to find ways that build on your strengths and that are effective in your current and developing social networks. How do you recruit clients for your specialization? It can be done by directly contacting them or by making contact with those who would refer clients to you.

Directions for Marketing

Marketing methods that are aimed at other professionals or at the community at large are covered here. Who are the contacts, gatekeepers, and referral sources who will send you clients? How do you join the social networks and spread the word about your availability? What are the most relevant organizations and social groups? What works best for this specialization: advertisements, mailed letters of introduction, brochures, presentations to groups, or other approaches unique to this area? We offer the advice and experience we have gathered personally and from others.

Increasing Your Formal Knowledge Base

Under "Increasing . . . ," we offer the best resources we could find for improving your clinical abilities in each specialization. These resources are categorized by their formats as follows: "Core Readings," "Journals," "Online Resources," "Professional Organizations," "Clinical Tools," "Packaged Programs and/or Franchises," and "Patient Education Materials" (including online resources, printed resources, and organizations).

In the next section of this Introduction to the Book, we support your moving into a more specialized practice by helping you analyze your needs, interests, and resources that form the bases for change, and then begin to narrow the field of opportunities.

WALKING YOUR PATH TO SPECIALIZATION

> *Learning is what most adults will do for a living*
> *in the 21st century.*
> —SIDNEY JOSEPH PERELMAN

A basic tenet of this book is that you can learn how to anticipate practice opportunities by paying attention to changes in your world, starting with yourself.

Your History

Your feelings and experiences can be a source of guidance for the path ahead.

- As an undergraduate, did you have a concentration in another area outside psychology, and can this knowledge and interest be combined with your present expertise in psychology?
- If you are just starting your practice, what courses or topics did you find most interesting in graduate school? On what topics did you choose to write papers? During your internship, what types of clients or problems did you find most absorbing and challenging? What kind of feedback did you get from your supervisors and mentors about your skills and strengths?
- Do you have relevant life experiences that can form the basis for a specialty?

- Do you have an interest, hobby, or avocation that you can combine with clinical work?
- Do you still have, or can you remember when you regularly had, a sense of "mission" and were excited by your work? Which aspects of your work still excite and energize you? Start there and build upon them.
- When you attend a conference, seminar, or continuing education class, which topics are you drawn to? What are the subjects of the books you have read recently? Do these speak to important themes in your life?
- You may already be a specialist. Consider the kinds of clients and problems you see frequently and work with successfully. Can you expand the populations you serve and the range of your services?

Degrees of Preparation

Finding, exploring, and specializing in a niche may require only minor modifications of your way of practicing, or it may require major life and practice changes. In the simplest change, a "recycling" of skills, a clinician continues to use more or less the same skills; however, they might be applied in a different setting or locus of service, on different problems, or with different populations. A larger kind of professional change is what we call "retreading." Here the clinician needs to acquire some specific skills and credentials on top of current ones through programmatic reading, continuing education, and workshop attendance. Lastly, more effort and learning are required to enter some specializations, and so we call this process "retooling"—acquiring a whole set of new tools and mastering them. These types of specializations will require certification, academic coursework, and supervision.

For each specialization in the book, we include information on what kind of preparation is needed to perform it professionally and ethically. We have chosen mostly those that require recycling of clinical skills. Some niches in this book do require more training—retreading. They are included because of their value for the future, for the widening opportunities they offer, or for the expanding population or needs they serve. We have generally not included those requiring retooling, as the resources to make the transition are not widely available to the audience of readers we imagine. Whether you need to recycle, retool, or retread will depend on what skills you already have. We discuss this next.

What Does It Take to Specialize?

This book can help you answer an important question: "What investment of effort and time would be required for me to become a specialist in a particular niche of practice?" This question is a challenge for us to answer, because we believe that you, the readers of this book, vary greatly in terms of the resources you bring to the table. Even among those of you who are licensed doctoral-level psychologists, training and experience vary widely. Theoretical orientation (psychodynamic, cognitive-behavioral, family systems, etc.), coursework, internship experiences, and postgraduate training all make it difficult to come up with generalizations about preparation for particular niches. In addition, for most of the niches we discuss, there are no agreed-upon qualifications conferring specialist status. We see this as a positive state of affairs, in the sense that most of the niches can be entered without completing a formalized training program. This does not mean that no preparation is required, or that any preparation might do—only that you will probably be able to adapt your particular preparation to the niche activities, rather than the reverse process that is often made necessary by certification programs.

In interviewing niche practitioners and in reading the books they have written, we found much information validating our belief that it is not possible to map a singular path to becoming an expert in a particular area. For example, many of the niche practitioners with whom we talked, whose seminars we took, or whose writings we read did not achieve their specialist status through a formalized program (often programs do not exist for the newer niches), but by a patchwork quilt of formal coursework and training, self-study, mentoring and comentoring, supervision, and on-the-job training. We were also impressed by the fact that personal qualities and individual experiences outside of the field of professional practice were often cited as key factors in becoming an expert in a particular niche area.

The question of what is required to become a specialist in a particular area is one that has traditionally been answered by professional boards, by associations, by postgraduate programs, and of course by APA and its divisions. Yet for most of the niches we describe, guidelines have not yet been devised. Even when they are available, they are often flawed: They may be outdated, reflect only a single theory, or be products of the special interests of their promulgators. For a fuller discussion of some of the problems with guidelines, we recommend an article appearing in the *American Psychologist* (Beutler, 2000, p. 1001), which concluded, in part, "Most guidelines are based on the subjective interpretation of research literature by a small number of individuals who serve as authors of books and articles."

Nonetheless, it is axiomatic that specialists in a given area must possess expertise in the subject matter of their specialty area. Therefore we will point you to books, articles, journals, and other resources that will orient you to the niche. We will also point you toward professional organizations, where you may find colleagues who can provide supervision or mentorship.

Your Current Levels of Expertise

Might You Already Be an Expert?

If you are a professional in midlife, it's possible and even likely that you are an expert or at least are well on your way to becoming one. Decades of research have shed light on the qualities or common factors possessed by experts across a variety of fields. We suggest assessing your expertness by these "gold standard" common factors, offered by Meichenbaum and Biemiller (2000). In addition to having an excellent command of the content area, experts have the following qualities:

- They possess knowledge that is organized efficiently and easily retrievable, so that it can be used to identify goals, patterns, and task features and in planning task solutions
- They perform tasks in a deliberate and strategic way that can be thoughtfully monitored on an ongoing basis, and that is highly adaptable to the changing demands of the situation.
- They have the ability to automate some aspects of task performance in order to perform effortlessly. Such aspects of performance are "second nature," so that attention can be directed to other aspects of the task.
- They have the ability to describe their knowledge and processes to instruct others.
- They are put in a consulting role by others.
- They invent new ways of performing tasks.
- They are motivated to persist.
- They are motivated to undertake new challenges.
- They engage in extensive, deliberate, and effortful practice, including self-monitoring.
- They have benefited from a mentorship or apprenticeship with another expert.

Multiple Perspectives and Versatility

Well-trained clinical and counseling psychologists have many skills and have the ability to understand a problem from different perspectives. They know when and why to shift to a different approach. This is an enormously valuable and yet often underappreciated skill—versatility. Your educational background and the efforts you made to achieve it have equipped you to undertake and enjoy lifelong learning, midlife course corrections, exploring, and moving on. Tim Tumlin (personal communication, February 22, 2000) contributed the following (which we use with his permission) to a mailing list discussion of what psychologists do well:

... a broadly trained psychologist can do a good assessment with great testing, write a good report, develop coherent treatment plans, know how to talk to other professionals, manage a difficult and complex case, offer skilled psychotherapy, know about a lot of other therapies and theories when therapy gets stuck, talk research and statistics, keep current on the literature and know how to judge it, be able to analyze his/her own practice and patients and be able to understand them in more dimensions and communicate about them more clearly than anyone else.

Credentials and Training of Our Intended Audience

We have designed this book with several kinds of professionals in mind:

- Newly minted psychologists—that is, recent graduates from PsyD, EdD, and PhD programs in clinical, counseling, and similar applied areas who are about to finish internships and obtain licenses, and who want information and guidance on the realistic opportunities for clinical work because they have been exposed only to conventional and traditional areas of practice.
- Graduate students in doctoral programs who are worried about their futures because they have been told that managed care has killed independent practice, and who hope that this is not true. (It isn't.)
- Seasoned clinicians, licensed and working in the field, who are feeling a little stale or whose practices are shrinking rather than expanding. They are chafing under managed care's strictures and are looking for guidance on where to direct their energies and find inspiration and excitement.

The "Modal Practitioner" Concept

Above, we have described our intended audience in terms of credentials and training. However, in selecting and exploring the specializations we offer in this book, we needed to understand in much more detail what our readers are bringing to the table.

To articulate these strengths, we developed the concept of the "modal practitioner," who possesses a certain core of skills and experiences expected of someone who has completed a good graduate program in clinical or counseling psychology or a closely related area (including an internship), and who is licensed or license-eligible. Such core competencies are listed below, to enable you to understand what we were assuming when we rated the niches in terms of the preparation needed to specialize. If you are not a perfect fit to our modal practitioner, don't stop reading; we believe that specialists come by their expertise in very individualized ways. Also, intangibles such as talents, interests, and personal experiences can elevate the quality of services from "qualified" to "gold standard" (Haber et al., 2000). Furthermore, bear in mind that not every characteristic or quality described is necessary for every specialty.

Core Competencies of the Modal Practitioner: I. Background

- Completing a clinical, counseling, or related doctoral program, and holding or being eligible for a license to practice with adults, children, teens, and/or older adults.
- Knowledge, training, and experience in diagnosis, using the *Diagnostic and Statistical Manual of Mental Disorders*, fourth edition (DSM-IV) and several methods of assessment.
- Knowledge, training, and experience in basic psychological interventions, particularly supportive, expressive, cognitive, and behavioral approaches as utilized in counseling and/or psychotherapy.
- Knowledge, training, and experience in at least some of these: stress management, assertiveness training, communication skills, parenting skills, family dynamics, group dynamics (although not necessarily group "therapy"), grief work, crisis responding, triage, and so on.
- Knowledge, training, and experience in couple treatments.
- Knowledge and training (although not necessarily experience) in substance abuse treatments.
- Being an excellent communicator in at least one of these channels: professional writing or other ways of communicating with other professionals, speaking to the public or other groups, and communicating with patients.
- Knowing how to provide a "climate for growth" for clients.

Core Competencies of the Modal Practitioner: II. Attitudes and Values

In addition to formal training, qualifications, and experience as outlined above, we also assume that you bring the following values, attitudes, and/or interpersonal perspectives to the table:

- Understanding the relevance and importance of very basic therapeutic issues, such as a client's history, trust level, readiness for change, and culture.
- Being ethically sensitive and informed, cognizant of practicing within your areas of competence, aware of boundaries, and protective of clients who do not have clear boundaries.
- Being intellectually curious; being capable and desirous of learning more from mentors, supervisors, role models, teachers, and books.

- Being introspective and aware of the impact that your personal issues can have on a therapeutic relationship.
- Being curious about and interested in others—in your own society and culture, and in the cultures of others.
- Receiving important gratification from helping others.
- Conversely, not wanting to do harm, create dependency, or encourage iatrogenic symptoms.

How well did we describe you? Where did we go wrong? Make some notes in the margins for later consideration.

An Exercise: What Business Are You In?

Because applied psychology training and education over the last 30 years have focused primarily on psychotherapy, psychologists are highly identified with their role as psychotherapists. Their goal is to help others. Many practicing psychotherapists have also had good therapy themselves and want to provide that same valuable experience to others. Because of all this, it is often hard for psychologists to consider role diversification. "As a consequence, decreasing opportunities and decreasing rewards for a career based exclusively on providing outpatient psychotherapy have resulted in a crisis of identity for many practicing psychologists" (Levant et al., 2001, p. 83).

Take a moment: Do you consider yourself to be *primarily* a therapist? A facilitator? A consultant? A psychologist? An entrepreneur? A change agent? A _____? Pick just one now.

Recent history is full of examples of enterprises that defined their business suicidally. The railroad companies were in the business of "running railroads," and missed out on trucking by not defining themselves as "transporters of bulk freight." The Swiss "watchmakers" failed to define themselves as "manufacturers of timepieces" and missed out on the Japanese-made computer clock chip. (Look at your wrist. Does your watch have a battery or a watchspring?) Conversely, companies that have diversified their operations have stayed in business. The Singer Company doesn't just make sewing machines, but manufactures other home products. 3M, a company that mainly made sandpaper and cellophane but encouraged innovation, has made millions of dollars on a glue that doesn't stick very well but is used on Post-it Notes. So do you want to change your answer to the question of "What business are you in?"

Core Competencies of the Modal Practitioner: III. Practice Skills

If you are "only" a therapist, you are being constrained by the shrinking funding for psychotherapy, especially the more traditional types of therapy.

However, if you are a psychologist, you should do fine, because you have learned skills that are highly adaptable. In Figure 1, we list many common skills possessed by practitioners. Consider making several copies of this figure, so that you can rate yourself and also ask others to do so (see below). Take a moment now to rate your proficiency in each.

We often take our already acquired skills for granted, and it therefore might be helpful for you to ask one or more close colleagues, mentors, and/ or supervisors to rate your specific strengths/competencies. Ask each rater to consider your training, talents, and experience and to rate your competency in each function or area. Similarly, since we aren't experts in every niche area, you will benefit from the advice and feedback of a supervisor or mentor who is well versed in the niche and will be able to help you customize your path to becoming a specialist.

Your Unique Resources

Figure 1 lists common skills, but we are all individuals who bring special strengths to our professional work. These can contribute enormously to our becoming specialists. On a separate piece of paper, begin making some notes in response to these questions:

- What uncommon abilities, important values, particular interests, life experience or hobbies, unusual backgrounds, or relationships do you have that might be relevant to your developing a niche practice? For example, did you grow up in a family-owned business?
- Do you have a friend, neighbor, peer, sibling, relative, or spouse/ partner who could provide networking or mentoring opportunities for you?
- Have you had a life experience dealing with a particular problem, such as being a caregiver or overcoming a personal limitation, that you can apply to a particular specialty area?
- Do you have a talent or ability in another area that you can combine with your professional skills to form a specialty area?

THE BASICS OF MARKETING

> *We are continually faced with a series of great opportunities brilliantly disguised as insoluble problems.*
> —JOHN GARDNER

Specialized services require, by definition, marketing of those services. Did you flinch at the word "marketing"? We understand. Lots of us went into private practice expecting to avoid the messiness and compromises of the

RATING OF PRACTICE SKILLS

Name: Rater: Date:

Rating scale:

1—No knowledge or experience in this skill area.
2—Developing capability; some knowledge, ability, or experience.
3—Good command of this skill area.
4—Mastery of this skill area; solid background, experience, ability.
5—Expert.

Practice skill areas:

_____   Assessment and testing

_____   Evaluation, diagnosing, triage

_____   Career counseling

_____   Stress management

_____   Consultation and liaison

_____   Neuropsychology

_____   Child development

_____   Writing and editing

_____   Teaching and training

_____   Supervision

_____   Clinical hypnosis

_____   Ethics issues and consulting

_____   Legal issues and forensics

_____   Medical diseases with psychological aspects

_____   Rehabilitation and physical injuries

_____   Biofeedback

_____   Pain management

_____   Program evaluation and consultation

_____   Drug and alcohol treatment

_____   Team building, project management

_____   Leadership and self-motivation

(continued)

FIGURE 1. A form for rating your practice skills (this can be completed by yourself or by another rater). From *Rewarding Specialities for Mental Health Clinicians* by Rona L. LoPresti and Edward L. Zuckerman. Copyright 2004 by The Guilford Press. Permission to photocopy this figure is granted to purchasers of this book for personal use only (see copyright page for details).

_____   Behavior modification or therapy

_____   Computers and the Internet

_____   Anger management

_____   Crisis assessment and management

_____   Culturally informed, diversity-sensitive assessments, evaluations, and interventions

_____   Psychopharmacology

_____   Communication methods

_____   Relaxation techniques

_____   Mobilizing psychosocial supports and community resources

_____   Negotiation and mediation strategies

Other skill areas or experiences of any kind that may be relevant to specializing (fill in as appropriate):

_____   _____

_____   _____

_____   _____

_____   _____

_____   _____

retail business world. Well, both worlds have changed a lot. Thanks to managed care and the "oversupply" of clinicians it has induced, long gone are the days when hanging out your shingle was enough to direct a steady stream of clients to your door.

On the other hand, there is ethical marketing. Think of it as "reaching out to those in need," "educating the consumers of our services," or "standing out from the crowd of less skilled practitioners." How about "getting the word out," or "not hiding your light under a basket," or even just "offering to provide services"? To practice your profession now, you have to understand and communicate what you have to offer. Today, health care professionals of all stripes avail themselves of the competitive advantage of marketing.

In 1999 the American Medical Association (AMA) and six other "stodgy" medical societies formed the for-profit e-commerce company Medem, whose mission is to help its 27,000 physician members market their practices online (Guglielmo, 2001). The APA now regularly extols the benefits of marketing in its continuing education offerings and convention presentations; the *APA Monitor* regularly offers examples of marketing approaches; and in 1996 the APA Practice Directorate, with Coopers and Lybrand, LLP, published *Marketing Your Practice,* one in a series of publications aimed at helping practitioners adapt to a changing practice environment. The introduction to that book states that "marketing is simply communicating one's skills to potential clients and may be viewed as a process by which a behavioral health practice systematically *determines the needs of its patients and potential patients* and *then develops a plan to meet those needs*" (APA Practice Directorate with Coopers and Lybrand, 1996, p. x; emphasis added). In a foreword by Russ Newman, JD, PhD, executive director of the APA Practice Directorate, the rationale is expanded:

> Informed consumers expect to know enough about the services they seek to feel comfortable that help for their problems will be forthcoming. Third-party payers, whether employers, insurers, or the government, reasonably expect to know what services their beneficiaries will receive and the likelihood that treatment will be clinically effective and cost effective. The success of a psychologist's practice will, in large part, be contingent upon the psychologist's ability to communicate this information to prospective purchasers . . . (APA Practice Directorate with Coopers and Lybrand, 1996, p. vii)

Take a moment to review this logic. Don't these goals seem completely reasonable? Discovering effective ways to discern and meet client needs and to make the public aware of your services is essential to the development, growth, and health of your practice.

Become a Rainmaker

In the practice of law, "rainmaker" is the appellation bestowed on a person who regularly produces new clients for a firm, and without whom the firm's fortunes would be greatly diminished. Without some rainmaking for your practice, all of the fruits of your training and experience—the wonderful skills and valuable services you have cultivated and nurtured—will surely shrivel on the vine.

Although a thorough review of marketing is beyond the scope of this book, the following sections offer some ideas to stimulate your thinking about getting the word out on your practice specialization. Some of the marketing tools we find particularly powerful, easy, inexpensive, and natural for clinicians are described below. Many are simply extensions of our clinical expertise as listeners, evaluators, problem solvers, and helpers. A few "stretch the envelope" and are suggested for the more adventuresome among you.

Marketing Know-How

According to Martin (1996), your clinical experience and training have already given you many of the skills necessary for marketing your services: "There are no better sales skills than the ability to bond, listen, and empathize with a potential client" (p. 69). Intrinsic to your role as a therapist are the processes of listening objectively to the problems of clients, analyzing the possible causes, and creating attainable solutions. These precious skills not only are key to establishing a positive relationship with clients, but will help you to learn about and evaluate the clients' needs, and thus develop and customize your services.

Ready, Set, Communicate

Your enthusiasm for your services and your belief in their efficacy are fundamental to creating positive expectations on the part of clients. Describe the benefits they will receive from you, not your assets, services, or other qualities. Define your services in terms of easily understood, memorable, positive outcomes that potential clients can expect. Rehearse delivering a succinct vision of your business that is accessible to a lay audience.

Do Your Homework: Assessing Client Needs

We have already done some of the legwork for you in choosing and describing the niches, but you need to assess whether a particular niche has a good probability of meeting with success in your particular neck of the woods. This will depend upon many factors, including local need, demand, competition, and payers, as well as other local realities (such as socioeconomic factors, cultural acceptance, and population density). Here are some places to start:

- Spend some time observing trends. The self-help section of your local bookstore or public library can provide information about current areas of concern or interest in your community. What's popular in nonfiction, particularly self-help? The local newspaper can also be a good barometer of concerns. Don't just read the headlines; concerns and interests can be gleaned from the editorial page, the classified ads, community events (such as support group meetings), announcements of public presentations, and the weekly columns. Call-in radio programs can also provide insights about the ways needs are currently formulated and the concerns of those within your practice area.
- If you live in a geographic area that has its own Web portal, information about needs may be available there. What concerns do people express in the discussion groups? What special-interest groups have formed, and what do they tell you about local needs?
- Surf the Web to see the proliferation of local support and discussion groups on psychology topics. Topica (at http://www.topica.com) is a directory of Internet discussion groups with a search function that will allow you to locate discussion lists by keyword. There are others that can search discussion lists by individual messages (e.g., Deja-News, now part of Google.com). Pay particular attention to any discussions that relate to dissatisfactions or obstacles faced by the potential client population. Overcoming these can create a practice niche in itself.
- Get the scoop on your competitors. Start with the Yellow Pages and look under the headings "Counselors," "Psychotherapists," "Psychologists," "Marriage counselors," and "Social workers." If your state psychological association (or related professional groups) publishes membership lists, see what services practices in your area offer in the niche you are considering. Go to the Web sites of practices to see what populations they identify and which kinds of services they offer.
- Make a list of the possible local payers for the niche you are considering. If you are considering concentrating only on self-pay, will the economic conditions in your area support this as a direction? What are the trends in family income and expenses that you feel will support your self-pay niche? Or, if payers are managed care organizations, how would your new services be covered?

- Seek feedback from previous clients. Questionnaires should focus on satisfaction with services, perceived improvements, and unmet needs. Follow up on nonresponders. Use the results to refocus your efforts.

Under each specialization's "Reaching Clients" heading, we provide specific suggestions for marketing. In addition, important information relevant to marketing can be found throughout each niche, especially under these headings:

- "Overview and Opportunities," orienting you to the needs and demands in each niche.
- "Prospects and Prospecting," containing information on potential client populations, competition, and reaching clients that will be useful in designing your marketing strategy.
- "Core Readings," containing information on treatment outcome that can be used to develop marketing materials.

Marketing Strategies: A Sampler

Below is a list of basic methods (you will have heard of some, and you may already do others) to get the word out about your services. Doing more of them will also affirm, reinforce, and articulate your beliefs in your value— always a good experience.

- Create a business card, practice brochure, and/or newsletter that focus on the benefits of your services and supply these to every potential referral source and client. If you have a Web site, make sure to note its address, or uniform resource locator (URL). See Dean (1999) for examples of some approaches to creating practice newsletters.
- Don't miss opportunities to cast a positive light on your practice and to create client enthusiasm. Your office decor; your telephone answering message; your waiting room's magazines; your office's location; your business cards, stationery, and brochures; and your personal appearance are all opportunities to present your services as approachable, accessible, comfortable, and client-centered. Keep your waiting room stocked with information about your practice specialties and other materials of interest to clients. Make the most of your telephone answering machine message. List all of your services on your business cards and stationery. Emphasize benefits, not just features like credentials.
- Follow up every referral, call, question, or other sign of interest by phone, by e-mail, by letter, or in person, and do it in 24 hours or less.

- Track and cultivate your present and past referral sources. Always call and personally thank referral sources for their confidence in you.
- *Ask* for referrals when you speak to any potential referrers. Don't just tell them what you do, but tell them you have openings, would be happy to see any clients, can do evaluations and make recommendations, and so forth. I (ELZ) did a radio show for some years and never got a client to call unless I specifically said I was taking patients.
- Build relationships with physicians. With the permission of your clients, provide feedback to their primary care physicians about your assessment and recommendations, and any other issues of mutual concern regarding the clients.
- Go beyond competency (Grodzki, 1999) to "gold standard" levels (Haber et al., 2000) of capabilities, and be sure to communicate this to potential clients.
- Present and former clients can be your best referral sources, because they are "living proof" of the value of your services and are completely believable. Make sure your clients have access to information on all of your practice offerings. As noted above, your waiting room should have an ample supply of brochures, business cards, and copies of any articles you've written for the public. When terminating treatment with clients, we all mention that we would be happy to see them again if they are in need—but we can also ask them, if they are satisfied with our services, to refer their friends, neighbors, coworkers, and relatives.
- "Give psychology away." Host a screening event for depression, anxiety disorders, or ADHD. A Web site has more information (http://www.mentalhealthscreening.org/reg).
- Create, borrow, or rewrite press releases, or letters to the editor in newspapers that reach your potential clients.
- Offer to write a column for your local paper. Heller (1997) believes that this is one of the most effective marketing techniques. Provide an attractive and professional picture for the publisher.
- Propose stories to reporters at your local newspaper. Members of Division 42 of APA (http://www.division42.org) have access to professionally written letters customizable for these contacts.
- Seek newspaper, radio, or television appearances or interviews. Haber et al. (2000), Lawless (1997), Heller (1997), and Kolt (1999) all provide good ideas on this. Division 46 of APA, Media Psychology, provides excellent resources for those interested in pursuing this avenue. Its Web site (http://www.apa.org/divisions/div46/) contains back copies of its newsletter and instructions on how to join its e-mail list.
- Become active in state and/or national level professional organiza-

tions. As media chair for the New Jersey Psychological Association and Web site editor for Division 42, I (RLL) have been afforded many opportunities to network with individuals who have been helpful to my practice.

- Develop and pay for advertisements in local newspapers or similar media. Many of the books cited here offer suggestions and advice on designing effective ads and campaigns.
- Create a Web site with resources and links. Some ideas from *Psychotherapy Finances* are available at ("Technology: 9 Steps for Building . . . ," 2002).
- Give a course at an adult school on a topic related to your specialty. I (RLL) did this for several years, and this resulted in a steady stream of referrals to my practice.
- Add value to your services. Create lists of recommended books, relaxation resources, community resources on various topics, and so on, and give these to patients and anyone else you think would benefit. Of course, these would be on your stationery.
- Create additional services for clients, so that once you have helped them resolve their initial problem (and built goodwill, trust, and confidence), they can utilize your services to meet different needs.
- Become known in your town through volunteer work. Serve on boards and get to know the movers and shakers. I (RLL) volunteer for crisis counseling, and this has led to great networking opportunities in my town. I have met those who work behind the scenes in town management. Volunteer for community activities that use your psychological expertise and perspectives.
- Speak on psychological topics at civic organizations, schools, churches, and other local groups. For more than 10 years, I (ELZ) presented a 2-hour workshop on overcoming one's fears of rejection to a church-sponsored job-finding club.
- Network through friends, acquaintances, and relatives.
- Initiate conversations with nonpsychologist professionals who might refer clients. Talk to your dentist, lawyer, tax advisor, and others.
- Network with other professionals and business people in formal networking settings such as the Rotary Club and similar civic organizations.
- Network at interdisciplinary or mental health meetings and activities. Offer everyone you talk to some idea of what you do and can do, so they have a "hook" on which to hang your name.
- Meet face to face with referral sources. Ask for just 5 minutes and stick to that. If interest in your further services develops, set up a second meeting.
- After you talk to someone about your practice, follow through by

sending written materials about your specialty that the person seemed interested in, or send a business card and a brochure with a note. "Take advantage of the Recency Effect. Follow-up brilliantly" (Beckwith, 1997, p. 91).

- Make "cold calls" to potential referral sources. Rose Piper LaCroix (1998), who has 10 years of experience in marketing mental health practices, believes that this is the most effective marketing tactic. Read her recommendations (http://www.shpm.com/ppc/mar/qamktyp. html).
- Learn to describe your practice activities succinctly when you are asked about your work. Practice your wording until you are comfortable and the message is complete and clear. If you stumble, potential clients and referrers may suspect incompetence or dishonesty.
- Reevaluate your Yellow Pages ad, if you have one. See Haber et al. (2000), Heller (1997), and Crandall (1998) for some ideas.
- If you measure outcomes, use this information to market and shape your practice. If you don't yet, set up a simple outcome measurement program (see, e.g., Clement, 1999).

Suggestions for Using This Book

You can focus your reading of this book by using the Quick Guide to Finding a New Practice Specialization (Table 1), or you can simply flip through the sections of niches and stop wherever an idea draws you on to read more. If you do the latter, please attend to when you get excited—and, especially, to how exactly you shut down your excitement and go on to something else. This is important information for your decision making.

If you find a niche that is of interest but is not exactly right for you, look at the cross-references to other niches that may be a better fit. This may be a useful approach if you are curious about what is available in an area you have been considering, such as medical, legal, or business consulting.

Good luck and good hunting!

TABLE 1. Quick Guide to Finding a New Practice Specialization

My orientation is best described as:	Turn to niche #:
Generalist therapist	You can use all of this book.
Cognitively and/or behaviorally oriented therapist	1.1. Treating Sleep Dysfunctions 1.4. The Psychological Management of Chronic Pain 3.1. Treating Public Speaking Anxiety . . .
Dynamically oriented therapist	1.2. Supporting Caregivers . . . 1.3. Working with Dying and Grieving People 2.4. Competent and Resilient Girls 5.6. Pet Loss Work and Animal-Assisted Therapy
Family therapist	1.2. Supporting Caregivers . . . 2.1. Relationship Enrichment Programs 2.2. Assisting Stepfamilies and Blended Families
Group therapist	2.1. Relationship Enrichment Programs 3.1. Treating Public Speaking Anxiety . . . 4.1. Treating Shoplifting 4.2. Working in Correctional Facilities
Tester/assessor/evaluator	2.3. Gifted Children 3.3. Improving Work Performance 5.1. Gerontology and Services to Aging Individuals
Specialist in women or minorities	1.3. Supporting Caregivers . . . 2.4. Competent and Resilient Girls 3.3. Improving Work Performance 5.3. Culturally Informed, Diversity-Sensitive Practice
Child and adolescent therapist	2.2. Assisting Stepfamilies and Blended Families 2.3. Gifted Children 2.4. Competent and Resilient Girls 2.5. Clinical Interventions for Students and Schools
Substance abuse specialist	3.3. Improving Work Performance 4.2. Working in Correctional Facilities 5.2. Clinical Practice in Rural Areas 5.4. Sport Psychology, Exercise, and Fitness
Educational or school specialist	2.3. Gifted Children 2.4. Competent and Resilient Girls 2.5. Clinical Interventions for Students and Schools 5.4. Sport Psychology, Exercise, and Fitness
Rehabilitation specialist	1.5. Treating Survivors of Motor Vehicle Accidents 4.2. Working in Correctional Facilities 5.1. Gerontology and Services to Aging Individuals
Clinician with an unusual background	Turn to the whole book.

Note. If you want to build on your present discipline, tradition, or orientation rather than leave it, choose the statements in the left column that best describe you. Then turn to the niches given in the right column to locate specialties that are likely to fit you.

Section 1

The Psychological Sides of Medical Illness

Introduction, Overview, and Commonalities

In this section, we present some ways for you to partner with physicians, with other medical caregivers, and directly with patients to provide psychosocial interventions for physical illness. Depending on your interests, training, and experience, opportunities exist in such diverse areas as working collaboratively in primary care settings, intervening with dental patients, being a member of a team treating chronic pain, providing or consulting in palliative care, supporting chronically ill individuals and their caregivers, treating the survivors of motor vehicle accidents, treating sleep disorders, and providing support for dying persons and their survivors.

THE VALUE AND NEED FOR PSYCHOLOGICAL INTERVENTIONS IN MEDICAL ILLNESSES

For decades, research has delineated the powerful interactions between physical health and psychological well-being, as well as physical, psychological, familial, community, cultural, and spiritual aspects of illness and its impacts. Hundreds of studies support the health benefits and cost reductions to be gained from providing psychosocial services to physically ill people (Sobel, 1995; Pallak et al., 1995, Chiles et al., 1999). We use the term "behavioral health" to describe studies and interventions that address these biopsychosocial interactions.

Despite this expanding knowledge, there are vast areas of unmet needs:

- Of the chief causes of serious illness, disability, and death in the United States today, *all* have substantial psychological and/or life-

33

style causal components, such as smoking, obesity, drug and alcohol abuse, interpersonal violence, or stress—and all of these can be lessened by the interventions we are trained to use (Cooke, 1995).

- Research has repeatedly demonstrated causative relationships between psychological or cognitive factors such as perceived life stress, depression, and pessimism on the one hand, and the development, course, outcome, and/or relapse of physical illnesses on the other (Peterson et al., 1988).

- The majority of visits to primary care physicians (PCPs) are actually related to mental health issues. Patients with untreated (and often undiagnosed) emotional disorders often seek treatment for physical complaints that are stress-related (Kroenke & Mangelsdorff, 1989; Lechnyr, 1992) or biopsychosocially caused (i.e., the results of lifestyle choices, injuries related to domestic violence, child abuse, preventable accidents, or drug and alcohol use) (Cooke, 1995).

- Even more striking is the fact that as many as one-third of patients seen by PCPs meet criteria for a *Diagnostic and Statistical Manual of Mental Disorders* (DSM) diagnosis, and these patients average twice the frequency of doctor visits as those without mental illness (Eisenberg, 1992). Among over 1,200 primary care patients in an urban practice, Olfson et al. (2000, p. 876) found that "major depression (18.9%), generalized anxiety (14.8%), panic (8.3%), and substance use (7.9%) disorders and suicidal ideation (7.1%) were highly prevalent," with many patients suffering from more than one disorder. Physicians are aware of the need to address behavioral issues affecting health, but feel unprepared to do so (Longlett & Kruse, 1992), and express difficulty and frustration in responding effectively within the constraints of the primary care setting (Alto, 1995).

These days, need alone does not justify providing services; the financial logic and benefits of intervention must also be demonstrated. Fortunately, numerous studies (for reviews, see Friedman et al., 1995; Chiles et al., 1999; American Psychological Association [APA] Practice Directorate, 2001) have demonstrated a "medical cost offset"—that is, the reduction of inappropriate demand for (typically more expensive) medical services, and overuse of (unproductive provision of) such services, which occur when psychological treatment is provided to patients with emotional disorders. For persons with physical illnesses, such psychological services as pain management in chronic conditions, pre- and postsurgical counseling, and support groups for patients with cancer have demonstrated substantial savings by reducing the use of high-cost medical services. Savings can result from lessened direct costs—the reduced use of all medical services; use of less costly services (such as office visits instead of emergency room visits); avoidance of inappropriate services (e.g., fewer expensive workups for psychological conditions masquerading as medical disorders, such as anxiety attacks mimicking heart attacks); and use of appropriate providers when needed (psychotherapists, not MDs). The indirect economies resulting from increased productivity, decreased disability, and lessened caregiver burden are harder to assess but also important.

Although cost concerns have been an impetus for behavioral health interventions, the improved quality of life resulting from them has also driven their adoption within the medical care system. Research presented in this section shows that such interventions can speed healing and recovery, reduce disability, improve coping, and diminish caregiver burden, all without increasing overall costs, and frequently by reducing them.

WORKING WITH THE MEDICAL SYSTEM

It is well established that few of the medical patients who could benefit from behavioral health interventions are appropriately diagnosed; fewer still receive treatment; and among those receiving treatment, noncompliance with medication and follow-up are serious problems. Moreover, only about 5% of those with a mental illness ever receive psychotherapy services, and most mental illness is treated by nonpsychiatric physicians working within or alongside the medical system. This situation offers mental health clinicians the opportunity to access a large underserved client base while offering patients easier access to beneficial services.

In order to make mental health referrals, PCPs and other providers[1] need to know that interventions of proven efficacy exist to help their patients. However, many physicians do not have current information regarding, or may be skeptical of, the psychosocial interventions available. If you are willing to present this kind of solid information to physicians in formal (seminars, professional meetings, newsletters, case consultations, rounds) or informal (networking, lunches) formats, you will help physicians overcome a major obstacle to mental health referrals and benefit all involved.

Among physicians who report that they would refer more patients to mental health care providers, many do not know of accessible and responsive clinicians to whom they can refer. If you are willing to network actively with physicians in your area, and to comply with their needs for communication, you will help them resolve these deficits in their referral network. Finally, referrals to specialist mental health clinicians often do not result in actual follow-through by the patients. Physicians are not always comfortable

[1]Other medical care providers include nurses, dentists, podiatrists, chiropractors, physical and occupational therapists, and the like, all of whom can refer the patients they see and follow.

or adept at making mental health referrals. You may be able to teach physicians when and how to make appropriate and effective referrals to the exact services you offer and how to follow through. If you are also willing to adapt your way of practicing to expedite access, you can help patients overcome the obstacles to care that they encounter during a typical referral process.

Differences in the professional cultures of medicine and mental health result in differing expectations and practices on the part of physicians and mental health practitioners. If you are willing to adopt a consultative, collaborative, or team approach with physicians and to provide, for example, succinct and timely progress feedback and on-the-fly consultations, physicians will be more likely to seek you out as a resource.

However, if you wish to maintain an office-based private practice model, it is possible to work directly with medical patients but outside the usual medical care system. Patients and their caregivers are becoming more sophisticated regarding services beyond the physician- and hospital-based system. People are quite willing to commit their resources (time and money) to access all systems of care that they consider efficacious. This is particularly true for patients dissatisfied with the treatment options within traditional medicine (e.g., for chronic pain), or those who wish to avoid medication's side effects or costs, or those for whom drug interactions or physical conditions make traditional treatments undesirable. These represent substantial groups of patients who can benefit from psychological services.

A SKILL SET FOR BEHAVIORAL HEALTH INTERVENTIONS

Basic skills and experiences that we expect most clinicians to draw upon for these niches include high degrees of facility with the following:

- Conducting psychological interviews, taking relevant kinds of histories, performing mental status and other assessments, integrating diagnostic conclusions into physicians' reports, and communicating results effectively and quickly to referral sources.
- Treating habit disorders with motivational interviewing; harm reduction and relapse prevention; and functional analyses, behavior shaping, and contingency management.
- Conducting effective psychoeducation to support all other behavioral health interventions, including those aimed at increasing self-management and assertiveness.
- Stress management, using a variety of relaxation and cognitive methods.

- Offering individual, family systems, and group psychotherapy approaches.

Specialized skills clinicians should have or may need to develop to work in behavioral health include these:

- Familiarity with the culture and norms of health care.
- Evaluation from a behavioral health (biopsychosocial) perspective, including familiarity with illnesses, disabilities, treatments, medications, and neuropsychological and developmental issues.
- Biofeedback and hypnosis for stress management and self-regulation of bodily functions disordered by disease or the effects of treatments. Particularly successful have been treatments for Raynaud's syndrome and incontinence.
- Dealing with terminal illness and bereavement.
- Providing supportive interventions to clients, relatives, and caregivers to enhance treatment compliance/adherence, coping with losses, active participation in rehabilitation, and overall recovery.
- Medical crisis management and interventions.
- Awareness of the medical, legal, financial, and social support network of one's community.
- Application of cognitive-behavioral therapy (CBT) techniques in the health area.

INCREASING YOUR FORMAL KNOWLEDGE BASE

You can develop your own study program, which should include reviewing the literature in the specialty area, taking courses and attending conferences, and receiving consultation or supervision from another clinician who has experience working in that specialty setting. Many of the organizations listed under the "Professional Organizations" heading for each niche offer training and seminars, mentoring opportunities, newsletters, journals, and online information that will help you recycle or retread your skills.

REACHING CLIENTS/DIRECTIONS FOR MARKETING

Relationship building with physicians is essential. In a survey of 5,000 PCPs by the Center for Studying Health System Change of the Robert Wood Johnson Foundation, 70% of respondents reported that they could not find high-quality mental health referrals for their patients ("Primary Care Docs Report Poor Access," 1997).

- Coordinate care with your clients' PCPs, and let them know you are available to discuss areas of mutual concern. Regularly send reports on your diagnoses, plans, and client progress to every client a physician refers to you (with the client's permission, of course).
- Get on the associate medical staff of local hospitals. Membership usually allows you to rent (or sublet) office space in a medical arts building. You will need to be recommended; if an opportunity is not obvious, ask your personal physician to recommend you (supply him or her with solid credentials and recommendations).
- Make friends with the medical staff secretary, who is crucial to your happiness and prosperity. For example, she (this person is almost always a she) will have the list of the local "detail" persons (pharmaceutical and other companies' representatives). She will be the best-informed person in the hospital about its politics and plans, but do not expect her to share secrets or gossip, although you can use her knowledge to clarify misunderstandings.

Staff membership will keep you informed of what is happening and let you in on the politics of the hospital. If you dislike managed care, you have that in common with nearly everyone. My (ELZ) recommendation is to make it clear that you do not want prescribing privileges (your methods are better than medications in many cases) or admitting privileges, but would like to continue to see patients of yours who are admitted to any service (not just to psychiatry). Although nonpsychiatrist clinicians should not expect any support from psychiatrists, do your best to be friendly and honest with them, at least. Do not let yourself be provoked or defensive.

Learn the abbreviations of medicine, such as DRG (for "diagnosis-related group"), as well as everyone's degrees. (Any standard medical dictionary, and many Web sites, will give these abbreviations.) Hang out in the medical library and introduce yourself. Make friends with the librarians; they love to be helpful, and often can benefit from your specialized knowledge. Offer to consult with them on purchases concerning psychology. Meet the staff members in the records room and their boss (the registered records librarian). Visit the nursing department and offer to do some lectures, professional education, or consultations. You will have to be flexible, but nurses are the best sources of referrals in the health care system. Go to all the holiday parties and bring lots of food and business cards. Be especially nice to the president of the medical staff. Get to know others in the building, and make yourself available for brief (and immediate, if possible) assessments and consultations, and you will be appreciated by the overworked staff. If your skills and the situation allow it, consulting to the emergency department on psychiatric crises is always needed.

Other referral and marketing tips include the following:

- You can make it easier for physicians to refer by providing them with brief assessment instruments (e.g., Primary Care Evaluation of Mental Disorders [PRIME-MD; Spitzer et al., 1995, 1999]) and handouts about your practice and about the effectiveness of your interventions. If you are a member of the APA, Divisions 29 and 42 have produced brochures on behavioral health topics such as cancer, heart disease, dental anxiety, and serious illness, which can be personalized for use in your marketing efforts with physicians. Fact sheets related to the benefits of a behavioral health approach that will be useful in your marketing efforts include one by the APA (2000) and another by the National Association of Psychiatric Health Systems (2000).

- When you find a companionable physician or other practitioner, consider subletting office space from this professional, and work on establishing collaborative relationships. Perhaps arrange to use an office outside regular office hours to meet with small groups of patients and/or caregivers. For many years, I (ELZ) sublet space from a speech therapist who was associated with the rehabilitation department of a hospital, and so I was able to get staff privileges through him and this department.

- Physicians are becoming more aware of the importance of psychological and relationship factors in the practice of medicine (see, e.g., Novack et al., 1997). Consider offering presentations on this topic and others of possible interest (e.g., burnout, giving bad news to patients) at your hospital's meetings or those of the local medical society. Medical care has dozens of allied fields, and all of them have meetings and can refer patients. I (ELZ) have made presentations to associations of hospital financial administrators, dental societies, and geriatric and public health nurses.

- Community screening programs are available for anxiety, depression, eating disorders, and substance abuse. In addition to helping those in your community, these can be practice builders. The hard work (developing marketing and assessment materials, etc.) has already been done for you. Just add some of your time and effort, and avail yourself of an excellent, professionally developed marketing opportunity.

- National Doctors' Day (usually March 30) and Patient Recognition Week in February are both opportunities to offer materials or presentations to physicians on topics of concern or techniques they could utilize with their patients. There is an online list of specific mental health observance days (http://www.healthieryou.com/advocacy/observe.html).

THIRD-PARTY PAYER ISSUES

Since many of the specialties in this section of the book concern disorders that are covered by medical insurance, this is clearly not a managed-care-free area. The journal *Medical Economics* (http://www.medec.com) will help you to keep pace with managed medical care, coding, insurance reimbursement, and other practical aspects of real-life medical practice. If you work in concert with physicians, you will want to be on the same panels so you can accommodate referrals.

The AMA has recently added six new *Current Procedural Terminology* (CPT) codes covering psychosocial services to patients with medical diagnoses. These codes do not require a DSM diagnosis and thus will provide services for many more clients. See Foxhall (2000) for more on this. Although using these codes will not guarantee payment, it is an essential step in that direction. In addition, according to William Deardorff, PhD, some third-party payers presently accept psychologists as providers for certain medical CPT codes, such as Evaluation and Management (E&M)[2] codes for physical disorders. We quote his contribution to an e-mail list discussion here, with his permission:

> In my practice, I bill for the initial consultation using the codes 99244 or 99245 depending upon the complexity. The initial consultation includes the interview (presenting problem, [mental status exam], history, etc.). In addition, I will review all available medical records and talk with the referring physician. Also included, as necessary, is testing that is focused upon assessment of the medical problem (for example, the Multidimensional Pain Inventory). I will always dictate a narrative report to substantiate what was done in the consultation. My billing includes the consult code (e.g., 99245) using the medical diagnosis provided by the referring doctor. I do not use a psychiatric diagnosis since in the majority of my patients, there either isn't one or it is not the focus of my treatment. Many of my cases have their own psychotherapist or psychologist they are seeing for other things. (Deardorff, 2002)

---

[2]Six E&M codes have been developed and were implemented for psychologists by Medicare starting January 1, 2002. However, each region's Medicare administrator and each insurance company or managed care organization will decide when and how to implement payment for these codes.

ATTENDING TO TRENDS

- Managed care and insurance reimbursement trends will affect physicians' practices and behavioral health practices as well. Keep abreast of developments that affect third-party payers by subscribing to newsletters and checking Web sites concerned with these topics, such as the managed care section of the New York chapter of the National Association of Social Workers (online at http://www.naswnyc.org/managed.html) and the newsletter of the National Coalition of Mental Health Consumers and Professionals at (http://www.nomanagedcare.org).

- Online patient resources, such as Web pages and bulletin boards, are a way of learning about patient issues and making a contribution. Medscape.com is especially valuable for its breadth.

- Don't forget to explore the best-selling mass market health publications, to acquaint yourself with the concerns of patients and their families.

Treating Sleep Dysfunctions

OVERVIEW AND OPPORTUNITIES

There may be no better way to extend your practice into the medical arena than treating sleep problems. Since help with sleeping is one of the most common reasons people consult physicians, this specialization is an opportunity to work with PCPs—either to provide consulting evaluations, to accept referrals for treatment, or to be part of a team. You might also be interested in working in a multidisciplinary environment, such as a sleep clinic or multidisciplinary group practice. Sleep dysfunctions are common problems suffered by millions, whose treatment has not been claimed by another profession. There are fairly simple psychological treatments of proven effectiveness, whereas medical interventions can have significant side effects, including the risks of addiction. What could be a better basis for offering psychological treatment?

Sleep problems are nearly always self-diagnosed, and so self-referral is likely. Of adults who responded to a Harris Poll in 1997 (National Sleep Foundations, 1997a), almost 50% reported being troubled by sleep problems. Sleepiness affects every aspect of the waking day, from reaction time to coordination, mood, alertness, and short-term memory. According to another poll (National Sleep Foundation, 1997b), approximately 36 million U.S. workers believe that lack of sleep negatively affects their job performance, particularly with respect to decision making, problem solving, and the ability to handle stress.

Psychological treatments for sleep problems are impressively effective, and beneficial outcomes are easily demonstrated (Jacobs et al., 1996; Lacks & Morin, 1992; Murtagh & Greenwood, 1995). According to Michael Perlis, director of the University of Rochester Sleep Research Laboratory, "At this point, there's no question about the potency and the power of CBT for insomnia. . . . This is one of the places where psychology really shines" (quoted in Smith, 2001, p. 37). Morin et al. (1999) compared CBT alone with drug treatment, combined drug treatment and CBT, and placebo. Although the three active treatments were all more effective than placebo in the short term, at a 2-year follow-up only the treatments employing CBT sustained their effects. Morin et al.'s conclusion was that "insomnia is best treated with a behavioral approach alone" (1999). With behavioral treatments, gains sometimes even increase over time—a possible "sleeper effect" of treatment ("Psychological Treatments for Insomnia," 1995). In fact, Hauri (1997) concluded that patients who received only behavioral interventions had better outcomes than those who received a combined drug–behavioral intervention.

The most common interventions—medications—are problematic. Sleep medications increase light sleep, but decrease deep sleep, which is essential. Moreover, sedative/hypnotics create daytime psychomotor and cognitive impairment, daytime drowsiness, and/or anxiety. In fact, they impair daytime performance more than sleeplessness itself does. And they present significant risks of overdose (deliberate and accidental), physiological dependency, and problematic drug interactions.

YOUR POTENTIAL SATISFACTIONS

- There are effective psychological interventions for sleep disorders, so you can really help your clients. Total failure is very unlikely, and you can benefit almost everyone you see.
- Patients are grateful and satisfying to work with.
- There are no emergencies; confidentiality and consent are not problems; and there are generally few difficult comorbid conditions, family issues, or the like with which to deal.
- This area of treatment may thus provide an easy entrée into working with physicians and with mind–body interactions in general.

YOUR SKILL SET

Recycling Your Current Competencies

- You should be familiar with and skilled in cognitive interventions, to address the repetitive and dysfunctional thought patterns producing most sleep functions.
- You should have skills in functional analysis and contingency management methods.
- Training in hypnosis and other relaxation methods is valuable for this work.

Retreading for Added Skills

- You must know the terms and diagnostic system for sleep disorders; the typical pharmacological and nursing treatments, and their risks and benefits; what sleep studies consist of, and their findings; the nature and physiology of sleep; and the relationship between physical illnesses and sleep.
- You should be familiar with the comprehensive treatments that are well described in books and treatment manuals (e.g., Morin, 1993; Morin & Colecchi, 1994; Pressman & Orr, 1997).
- No special credentials are needed, but training and certification are available. According to an *APA Monitor* article (Smith, 2001) practicing psychologists can get up to speed through training at national sleep meetings or by putting in some learning time at a local sleep clinic.

NATURE OF THE WORK

The nature of sleep difficulties is understood well enough for productive interventions. The dynamics are almost always discoverable, and the rationales for treatment are easily taught to patients. Assessment is straightforward and involves simple, well-validated tools, many of which are easily available in books (e.g., Morin, 1993) and journal articles. The diagnoses fit the data well and are logical, well accepted, and noncontroversial. These make the treatment of sleep disorders rather straightforward.

Approaches and Techniques

Psychological and behavioral approaches to sleep disorders need to be comprehensive in order to be effective because no single approach alone has been found to be as effective as a combination of approaches (Jacobs, 1999; Morin & Colecchi, 1994). Thus most practitioners working in this area have adopted a multicomponent approach to treatment.

Client compliance with the treatment regimen is crucial for the success of the treatment. Diary keeping, confrontation of noncompliance, motivating, teaching, and other patient-centered approaches are necessary.

The usual techniques include the following:

1. Sleep hygiene and lifestyle changes (exercise rescheduling, changes in diet and mealtimes, ceasing or limiting alcohol and caffeine use, etc.), as well as stimulus control techniques (e.g., using the bed only for sleep and sex, and other ways of standardizing the sleep environment). Behavioral changes include sleep restriction, bedtime–rising

scheduling, eliminating naps, and rising when unable to fall asleep in 15–20 minutes.
2. Relaxation training, because sleep requires physical and mental calmness. All the common psychological methods for such training can be effective.
3. Stress management techniques aimed at lessening worrying, rumination, and so forth.
4. Relapse prevention methods. (However, only 10% of psychologically treated patients relapse!)
5. Withdrawal from medications, which should be implemented in concert with the patient's physician.

Cross-Reference to Related Specialization

Niche 1.4. The Psychological Management of Chronic Pain. (Chronic pain greatly interferes with sleep for many.)

Subspecializations

Narcolepsy

Between 0.5% and 1% of people suffer from narcolepsy—sudden, involuntary, deep, but brief sleep, which becomes very life-limiting. Psychologists can help patients manage this disorder (Goswami et al., 1996). See also "Young Adults with Narcolepsy" at http://www-med.stanford.edu/school/psychiatry/narcolepsy/index.html, which offers information and support for patients.

Late-Life Insomnia

Late-life insomnia is another area of often-neglected need, even though it has been demonstrated that behavioral interventions are effective with geriatric patients (Morin et al., 1993). Other populations that have been shown to benefit from sleep interventions include patients with cancer, those with chronic pain, and psychiatric patients.

Practice Models

Working in collaboration with physicians in different settings is the standard. See the introduction to this section for more on this. Support and CBT can take place in a group format or in individual sessions. At the Harvard Mind/Body Institute, the behavioral interventions use a 2-hour group format, following an initial diagnostic workup. The group sessions focus on support, motivation, relaxation practice, stress management, and cognitive restructuring (Jacobs, 1999).

Financial Considerations

The National Institutes of Health (1995) have called for the integration of behavioral approaches in the treatment of insomnia. They recommend that psychosocial interventions for pain and insomnia should be reimbursed as part of comprehensive medical services at rates comparable to those for other medical care, particularly in view of data supporting these interventions' effectiveness and data detailing the costs of failed medical and surgical interventions.

Although some patients seeking help for sleep problems may meet criteria for adjustment disorder, depression, or anxiety disorders, many will not. In some cases, services to patients with medical problems can often be billed with medical CPT codes, not psychiatric ones. Patients are often willing to pay for treatment even when it is not covered, because they see the immediate reduction of symptoms, and the treatments are of brief duration and so can be of lower cost. In addition, it is possible to do group work to reduce your costs further.

Cautions, Ethical Dilemmas, Culture Clashes, and/or Managed Care Issues

A comprehensive physical exam is routinely necessary to rule out competing diagnoses. Sleep studies at an overnight sleep laboratory is often used for diagnosing and ruling out other disorders.

PROSPECTS AND PROSPECTING

Where Is the Need?

Almost half of all adults have trouble sleeping at one time or another, and 12% suffer from frequent insomnia. According to the National Sleep Foundation (1998), 27% of adults have used a medication to help them sleep in the past year: 10% have used prescription medications, 16% have used over-the-counter medications, and 1% have used both. As a result of poor sleep, 9% of adults report using medications to help them stay awake in the past year.

Competition

Considering the prevalence of sleep disorders, there are remarkably few clinicians providing interventions for them. Physicians receive less than 2 hours of training in sleep disorders in medical school (Jacobs, 1999; Rosen et al., 1993), and no other profession treats this problem. The medical sleep labs rarely do treatment and will make referrals.

Reaching Clients/Directions for Marketing

As noted earlier, self-referrals are common, because the public knows the significance of sleep problems and recognizes the need for effective, non-medical treatment that is easy to explain and demonstrate. The relationship between daily stress and sleep disruption is recognized, even by the lay public. In one survey (National Sleep Foundation, 1997a), for example, 34% of employees identified stress as the reason they were unable to sleep, and 14% blamed anxiety/worry as the cause of their sleeplessness. Almost all adults responding to another survey (National Sleep Foundation, 1999) agreed that sleep is as important to health as nutrition and exercise. And 70% of adults surveyed knew that most sleep problems will not get better without treatment.

Physicians are often quite willing to refer patients. Insomnia is the third most common complaint in visits to physicians (Jacobs, 1999). They recognize that medications are ineffective for chronic sleep disorders and potentially addictive. But physicians may need education in recognizing both the symptoms and effects of these disorders. A good article on signs and symptoms of sleep disorders for physicians can be found on the Web (Doghramji, 2000).

Here are some approaches to marketing your sleep disorder niche:

- Corporations—particularly those with shift work, those requiring long hours, and/or those with high accident rates—may be interested in presentations about the effects of sleep deprivation on productivity, accidents, creativity, and health. The National Commission on Sleep Disorders Research (1993) reported that sleep disorders cost about $15.9 billion a year in the United States, along with an estimated $50 to $100 billion in indirect and related costs due to reduced productivity, lost wages, or injuries resulting from drowsiness. Individuals who sleep less than 6 hours per night are in poorer health and face a higher risk of developing mood or anxiety disorders. Symptoms of their sleep deprivation (such as fatigue, irritability, and accident-proneness) affect their physical health and ability to perform at work, costing businesses billions of dollars.
- Research has established that people with insomnia have twice the number of car accidents as those whose sleep is normal. A survey of adults by the National Sleep Foundation (1998) found that 62% admitted to driving while drowsy in the prior year, and 27% said they had actually fallen asleep while driving in the prior year. A National Transportation Safety Board (1990) study found that fatigue is involved in 30–40% of truck accidents, and in 31% of accidents that resulted in the driver's death. Professional and citizens groups concerned about the effects of insomnia, include Citizens for Reliable

and Safe Highways (CRASH), a grassroots organization concerned with truck safety, and the Automobile Association of America Foundation for Traffic Safety (AAAFTS), concerned with accidents related to drowsy driving. Annually, 100,000 traffic accidents are caused by drivers who fall asleep, claiming 1,500 lives each year. Partnering with the AAAFTS and other groups interested in traffic safety, "piggybacking" on their events, or providing materials for newsletters of groups interested in the topic of safe driving can also provide positive exposure for your practice.

- For those who would like to work with child and adolescent sleep disorders, schools and pediatricians could be good referral sources. Children's night terrors and nightmares can be very distressing. Most adolescents are chronically sleep-deprived, with 2 hours of sleep debt per school night; the results are widespread drowsiness and impaired performance. Thirty percent of students fall asleep in school at least once a week (Maas, 1999). Wolfson et al. (1998) found an association between sleep debt and lower grades in school, as well as a relationship between conduct/aggressive behaviors and shorter sleep. Interestingly, although they sleep more than older adults, young adults are more likely to suffer from daytime drowsiness, are more likely to drive when drowsy, and are more likely actually to fall asleep while driving. Maas (1999) has noted the effects of sleep debt among college students; these, combined with the possibility that some children and adolescents may be more susceptible to problems resulting from sleep debt, may provide opportunities for clinicians to explore interfaces with both schools and pediatricians in this developing area.
- National Sleep Awareness Week (usually the first week in April) occurs in concert with the change to Daylight Savings Time, and is an excellent opportunity to submit an article to your local newspaper on behavioral treatments for insomnia or the effects and dangers of sleep deprivation.

INCREASING YOUR FORMAL KNOWLEDGE BASE

Core Readings

Morin, C. M. (1993). *Insomnia: Psychological assessment and management.* New York: Guilford Press.

Perlis, M. L., & Youngstedt, S. D. (2000). The diagnosis of primary insomnia and treatment alternatives. *Comprehensive Therapy, 26*(4), 298–306.

Pressman, M. R., & Orr, W. C. (Eds.). (2000). *Understanding sleep: The evaluation and treatment of sleep disorders.* Washington, DC: American Psychological Association.

Reite, M., Ruddy, J., & Nagel, K. (1997). *Concise guide to evaluation and management of sleep disorders* (2nd ed.). Washington, DC: American Psychiatric Press.

Stepanski, E., & Perlis, M. (2001). Behavioral sleep medicine: An emerging subspecialty in health psychology. *Journal of Psychosomatic Research, 49,* 343–347.

Journals

Journal of Sleep Research

Sleep (the journal of the American Academy of Sleep Medicine)

Online Resources

Stanford University Center of Excellence for the Diagnosis and Treatment of Sleep Disorders
http://www-med.stanford.edu/school/psychiatry/coe
—This is an information mine for sleep and sleep disorders by one of the original sleep researchers in sleep, Dr. William C. Dement. Departments at the school encompass disorders, surgery, research projects, and public education.

Journal Sleep (online version of *Sleep*—see above)
http://www.journalsleep.org

Silent Partners: Sleep Clinic
http://www.silentpartners.org
—A rich site for professionals and patients from the University of Toronto. The links page is of especially high quality and size and is completely current. There are links to organizations of all kinds, sleep schools, medical companies, and online multimedia educational programs. This can well serve as your primary source for online materials and resources.

Stanford Primary Care Sleep Education Project
http://www.go2sleep.com
—This project is dedicated to educating physicians on the diagnosis and treatment of sleep disorders. This site will provide you with information on the needs and knowledge set of the average PCP.

New Abstracts and Papers in Sleep (NAPS)
http://www.websciences.org/bibliosleep/naps

Sleep, Dreams and Wakefulness
http://ura1195-6.univ-lyon1.fr
—This site offers full text papers online, as well as an extensive database of abstracts. Although in French and English, it is easily searchable.

American Family Physician
http://www.aafp.org/afp/20010115/277.html
—A helpful article for physicians on childhood sleep disorders.

Pediatrics
http://pediatrics.aappublications.org/cgi/content/full/107/4/e60
   —Another helpful article for physicians on childhood sleep disorders.

Professional Organizations

American Academy of Sleep Medicine (AASM)
http://www.AASMnet.org

American Sleep Disorders Association (ASDA)
http://www.asda.org

The Canadian Sleep Society (CSS) / Société Canadienne du Sommeil (SCS)
http://www.css.to/about/index.htm
   —Based at Laval University, this site has links to its journal Vigilance, an excellent set of public education materials, under "Information & Education." The link to sleep journals is especially good because of its instruction on access.

Clinical Tools

Morin and Colecchi (1994) and Morin (1993) provide clinical guidelines and treatment protocols for the treatment of insomnia that can be adapted to your practice.

Patient Education Materials: Online Resources, Printed Resources, and Organizations

Sleep Home Pages
http://www.sleephomepages.org
   —The richest site on the Web, with materials for the public, clinicians, and researchers. Lots of ways to keep up with the developing literature, find authoritative information, and discuss problems.

The National Sleep Foundation
http://www.sleepfoundation.org
   —A nonprofit organization that promotes public education about sleep disorders and prevention and/or remediation of health and safety problems associated with sleep disorders. They also provide brochures on such topics as women and sleep, sleep and aging, drowsy driving, and a sleep quiz. These are available for purchase in bulk, and could be utilized both in your practice marketing and as patient handouts.

Shuteye Online
http://www.shuteye.com
   —Although sponsored by a drug company, the site offers the public an interactive questionnaire, a sleep diary, a checklist to prepare for a physician visit, and lots of good readings.

Dement, W. C., & Vaughn, C. (2000). *The promise of sleep: A pioneer in sleep medi-cine explores the vital connection between health, happiness and a good night's sleep.* New York: Dell.

   —Dement teaches how to measure, assess, and reduce sleep debt. Their "sleep camp" program provides strategies for a comprehensive battle plan to combat sleep debt.

Jacobs, G. D. (1999) *Say goodnight to insomnia.* New York: Holt.

   —Stimulus control, sleep scheduling, and CBT are covered in a comprehen-sive approach to better sleep from Harvard professor Greg Jacobs.

Maas, J. B. (1999). *Power sleep: The revolutionary program that prepares your mind for peak performance.* New York: HarperCollins.

   —An excellent resource from Cornell sleep research pioneer James Maas, this book tackles the subject of sleep debt and its effects on daytime alertness and performance, and provides effective strategies for better sleep.

Supporting Caregivers and Working with Chronic Illnesses

OVERVIEW AND OPPORTUNITIES

Family members, not organizations, provide the vast majority of care for those with chronic diseases, developmental disorders, traumatic brain injury (TBI), severe and persistent mental illness (SPMI), cystic fibrosis, AIDS, spinal cord injury, Alzheimer's disease, and other serious or terminal conditions. Caregivers also suffer as a result of these conditions, and their problems are too often overlooked.

A survey of persons caring for a family member with SPMI found that this has a "profound" impact on caregivers: "The mental health of many family caregivers borders dangerously close to clinical depression, due to the stressful demands of treating and living with a person suffering from schizophrenia" (Michigan Adult Foster Care, n.d.). Respondents in a caregivers' survey conducted by the National Family Caregivers Association (NFCA) cited lack of understanding from others (43%), sleeplessness (51%), and frustration (70%) as problems, and 41% said that changes in family dynamics and the sense of isolation that accompany caregiving were debilitating (Mintz, 1996).

The problems of caregivers in dealing with the chronically ill and disabled population have been neglected, according to Suzanne Mintz, president and cofounder of the NFCA:

> Family caregivers are ill-served by our current healthcare system. I suspect this isn't intentional, but rather a by-product of neglect. The symptoms of our dis-

tress and common illness are not categorized. We are not the subject of on-going medical research, nor are articles typically written about us in medical journals. There is not a known disease or condition called "Caregiver Disorder." We are for all intents and purposes invisible to the formal healthcare system. We are seen as the sad-faced people who come to visit our loved one in the hospital. We are the ones who drive them to physical therapy, administer medicine at home, have power of medical attorney. We are family. We are not considered to be another patient. (Mintz, 1996)

Another indicator of caregiver stress is elder abuse or neglect. The Administration on Aging of the U.S. Department of Health and Human Services (1998) reports estimates that at least 500,000 older persons were abused and/or neglected, or experienced self-neglect, during 1996 (the study period). It also estimates that for every report of abuse or neglect, five go unreported.

As a mental health practitioner, you can provide effective and often unique supportive services to those caring for people with chronic and severe conditions, illnesses, and disabilities of all kinds. You can thus reduce the burdens and other negative consequences for those cared for, the caregivers, and society at large.

YOUR POTENTIAL SATISFACTIONS

There are several effective interventions to offer to caregivers beyond simple information giving and generic comforting; these include stress management, cognitive restructuring, and therapy. Also, most caregiving occurs in families, and so you can experience the joys and sorrows, histories and futures of life in other families. Lastly, payment is available for providing these needed and valuable services.

YOUR SKILL SET

Recycling Your Current Competencies

- The condition of caregivers is usually not assessed by medical professionals, who focus on the people receiving care. Your assessment skills can rebalance this equation as you evaluate depression, perceived stressors, anxiety, anticipatory grieving, dependency and passivity, frustration levels, and so forth. In addition, medical personnel are well known to underdiagnose psychological conditions, and you may be able to bring needed attention and services to bear on all concerned.

- Your skills in individual, couple, family, and group therapies can all contribute to successful treatments for caregiver stress.
- As with other medical specializations, you will need to work well with medical professionals and teams (see the introduction to this Medical section).

Retreading for Added Skills

If you can augment your skills with grief work, assistance in parenting disabled individuals (including a knowledge base in a particular disability), or geriatric experience and knowledge, your clients will benefit greatly.

NATURE OF THE WORK

Much of the work in this area concerns understanding and modifying the "burden" experienced by caregivers. Marsh and Johnson (1997) differentiate the subjective and objective burden of those caring for family members with SPMI. Both subjective burden (comprised of grief, symbolic loss, chronic sorrow, roller-coaster emotions, and empathic pain) and objective burden (consisting of family disruption, symptomatic behavior, caregiving role, and dealing with multiple service delivery systems) must be considered during interventions with these families. Psychologists are, of course, specialists in assessing and addressing these subjective experiences and in using techniques to modify perceptions of burdens.

Therapists can also address and ameliorate relationship problems, because these play an important role in explaining differences in experiences of caregiving burden. Several studies have found that greater affection or intimacy with the impaired relatives has been related to lower subjective strain or burden among caregivers (Horowitz & Shindelman, 1983; Walker et al., 1992). In particular, a better relationship quality prior to the onset of disability has also been found to predict lower subjective burden (Strawbridge & Wallhagen, 1991). Evidence regarding the importance of negative interactions suggests that these interventions have the strongest effect on perceived burden (Fiore et al., 1983; Sheehan & Nuttall, 1988).

Both the care recipient's degree of functional impairment and his or her degree of cognitive impairment have been found to be related to various psychological and physical outcomes in the caregivers—for example, depression, anxiety, and cardiovascular reactivity (see, e.g., Sheehan & Nuttall, 1988; Uchino et al., 1994). Over a 3-year period, Redinbaugh et al. (1995) found a substantial proportion of caregivers for patients with Alzheimer's disease to be either episodically depressed (33%) or chronically depressed (20%). Among caregivers who have experienced the death of care-recipients, depressive symptomatology has been found to continue for as long as 4 years after loss (Bodnar & Kiecolt-Glaser, 1994). Obviously, treating the depression and grieving would be very beneficial.

Approaches and Techniques

Most effective interventions offer three components: individual and family counseling sessions tailored to each caregiver's specific situation; weekly support group participation; and constant availability of counselors to caregivers and families to help them deal with crises and with the changing nature of the patients' symptoms over the course of the disease. An important component of the intervention is the involvement of other family members in addition to the primary caretaker.

Many interventions are appropriate for all caregivers. Intrieri and Rapp (1994) found that caregivers who used problem-solving strategies such as planning, identifying alternative solutions, and anticipating consequences, and who had the ability to delay gratification, displayed fewer symptoms of caregiving burden. These caregivers were able to utilize self-statements and cognitions to help them cope with the stresses of the caregiving role. Psychoeducational interventions that teach these skills can be helpful to caregivers who are experiencing stress as a result of their caregiving responsibilities. Rainer (2000) offers an overview of services we can offer to those caregivers suffering from "compassion fatigue." Other services of potential value to families include educational workshops, family psychoeducation (Lam, 1991), and grief interventions, as well as individual, couple, and family therapy.

Clinicians who are experienced in treating SPMI can provide a needed service to families through family consultation (Marsh & Johnson, 1997). The can offer expert knowledge and advice on issues related to management, living arrangements, traversing the service delivery system, and support issues. Psychosocial and psychoeducational family interventions have been found to be effective in reducing relapse rates and increasing medication compliance. Particularly promising are findings that family interventions that reduce expressions of hostility and criticism ("expressed emotions") greatly improve medication compliance and reduce rehospitalization among discharged patients diagnosed with schizophrenia (see, e.g., Hogarty et al., 1991; Kavanagh, 1992).

Parents and families of disabled children are an understandably overwhelmed population in need of support services throughout their children's development, yet they receive little clinical attention. They experience extreme caregiving burden, stress, and disruption from parenting children with pervasive developmental disorders, attention-deficit/hyperactuivity disorder (ADHD), cystic fibrosis, Down's syndrome/trisomy 21, or other serious childhood disorders. Particularly when occurring in the context of other unresolved issues, the subjective sense of loss related to having an "imperfect" child can lead to depression, guilt, grief, and anxiety in parents. Training skills, in parenting skills assertiveness skills, couple and family communication skills, and stress reduction techniques has proved useful. Fathers have rarely been addressed, but Naseef (1997) describes the mutative effect of a fathers' group on his coming to accept his autistic son. He comments that "men have a different tone of grieving. Men's intimacy is different from women's, but not defective. Connecting with other fathers can have a powerful impact" (p. 109). This is well worth exploring for a niche.

Among siblings, guilt, resentment, and anger due to being overshadowed by a disabled child is both common and debilitating, and child clinicians are needed for these problems. Children who are underappreciated for their achievements or placed in a parental role can be helped by strategic therapeutic interventions. For example, the Siblings That Are Really Special Program is an 8-week-long program for the 7- to 12-year-old siblings of children with cancer at Children's Hospital in Oakland (747 Fifty-Second Street, Oakland, CA 94609; 415-428-3589). The SIBSHIP program that is part of the Parent/Educator Partnership (Grant Wood Area Education Agency, 4401 Sixth Street S.W., Cedar Rapids, IA 52404; 319-399-6702) combines recreation with structured discussion opportunities for the siblings of special-needs children. The Sibling Support Project (http://www.thearc.org/siblingsupport) is a national program providing support groups and workshops for siblings of children with disabilities.

Cross-References to Related Specializations

Niche 1.3. Working with Dying and Grieving People
Niche 5.1. Gerontology and Services to Aging Individuals

Subspecializations

Working with Chronic Illnesses

A natural segue from working with caregivers is working with those who are receiving the care for their chronic illnesses. Over 45% of Americans suffer from chronic, recurrent, limiting medical conditions such as diabetes, bronchitis, arthritis, cardiac problems, asthma, and HIV (Hoffman et al., 1996). In addition, many more suffer from mental or emotional disorders.

Problems that can be addressed include decreasing the high rates of depression and anxiety among chronically ill individuals; increasing compliance with treatments; and providing help in making lifestyle changes, coping with role changes, pain management, assertiveness, and grieving for losses.

The chronic illnesses that have been found to respond positively to some form of psychosocial intervention include a roster of the most common and the most devastating disorders (Emmelkamp & van Oppen, 1993). Psychological interventions for chronic heart disease, diabetes, cancer, asthma, and rheumatoid arthritis (RA), as well as less life-threatening diseases (such as skin disorders, tinnitus, disorders of the bowel and lower intestine, and chronic headache), have yielded promising results.

Other Subspecialty Areas

- Family interventions for assisting end-of-life decisions.
- Assistance for grandparents raising their grandchildren.
- Support for long-distance caregivers.
- Working with secondary traumatization.

Practice Models

- Collaborative arrangements with physicians, rehabilitation facilities, physiatrists, or special education settings are avenues to explore. Assessment, psychoeducational programs, and clinical interventions for caregivers, and direct care services for family members who are not able to live on their own, are all areas of need. Direct care can be limited to brief home visits or group day programs, or can include more comprehensive services if needed.
- Private solo practice with an orientation to caregiver stress is possible. However, you might want to consider providing services in the home or by telephone. Telephone conferencing for psychoeducational interventions might be an approach to explore, as it would allow you to interact with a number of caregivers at one time.

Financial Considerations

Family social skills interventions and/or psychoeducational efforts that are adjunctive to treatment for mental and medical illnesses may or may not be covered by health insurance. However, because of the high rates of clinical depression among caregivers, some treatment will be reimbursable and so may involve managed care.

Cautions, Ethical Dilemmas, Culture Clashes, and/or Managed Care Issues

When working with individuals with chronic illnesses, obtain your patients' consent to coordinate care with their PCP and/or specialist physicians.

PROSPECTS AND PROSPECTING

Where Is the Need?

In 1995, there were more than 25 million caregivers in the United States (Mintz, 1996). According to the Robert Wood Johnson Foundation (1996), the demand and supply trends in caregiving are pulling in opposite directions. In 1970, there were 21 "potential caregivers" (defined here as people aged 50–64) for each very elderly person (age 85 or older); by 2030, there will be only 6 such potential caregivers for each very elderly person. By 2020, there will be 39 million people with a chronic condition that limits their ability to go to school, to work, or to live independently. Based on current trends, by 2020 up to 14 million elderly individuals will need long-term care—double the 7 million who need such care today.

Competition

For those caregivers with DSM diagnoses, there are the usual competitors. For psychoeducational and support interventions, caregiver support is a field in which many providers with lesser training participate. However, this is an area of enormous unmet need, with relatively few clinicians offering specialized services.

Reaching Clients/Directions for Marketing

Your biggest challenge is likely to be access, not competition. If you can develop strategies (such as providing a mixture of home visits, telephone conferencing, and access through physicians' offices in convenient locations) that address this barrier, you are likely to have little competition.

Contacts with health care professionals and organizations may be quite productive. Gerontologists, family physicians who treat all kinds of chronic conditions, physiatrists, and rehabilitation professionals all know of the needs of caregivers.

You can reach out to caregivers through grassroots organizations (see below). You will find that you are one of the few who does so, and your efforts will be greatly appreciated.

An illuminating and useful market research report from December 2001, available from NFCA at their Web site (http://www.nfcacares.org), will inform your marketing efforts.

National Family Caregivers Month (November) is an opportunity to let your community know about your services through letters to the editor or advertising. The NFCA (see below) is a sponsor and you can subscribe to their mailing list to receive information about activities and order National Family Caregivers Month materials.

INCREASING YOUR FORMAL KNOWLEDGE BASE

Core Readings

Brody, E. M. (1990). *Women in the middle: Their parent-care years.* New York: Springer.

Figley, C. R. (Ed.). (1998). *Burnout in families: The systemic costs of caring.* Boca Raton, FL: CRC Press.

Lefley, H. P. (1996). *Family caregiving in mental illness.* Thousand Oaks, CA: Sage.

Light, E., Niederehe, G., & Lebowitz, B. D. (Eds.). (1994). *Stress effects on family caregivers of Alzheimer's patients: Research and interventions.* New York: Springer.

Olshevski, J. L., Katz, A. D., & Knight, B. G. (1999). *Stress reduction for caregivers.* Philadelphia: Brunner/Mazel.

Valle, R. (1998). *Caregiving across cultures: Working with dementing illness and ethnically diverse populations.* Washington, DC: Taylor & Francis.

Online Resources

Expert Consensus Guideline Series: Agitation in Older Persons with Dementia. A Guide for Families and Caregivers
http://www.psychguides.com/gahe.html
—A 15-page, comprehensive guide for families and caregivers.

The Caregiver's Handbook
http://www.acsu.buffalo.edu/~drstall/hndbk0.html
—An entire handbook of caregiving for Alzheimer's disease.

Patient Education Materials: Online Resources, Printed Resources, and Organizations

Caregiving Online
http://www.caregiving.com
—The publisher of *Caregiving Newsletter* offers many resources for caregivers of the aging.

National Family Caregivers Association (NFCA)
10605 Concord Street, Suite 501, Kensington, MD 20895-2504; 800-896-3650, 301-942-2302
e-mail: info@nfcacares.org   http://www.nfcacares.org
—NFCA publishes a quarterly newsletter and *The Resourceful Caregiver*, a resource guide for caregivers, and offers brochures. It also has a caregiver-to-caregiver peer support network and a bereavement program.

Family Caregiver Alliance
425 Bush Street, Suite 500, San Francisco, CA 94108; 415-434-3388; fax 415-434-3508
e-mail: info@caregiver.org   http://www.caregiver.org
—This organization provides information on caregiving for patients with Huntington's disease or TBI, information on how to form a support group for families of brain-impaired adults, and online support groups.

The Well Spouse Foundation
610 Lexington Avenue, Suite 814, New York, NY 10022-6005; 212-644-1241, 800-838-0879
e-mail: wellspouse@aol.com   http://www.wellspouse.org
—This group publishes a bimonthly newsletter, *Mainstay*. It also sponsors mutual aid support groups in many areas, letter-writing support groups, and an annual conference and other regional and weekend meetings around the United States.

Caregiver Network Inc.
561 Avenue Road, Suite 206, Toronto, Ontario M4V 2J8, Canada; 416-323-1090; fax 416-966-2341
e-mail: karenh@caregiver.on.ca   http://www.caregiver.on.ca
—This group provides information on all aspects of caregiving in Canada, including support services and support groups. It also publishes *The Caregiver*, a newsletter. Selected excerpts are available online.

Brandt, A. L. (1997). *Caregiver's reprieve: A guide to emotional survival when you're caring for someone you love.* San Luis Obispo, CA: Impact Press.
Edison, T. (Ed.). (1993). *The AIDS caregiver's handbook* (rev. ed.). New York: St. Martin's Press.
Heath, A. (1993). *Long distance caregiving: A survival guide for faraway caregivers.* San Luis Obispo, CA: Impact Press.
Heath, A. (1993). *Care log: A planning and organizing aid for long distance caregivers.* San Luis Obispo, CA: Impact Press.
—A three-ring binder of worksheets and forms to organize efforts.
Levin, N. J. (1997). *How to care for your parents: A practical guide to eldercare.* New York: Norton.
Mace, N. L., & Rabin, P. V. (1999). *The 36-hour day: A family guide to caring for persons with Alzheimer's disease, related dementing illnesses, and memory loss in later life* (3rd ed.). Baltimore: Johns Hopkins University Press.

—A new edition of the original book on caring for a loved one with Alzheimer's disease.

Smith, K. (1992). *Caring for your aging parents: A source book of timesaving techniques and tips.* San Luis Obispo, CA: Impact Press.

—Highly practical, focused advice on all aspects in 120 pages.

Wexler, N. (1997). *Mama can't remember anymore: Care management of aging parents and loved ones* (2nd ed.). Holt, MI: Partner's.

Williams, M. E. (1995). *The American Geriatrics Society's complete guide to aging and health.* New York: Harmony Books.

—A good introduction and overview with good advice on preparation for aging and healthcare. Useful for patient education.

Working with Dying and Grieving People

OVERVIEW AND OPPORTUNITIES

Hey, don't turn the page! Most of us have a "natural" or at least well-learned habit of avoidance when it comes to death and dying. Yet, since these events are universal, there are many opportunities for those willing to confront their own and others' avoidance, improve coping, and lessen death's psychological damage. Here are some examples of needs and services in this realm. You might design your practice to meet one or more of them.

- Although mourning is a normal process, it can become complicated, delayed, or aborted, resulting in pain, life constriction, and dysfunctions. These situations can benefit from psychotherapy.
- A terminal illness may be a death sentence—but dying can last many years, require many choices, and involve many others. Dying and death raise existential, spiritual, and religious issues, and the current interest in exploring these aspects in psychotherapy allows the development of a specialty practice.
- Those grieving for the loss of a child can suffer in unique ways. Children embody our hopes, and their loss is usually seen as bitterly unfair no matter the circumstances. Pregnancy or perinatal losses through stillbirth, abortion, or birth of a terminally ill child all require grieving.
- Hospices deal with the end of life, and psychologists can work effectively with families and the staffs of these organizations.
- Psychologists pioneered the "psychological autopsy" to understand the causes of a suicide. Although this has obvious forensic applica-

tions, families too can benefit from understanding the actual dynamics of a relative's death.

- Due to modern Western culture's denial and distortions of death, many people can benefit from what is bluntly called "death education," a worthwhile preventive effort.
- The clergy, funeral home personnel, and other "death workers" deal with a lot of grieving people, but often do not have the models and skills to handle many acute grief and loss patterns. Psychologist consultation and referral are possible for those cases.
- Suicide prevention efforts are almost always worthwhile. These efforts can involve educational interventions at all levels, clinical work with suicidal individuals, and interventions with the traumatized associates and relatives of a person who has committed suicide.
- There are many losses to be mourned besides deaths. Examples include the losses of jobs and careers, relationships, and various hoped-for outcomes. The dynamics of grieving, accepting, and moving on may be very similar in these cases.

Psychologists bring many effective tools to these painful situations, and psychology has much to contribute to bearing and growing from experiences with loss and dying.

YOUR POTENTIAL SATISFACTIONS

Doing this work is not depressing, but freeing. Most of us avoid the topic of death and dying out of denial, or the anxiety of confronting losses, or the fear of being exposed to raw and bottomless pain. Abandoning one's avoidance and confronting the inevitability of one's demise and the inevitability of losses can liberate us from these efforts. Participating in the ways others cope with their ending can be inspirational. Seeing others' lives come to a close can help us see the trajectory of our own lives and the impacts we have on others.

Western culture often discourages full grieving, and many confuse grief with depression and self-pity. Psychotherapists have always prized and worked to validate individuals' experiences, and in this area you will be working with the unique and intimate and against the culture's limitations and denials.

Death is elemental. It involves sadness, loss, hope, courage, terror, and tears; you will be touched.

All people want to have "a good death" or "to die well," and this mainly involves psychological processes and adaptations in which you are quite knowledgeable. Your credentials and techniques often will not matter as much as your humanity and openness.

YOUR SKILL SET

Recycling Your Current Competencies

- Familiarity and experience with effective treatments for anxiety and depression are basic needs.
- Personal experience in coping with losses is valuable.
- Presently, there are no special credentials required in this area.

Retreading for Added Skills

Skills and training in family systems, thanatology (the scientific study of death and dying), grief therapy, and knowledge of the dynamics and treatment of trauma are all valuable.

Some familiarity with the functional limitations of those with terminal illnesses, and the types of practical support they need, will be handy.

THE NATURE OF THE WORK

Normal mourning usually does not need therapy, but "traumatic grieving" or "complicated grief" does. Complicated grief is more than just longer-lasting or more severe grief. It is accompanied by significant depression and dysfunction in many spheres. Those experiencing protracted, intensely painful, or crippling mourning may include parents who lose a child (Rando, 1986; Murphy et al., 1998), elderly spouses who have been caregivers (Beery et al., 1997), suicide survivors (Silverman et al., 1994–1995), and bereaved children (Worden & Silverman, 1996). Jacobs and Kim (1990) concluded that, due to overlap with depression and anxiety disorders, "it is probable that 25% to 33% of acutely bereaved spouses suffer some complication of grief during the first year" (p. 316).

Areas of Practice

Grief Therapy: Psychotherapy with Those Mourning Losses

The rate of death among those bereaved during the previous year is many times that of peers matched for age, sex, socioeconomic status, and health (Lynch, 2000). Providing services to bereaved individuals can thus very significantly prolong and improve their quality of life. Losses of a parent, a child, a spouse/partner, or a sibling are all disruptions in the course of families. We can assist families to come to terms with the finality and impacts of members' deaths.

Deaths differ. Sudden or "premature" deaths seem more tragic and more difficult to cope with than those due to long illness. Deaths resulting from victims of accidents, homicide, or suicide have different meanings and may require different psychological interventions. Raphael et al. (1993) review therapeutic interventions to improve adjustment to loss, including "guided mourning" (Mawson et al., 1981), "regrief work," and "therapeutic rituals" (Van der Hart, 1988). It is generally accepted that working through feelings related to loss, making sense of the loss, reorganizing schemas, and finding new meaning in life are central to recovery (Mikulincer & Florian, 1996).

Adaptation in the Face of a Terminal Diagnosis

Psychotherapists are becoming increasingly involved in the care of dying patients, such as those with AIDS, Alzheimer's disease, and cancer (Hadjistavropoulos, 1996). Work with dying people and their families addresses communication, spiritual concerns, and practical matters. Mental health clinicians can help with coping with losses and adjustments to illness, accepting the trajectory of death, saying good-byes, and putting affairs in order. Choices about treatments and their outcomes, acceptance of "negative clinical outcomes," conducting rituals, enhancing communication, assisting with the unavoidable adjustments, and other functions can all benefit from psychological perspectives.

How therapy can help patients continue to live and even to grow in the face of a terminal diagnosis has received little research attention. In an early study, Linn et al. (1982) demonstrated that providing psychosocial support and other interventions improved quality of life in patients with late-stage cancer. Spiegel (1996) states that the "detoxification of death" is one of the patient's primary tasks. Other therapeutic tasks include the normalization of feelings, teaching how to grieve losses, finding meanings in one's life, and the restoration of hope within the necessarily shortened future (Rainer, 1998). For example, among women with advanced breast cancer, fighting spirit and emotional expressiveness appear to be associated with better adjustment (Classen et al., 1996), and Dobratz (1995) found social support to be critical for hospice patients facing the end of life.

Working with Hospices

Hospices offer tremendous benefits to the dying persons. To enter a hospice, one must have acknowledged one's terminal prognosis (with projection of a 6-month maximum lifespan for Medicare qualification) and be willing to forgo intensive life-sustaining procedures. The hospice model is family- and patient-based, is interdisciplinary, aims to control pain and distress, includes bereavement support both before and after death, encourages public education and access, and provides services mainly at home but also in a nursing facility.

Marwit (1997) provides a brief overview of the extensive and valuable contributions psychologists can make to hospice care:

- Pain management (through medication compliance, self-hypnosis, behavioral approaches, etc.).
- Stress reduction thorough relaxation and imagery to enhance quality of life, immunological response, and comfort.
- Family counseling around conflicts, communication, anticipatory grieving, and other typical family difficulties. Such counseling can moderate the morbidity and mortality of family members.
- Program evaluation and research for program development and justification of funding.
- Staff training and support around issues of loss, grief, coping, communication, decision making, and so on.
- Support and therapy for professionals and family members who, because of their personalities, family dynamics, death anxieties, or cultural norms, cannot communicate clearly about death with a client or family and yet need full knowledge to make informed and critical decisions.
- Teaching the skills for death education to others.

Psychologists can provide useful conceptual tools, such as an empirical orientation, a model of lifespan development, and biopsychosocial perspectives. "Approaching terminal illness from a biopsychosocial perspective provides a more complete, but more complicated, picture than was previously the case when diagnosis, course, and treatment were approached from a strictly biomedical perspective" (Marwit, 1997, p. 459).

Consulting with Funeral Home Directors and Staffs

Since we usually consult funeral home personnel only rarely in our lives, we can easily underestimate the size of this industry and the number of lives it touches. Funeral home directors and staffs deal with people at their most vulnerable, and most try to be as helpful as possible, although in many cases their profit motives dominate. These businesses are typically passed along in families, and so the level of sophistication and education in the humanities and biopsychosocial complexities can be quite low.

In addition to coping with bereaved individuals and preparing dead bodies for burial or cremation, morticians face financial pressures from the consolidation of national chains, the mandated need to control embalming chemicals, and their constant presence in the public eye. If you are willing to enter their realms and be respectful, you will find morticians and their work fascinating (see especially Lynch, 1997). You might start by offering to serve as a resource, such as being quickly available to see people suffering from severe traumatic loss. With accumulated trust, you might provide staff training or consulting, but these may not be billable hours. Do not be discouraged by initial rejection. Funeral homes are not uniform. Since many are linked through their ownership by one of the national chains, if you can establish a relationship with one funeral home, many others will quickly learn about you.

Helping Others Who Do "Death Work"

Other people who do "death work" besides funeral home personnel are often in need of psychotherapeutic consultation. For example, emergency workers and police may be traumatized by their contacts with death; those counseling bereaved or traumatized individuals may develop vicarious traumatization; and those dealing with survivors of disasters and crimes may benefit from therapy, as well as the survivors themselves. Kojlak et al. (1998) identified a subset of critical care health workers who felt they had inadequate support resources following the death of a patient.

Death Education

If the phrase "death education" strikes you as odd, that reveals some of your queasiness about death. If you like teaching, consider this specialization, which is not just for those currently grieving but for all of us. A good starting place is the Bereavement Education Center at (http://www.bereavement. org).

Psychological Autopsy

"Psychological autopsy" was originated by Edwin Shneidman and Norman Farberow in the 1950s (Shneidman et al., 1995). This investigation of the biopsychosocial context of a death seeks to determine, in ambiguous cases, the cause of death for forensic or insurance purposes. Practitioners seek to reconstruct the predeath circumstances and the person's thoughts, to offer an educated and professional opinion on the medico-legal cause of death.

Helping with End-of-Life Decisions

Psychological consultation can go beyond evaluating the competence of patients to make end-of-life decisions (e.g., advance directives or hastened deaths) or consent to treatments. Evaluating and treating the patients' almost universal depression in these cases; working with families struggling with withdrawal of unproductive interventions and their responsibilities; and coordinating accurate and complete communication are typical clinical duties.

Working with Grieving Parents and Children Who Have Lost Parents

Grieving parents and children constitute an obvious but underserved population, perhaps because of the poignancy and depth of loss experienced.

Cross-References to Related Specializations

Niche 1.2. Supporting Caregivers and Working with Chronic Illnesses
Niche 5.1. Gerontology and Services to Aging Individuals
Niche 5.6. Pet Loss Work and Animal-Assisted Therapy

Practice Models

Private practice and consultation models would constitute the mainstay approaches, although working collaboratively with specialist physicians (such as oncologists and geriatricians) is also a possibility. (See Niche 1.6.)

Financial Considerations

- Bereavement is a V-code in DSM-IV (V62.82), and so treatment for it is not usually covered by insurance. However, because the insurers haven't read Freud, they don't distinguish mourning from melancholia. If depression as well as complicated or traumatic grief is present, therapists can offer individual, family, or group psychotherapy and bill for treating the depression.
- Hospice care is covered by Medicare and most insurance plans. Your services could be covered as a consultant or as a staff member or upon referral.
- Consulting can be charged under your usual work policy.

Cautions, Ethical Dilemmas, Culture Clashes, and/or Managed Care Issues

Clinicians should be aware of the significantly greater risk of suicide among recently bereaved individuals. For example, Bruch et al. (1971) found that twice as many persons who completed suicide had lost their mothers in the previous 3 years and their fathers in the previous 5 years than had their matched controls. In a 12-year follow-up study, Li (1995) found that widowers, but not widows, were at a significantly greater risk of suicide following the loss of a spouse.

PROSPECTS AND PROSPECTING

Where Is the Need?

Many of the populations and needs have been identified above, but there is other evidence of significant need. Rando (1992) has shown that the incidence of complicated mourning reactions has increased over the years; she posits social and technological trends as the causes. In addition, she states that most clinicians are "unprepared and limited in their abilities to respond" to this increase (p. 43).

A dearth of grief counseling services in middle schools was noted by Carson et al. (1994–1995) in a survey of guidance counselors in one state, even before the current attention to violence in the schools and terrorism heightened awareness of needs for these services.

Kojlak et al. (1998) found that 48% of bereaved relatives of critical care patients were interested in receiving information on bereavement resources in the community. Marwit (1997) estimated that in the mid-1990s there were about 3,000 hospice programs in the United States treating about 450,000 patients a year, and that this number was growing by about 13% a year.

Competition

Many care providers understand dying and grieving from personal experiences, religious doctrines, or the treatment of depression, but psychologists can integrate multiple perspectives as well as offer empirically supported treatments.

Reaching Clients/Directions for Marketing

Many of those who need grief interventions have no idea where to obtain services, or even what to look for or where to start looking.

- You can contact hospices and other local organizations; health care providers who work with families of terminally ill patients; critical care workers; emergency medical technicians and other emergency personnel; funeral home directors; and grassroots caregiver and patient organizations to make them aware of your specialization.
- Offering brief noncredit courses in death and dying at local community colleges, or talking on local radio about the problems your cli-

ents have had in dealing with death, will often bring referrals. This is especially good for reaching small populations, such as those experiencing pet loss (see Niche 5.6) or the death of a child.

- Offer presentations at meetings of funeral home directors, teacher training programs, or local hospital in-service training sessions. Sending articles and newsletters every few months to these groups will keep your name in their awareness and so can be quite productive.

- Offer to teach courses on grieving, adaptation to loss, family counseling, and related topics at mortuary colleges or at schools for the health professions. These can lead to client referrals as well as to formal consultations.

- Holidays will be especially difficult for those who are grieving. Those who have lost parents or parents who have lost children are reminded on Mother's or Father's Day. Efforts that focus on helping bereaved individuals cope at these difficult times will be appreciated. Similarly, many suffer on the anniversary dates of other deaths. Writing about this in the public media will touch a chord in all readers.

INCREASING YOUR FORMAL KNOWLEDGE BASE

Core Readings

Death, Bereavement, and Grieving

Cook, A. S., & Dworkin, D. S. (1992). *Helping the bereaved: Therapeutic interventions for children, adolescents, and adults.* New York: Basic Books.
    —This volume provides a very comprehensive yet brief review of assessment and psychotherapeutic interventions from different orientations, implemented across different settings and cultures, for children and adolescents.

Doka, K. J., & Davidson, J. D. (Eds.). (1998). *Living with grief: Who we are, how we grieve.* New York: Brunner/Mazel.
    —How we grieve depends on our culture, religion, gender, and other variables; this volume offers a large set of perspectives for broadening your understanding.

Figley, C. R., Bride, B. E., & Mazza, N. (Eds.). (1997). *Death and trauma: The traumatology of grieving.* Washington, DC: Taylor & Francis.
    —If you already know the literature and interventions for treating the psychological aftermath of trauma (e.g., posttraumatic stress disorder), this book integrates these with grieving and its treatment.

Hendin, D. (1984). *Death as a fact of life.* New York: Norton.
    —A classic.

Kastenbaum, R. J. (1997). *Death, society, and human experience* (6th ed.). Boston: Allyn & Bacon.

—This is a textbook that can serve as an excellent introduction to the psychological aspects of death. It is best when it focuses on our "construction" of death.

Leick, N., & Davidsen-Nielsen, M. (1991). *Healing pain: Attachment, loss and grief therapy*. New York: Routledge.

—An elegant combination of empirical research and humane sensitivity for both professionals and educated laypersons.

Moller, D. W. (1996). *Confronting death: Values, institutions, and human mortality*. New York: Oxford University Press.

—This book is like a more academic and comprehensive version of Mitford's *The American Way of Death Revisited* (see below).

Piper, W. E., McCallum, M., & Azim, H. F. A. (1992). *Adaptation to loss through short-term group psychotherapy*. New York: Guilford Press.

—This volume details an effective approach to the consequences of unresolved grief.

Rando, T. A. (1984). *Grief, dying and death: Clinical interventions for caregivers*. Champaign, IL: Research Press.

—Rando offers both theoretical background and exercises for working with caregivers.

Rando, T. A. (1993). *Treatment of complicated mourning*. Champaign, IL: Research Press.

Wass, H., & Neimeyer, R. A. (1995). *Dying: Facing the facts* (3rd ed.). Washington, DC: Taylor & Francis.

—An excellent introduction to the data and issues of death, dying, and bereavement.

Worden, J. W. (2001). *Grief counseling and grief therapy: A handbook for the mental health practitioner* (3rd ed.). New York: Springer.

—Worden presents the "four tasks of mourning" (accepting the reality of the loss, working through the pain of grief, adjusting to an environment without the deceased person, and moving on with life) and the "seven mediators of mourning" (who the person was, the nature of the attachment, mode of death, historical antecedents, personality variables, social variables, and concurrent stressors). These constitute a very complete basis for intervening.

Hospices

Byock, I. (1997). *Dying well: The prospect for growth at the end of life*. New York: Riverhead Books.

—Dying well involves reaching landmarks: asking forgiveness, accepting forgiveness, expressing love, acknowledging self-worth, and saying good-bye. Also, pain must be controlled, and fear and loneliness must be reduced.

Ray, M. C. (1997). *I'm here to help: A guide for caregivers, hospice workers, and volunteers*. New York: Bantam Books.

Smith, S. A. (2000). *Hospice concepts: A guide to palliative care in terminal illness*. Champaign, IL: Research Press.

—Designed as a textbook for new staff or college classes, this book covers all the background information you need on history, context, disease, and family, grief, spiritual, and legal issues. A fine starting place.

Funeral Directors

Mitford, J. (1998). *The American way of death revisited* (rev. ed.). New York: Knopf.
  —Mitford's startling reportage and anthropological insights are presented in lively prose and with great humor. Her revelations in the original edition led to federal legislation limiting the worst exploitations.
Lynch, T. (1997). *The undertaking: Life studies from the dismal trade.* New York: Norton.
  —These essays by an articulate and sensitive man, who happens to be a mortician with scruples, take you inside his business and the lives of his small community.
Wolfelt, A. (1990). *Interpersonal skills training: A handbook for funeral service staffs.* Muncie, IN: Accelerated Development.
  —If you want to work with funeral home personnel, here is material to orient and structure your beginnings. Wolfelt has written many other useful books.

Journals

Psycho-Oncology: Journal of the Psychological, Social and Behavioral Dimensions of Cancer
Suicide and Life-Threatening Behavior
Death Studies
Loss, Grief and Care: A Journal of Professional Practice
Omega: Journal of Death and Dying

Online Resources

Death and Funerals

Death and Dying
http://www.dying.about.com/mbiopage.htm
  —You will find almost anything of value here—from funerals to euthanasia, organ donation to teen grief, inspirational quotes, attitude self-assessment, and the latest news. Click on "Results.about.com: Death" for more sites.

Sociology of Death and Dying
http://www.trinity.edu/~mkearl/death.html
  —Michael C. Kearl's site is a very rich and provocative one, well worth exploring to better understand death and the mass media, funerals, cemeteries, homicides, and "the American way of death." The access to the Growth House search engine is particularly useful. At the bottom, the Offbeat is fun.

Assisted Suicide/Euthanasia/End of Life
http://www.library.dal.ca/kellogg/Bioethics/webresources/specific_topics/
  euthanasia.htm
  —The links here address most of the issues, perspectives, and experiences of those on all sides of assisted-suicide and end-of-life decision. Good background reading; informative about situations you might confront.

National Funeral Directors Association (NFDA), 13625 Bishop's Drive, Brookfield,
   WI 53005; 800-228-6332; fax 414-789-6977
e-mail: nfda@nfda.org   http://www.nfda.org
   —NFDA is the largest funeral service organization in the world, with state chapters.

Hospices

Growth House
http://www.growthhouse.org
   —Probably the best place to start exploring and learning about care at the end of
one's life.

Hospice Web
http://www.hospiceweb.com
   —Very good information, frequently asked questions (FAQs), links, and so on.

Hospice Primer
http://www.thehomecarenetwork.org/e3front.dll?durki=4110
   —A brief but smart overview.

National Hospice and Palliative Care Organization (formerly National Hospice
   Organization)
http://www.nhpco.org
   —A good way to find an overview and to learn of training and consultation oppor-
tunities. Click on "Hospice and Palliative Care Information," and then "What Is
Hospice and Palliative Care."

Professional Organizations

The Association of Oncology Social Work
http://www.aosw.org
   —Here are links to professional resources: journals, organizations, lots of sites by
disease and by profession, sites for clinical information, and for support of professionals.

Patient Education Materials: Online Resources, Printed Resources, and Organizations

Grief Net
http://www.griefnet.org
   —It offers resources for the bereaved, including Kids Support Group (K2K) and
KidsAid for bereaved children (http://www.kidaid.com).

Before I Die
http://www.wnet.org/archive/bid
   —Based on an award-winning Public Broadcasting System presentation, it contains vast resources for the dying, their caregivers, and the bereaved on such topics
as palliative care, hospice, grief and loss.

James, J. W., & Friedman, R. (1998). *The grief recovery handbook: A step-by-step program for moving beyond loss* (rev. ed.). New York: HarperCollins.

Kushner, H. (1981). *When bad things happen to good people.* New York: Schocken.

McWilliams, P., Bloomfield, H., & Colgrove, M. (1993). *How to survive the loss of a love* (2nd ed.). Los Angeles: Prelude Press.

Rando, T. (1991). *How to go on living when someone you love dies.* New York: Bantam.

The Psychological Management of Chronic Pain

OVERVIEW AND OPPORTUNITIES

Pain is called "chronic" if it does not resolve in 6 months. It has been estimated that in the United States, over 80 million people suffer from chronic pain (Bonica, 1990). Yet it is now generally acknowledged that pain is almost always inadequately treated, leading to immense emotional suffering and disruption of all aspects of the sufferer's functioning (Mantyselka et al., 2001; Teno et al., 2001).

The treatment of pain with analgesics (with their side effects, interactions, and potentials for addiction, habituation, and overdose) was all that was available until the breakthroughs of psychologists. Ronald Melzack replaced the simple-minded "telephone circuit" model of pain (which assumed that pain sensors and nerves as conductors account for perceived pain, and that perceived pain is proportional to the amount of tissue damage/receptor stimulation) with the "gate control" theory of pain transmission (showing that the different kinds of pain nerve fibers interact, and that stimulating some can *inhibit* pain perception); he thus opened the door to such interventions as transdermal electric nerve stimulation (TENS units). Willard Fordyce, working with the physician John Bonica, reconceptualized subjective (and therefore unreachable) "pain" into observable and measurable "pain behaviors," and showed that these respond to reinforcement contingencies just like all other behaviors. Fordyce and Bonica's program at the University of Washington was the first modern, interdisciplinary, and effective pain clinic.

In subsequent years, many effective psychosocial interventions have been developed to decrease pain by helping patients change their perception of discomfort and control their emotional and physiological responses that can intensify pain. For example, although it may seem obvious that the greater the pain the greater the disability, this equation doesn't hold. The relationship is mediated by self-efficacy, social support, coping history, alternative vocations, and other variables. In a recent study, Arnstein et al. (1999) found that self-efficacy accounted for 47% of the variance between pain and disability. Pain intensity did contribute to disability, but much less. Arnstein et al. report that

> the lack of belief in one's own ability to manage pain, cope and function despite persistent pain, is a significant predictor of the extent to which individuals with chronic pain become disabled and/or depressed. Nevertheless, these mediators did not eliminate the strong impact that high pain intensity has on disability and depression. Therefore, therapy should target multiple goals, including: pain reduction, functional improvement and the enhancement of self efficacy beliefs. (p. 483)

Hundreds of studies now attest to the fact that psychological and behavioral factors play an important role in pain toleration (for a review, see Keefe et al., 1992). Personality and cognitive factors that have been found to affect reported pain intensity and tolerance include depression, passivity, locus of control, self-efficacy, patient beliefs about pain, and catastrophizing. Interpersonal stress has also been shown to be a factor in chronic pain (e.g., Schwartz et al., 1994). Even spouses' reactions to pain have been correlated with pain tolerance (Flor et al., 1987; Papas et al., 2001; Romano et al., 1991). Attention to these behavioral and psychosocial aspects of pain will help patients improve pain coping and reduce their burden of pain. Psychological treatment can also reduce the delays, costs, and risks of (unhelpful) medical and surgical interventions.

YOUR POTENTIAL SATISFACTIONS

- This is an opportunity to work in a multidisciplinary setting with proven techniques on a problem that has enormous personal, family, community, economic, and social costs. See Simon and Folen (2001) for a current and optimistic overview.
- Pain management is applicable to all segments of the population, all age groups, all economic levels, and all geographic areas, so that your present skills are likely to be relevant and your additional ones highly portable.

- As one writer has concluded, "Psychological interventions can save money and improve patient functioning by encouraging patients to stop looking for unrealistic medical solutions to their discomfort. This data supports [sic] the premise that psychotherapy can be useful in addressing the psychological problems that prevent chronic pain patients from getting on with their lives" (Cole, 1998, p. 30).

YOUR SKILL SET

Recycling Your Current Competencies

Relevant skills for a pain management practice include skill in performing functional analyses and behavior modification program design; familiarity with CBT, including cognitive restructuring; skills in assessing personality and psychological factors; and the ability to work well as part of a team.

Retreading for Added Skills

Additional skills include knowledge of physiology in illness and injury, and of rehabilitation procedures and the professionals involved in them. Skills in the assessment of pain and depression and the use of relaxation techniques (biofeedback, progressive muscle relaxation, hypnosis) are valuable. Certification in pain management is available and can be very helpful.

NATURE OF THE WORK

Any patient seeking treatment for chronic pain should be assessed both medically and psychologically before any intervention. Evaluations for depression, somatization, and a functional analysis are most common. There are two excellent guides to this kind of specialized assessment: Turk and Melzack (2001) and Camic and Brown (1989).

Comprehensive treatment is multidisciplinary and includes at least five elements:

1. Management (and usually withdrawal) of analgesic, hypnotic, and other medications (because they simply do not work for chronic pain).
2. Pain control education and training, using relaxation and stress management; imagery and meditation; muscle tension biofeedback; breathing training and yoga; CBT; and other approaches.
3. Extensive patient and family education and often family therapy to

discontinue the unwitting reinforcement of pain behaviors, revise the allocations of roles, and restructure the expectations of family members.

4. Vocational evaluation and training, with the goal of some kind of productive activity if not a return to previous employment. This training often includes work hardening and exercise programs.

5. Treatment of accompanying psychopathology, such as depression.

As an example of such efforts, psychologist Paul Arnstein and his colleagues at Boston College reported strikingly successful results of a CBT program for a most difficult group, those with severe chronic pain (Cheng, 2000). After a 10-week program, pain intensity had declined by 23%, disability by 19%, and depression by 27%. Importantly, pain intensity, disability, and depression continued to improve after 1 year; pain intensity had decreased by 27%, disability by 36%, and depression by 41%. These improvements remained significant even after controls for differences in pain intensity, use of antidepressants, or use of opiates for pain.

Areas of Practice

Below we offer an introduction to some of the disorders whose pain component has been successfully treated psychologically.

Headache

Blanchard and Diamond (1996) found well over 100 studies attesting to the effectiveness of nonpharmacological interventions in the treatment of benign headaches. Biofeedback, CBT, and relaxation training have all been shown to be effective (compared to placebo) for chronic migraine or tension headache management—with good follow-up at 5 years (Blanchard, 1992), with no side effects, and with a reduction of depression and trait anxiety associated with the headaches. These techniques are sometimes used alone and sometimes in combination. These results have been demonstrated for a variety of populations, including children (Larsson & Carlsson, 1966).

Rheumatoid Arthritis

Research going back 50 years has found that patients with RA rely on emotion-focused coping strategies to a much greater extent than patients with other forms of chronic pain (e.g., Felton et al., 1984), and that psychological variables (e.g., trait anxiety, depression, self-blame, helplessness, catastrophizing) and poor levels of compliance (Bradley, 1989) are additional factors to address in treating patients with RA. Young et al. (1995) showed decreased utilization of medical visits at an 18-month follow-up for a multi-component CBT–biofeedback treatment of RA.

Fibromyalgia Syndrome

The Arthritis Foundation (2002) reports that fibromyalgia syndrome (FMS) affects approximately 3.5 million Americans with disability rates up to 44%. Seven times more women than men are affected. It usually strikes in a person's mid-40s. FMS is characterized by generalized pain and musculo-skeletal fatigue, nonrestorative sleep, and morning stiffness.

Psychologists can contribute family and patient education about the nature and course of FMS and its reality (it is often denied or misdiagnosed because the sufferers don't look ill); can suggest ways of dealing productively with a family member who is sick, hurting, and often anxious and depressed; can explain the role of reduced physical and emotional stress to minimize or prevent flareups; and can assist with lifestyle changes, such as arranging sleep and rest schedules, making work adjustments, redistributing household responsibilities, and so on.

Chronic Low Back Pain

Chronic low back pain (CLBP) is the second most common reason for visits to PCPs (after upper respiratory infections), and so it has enormous costs both economically and personally. Despite its prevalence, medical and surgical treatment outcomes are poor (Gevirtz et al., 1996). Research has shown, however, that recovery from CLBP can be predicted from psychosocial variables such as job satisfaction (Williams et al., 1998). Although outcomes with psychological interventions such as CBT and biofeedback are somewhat mixed, Gevirtz et al. (1996) concluded that they are effective overall, particularly with younger patients.

Cancer Pain

Chronic severe pain in patients with cancer is widely undertreated with inadequate dosages of pain relievers. Although physicians are often advised to change this policy, they are still reluctant to do so (because of a fear of addiction or other untoward consequences), which opens a door for psychological interventions. Research on patients with cancer has shown that behavioral interventions can reduce the perception of pain and the discomfort and anxiety related to medical treatments (Suinn, 1997; Arathuzik, 1994). Jay et al. (1995) developed an intervention for pediatric pain management during bone marrow aspiration, which was more successful than was analgesic medication. As in patients with other disorders, it is important to assess for depression with pain in patients with cancer since relieving one appears to alleviate the other (Spiegel & Sands, 1988; Spiegel & Classen, 2000).

Geriatric Pain

Misconceptions regarding the "normality" of pain in elderly people may lead to undertreatment of debilitating pain in this age group. A review of the literature on geriatric pain treatment (Gagliese & Melzack, 1997, p. 3) concluded that "the elderly benefit from non-pharmacological treatment methods (biofeedback, relaxation training, and cognitive behavior therapy), and multidisciplinary treatment may be the most beneficial [for this group]." According to *Practice Strategies* ("Directions," 1998), CBT, caregiver education, and encouraging aggressive integrated treatment for geriatric patients are the key strategies in the latest clinical guidelines issued by the American Geriatrics Society.

Cross-Reference to Related Specialization

Niche 1.6. Collaborative Practice with Primary Care Physicians

Subspecialization

Pediatric Chronic Pain and Pediatric Surgery Preparation

Barbara Melamed's (Melamed et al., 1978) and Lizette Peterson's (Peterson & Shigetomi, 1981) pioneering work with children demonstrated the value of preparing children via videotape for what they would experience in the hospital, both before and after surgery. The results? Briefer stays, less medication, fewer complications—everything good that could be measured. For an update of work with medically traumatized children, see Bronfman et al. (1998). Schulz and Masek (1996) describe the use of behavioral techniques in medical crisis counseling in a pediatric acute care unit. Play therapy and family therapy modalities are useful for work with pediatric patients who have pain.

A Web site created by the IWK Grace Health Centre and the Psychology Department of Dalhousie University in Halifax, Nova Scotia, Canada, is of relevance. Pediatric Pain: Science Helping Children (http://is.dal.ca/~pedpain) offers a large "sourcebook" of pain management resources for professionals, a self-help section for parents and children, and links to journals specific to the field. The site is also home to the *Pediatric Pain Letter,* a quarterly newsletter with abstracts and commentaries on pain in infants, children, and adolescents.

Practice Models

Some psychologists in solo practice receive referrals from physicians who are familiar with their work, but most work in a group practice or a multidisciplinary pain service on a full- or part-time basis.

For collaborative practice, select physicians to work with who are already convinced of the utility of psychophysiological approaches. That's the advice of Joseph Cohen, a dentist working in a multidisciplinary practice that deals with pain management ("Directions," 1998). For pain management, this means going to doctors who specialize in soft tissue disorders, headache, and chronic pain, or who are already in a multidisciplinary setting with physical therapists. Physiatrists and orthopedic surgeons are also at the top of the list.

Jimmie Cole, PhD, and his wife, Mollie Cole, created Coping Skills Development, a psychoeducational group psychotherapy program that teaches patient self-management (Cole, 1998). It "focuses on restructuring the chronic pain patient's belief system by encouraging them to stop looking for medical solutions to their problems and move on with their lives" (Cole, 1998, p. 29). The Coles utilize CBT, relaxation, and assertiveness training, and they particularly target depression. Small groups meet for 16 weeks. They report improvements in Beck Depression Inventory scores and overall functioning (based on less medication use, reduction of health care visits, and progress on vocational goals) at 1-year follow-up.

Similarly, Jaylene Kent, PhD, a health psychologist at Kaiser Permanente Medical Center in Santa Teresa in San José, California, developed "Skills not Pills"—a 10-week program utilizing behavioral principles, psychotherapy, support groups, and cognitive skills for patients with chronic nonmalignant pain (Center for the Advancement of Health, n.d.). The staff includes a health psychologist, a physician, a licensed clinical social worker, and a registered nurse. Kent and her colleagues have demonstrated a 57% reduction in medical utilization among graduates of the program at a 1-year follow-up.

Financial Considerations

Patients with chronic pain are often depressed, and so health insurance may cover the cost of its treatment. Some pain management treatment is reimbursed by insurance, particularly in a multidisciplinary environment. Another route to reimbursement for your services is to become an employee of a rehabilitation team.

Cautions, Ethical Dilemmas, Culture Clashes, and/or Managed Care Issues

As noted earlier, patients with chronic pain should be assessed medically before behavioral health interventions begin, and you should obtain and interpret their records and inform their other treatment sources. This is especially important with these patients, who are more likely than most to have done a lot of "doctor shopping" or "doctoring," failed in pain treatment efforts, and misused analgesics.

PROSPECTS AND PROSPECTING

Where Is the Need?

The population for whom psychological pain management is appropriate is large and growing. It includes those with a history of or potential for addiction to analgesics. Even nonaddictive pain medications have drawbacks: According to Tamblyn et al. (1997), nonsteroidal anti-inflammatory drugs used for pain cause 7,600 deaths a year, due mainly to gastrointestinal bleeding. Bleeding and other adverse drug reactions send many patients looking for nonpharmacological solutions to pain. Other problems are the side effects of habituation, the need for higher dosages, and changes in cognitive functioning due to prolonged or high levels of some drugs.

Also, population trends should keep the demand for pain management strong. Those living longer are more subject to illnesses, and many illnesses have a major or chronic pain component. Because the economic cost of chronic pain can be so enormous, employers and insurers are interested in cost-effective approaches that can return employees to work. Pain management has been shown to be a cost-effective treatment (Caudill et al., 1991; Simmons et al., 1988) and to reduce nonmedical expenses, such as those due to absenteeism at work and reduced employee productivity. PCPs and other gatekeepers in capitated service programs, who need to keep costs down while providing effective treatment, should show a keen interest in these interventions (as should personnel in other managed care arrangements).

Competition

Some physicians are specializing in pain management, and some are opening free-standing pain clinics or pain services in health care centers. These physicians are generally neurologists, physiatrists, and orthopedists. Many patients find such services too mechanical and unproductive. Also, people who can do some hypnotism or some relaxation imagery may present themselves as experts in the management of pain, as do most chiropractors.

Reaching Clients/Directions for Marketing

- If you successfully treat a patient for pain or a coexisting depression, and the patient's physician hears of this, you are likely to get many referrals. All PCPs, internists, orthopedists, and neurologists accumulate a good number of patients in their caseload to whom they have nothing more to offer but cannot abandon.
- Lawyers and risk management specialists dealing with workers' compensation and other disability cases are sources of evaluation referrals and follow-on treatment.
- Many clients are referred to a team or clinic, of which you could be a member.
- Geriatric care facilities, elder care programs, and physical rehabilitation facilities are all likely sources of referrals.
- Free-standing pain management programs may cultivate workers' compensation and disability-insured referral streams, and you might see clients as part of a treatment team of employees or as a consultant.

INCREASING YOUR FORMAL KNOWLEDGE BASE

Core Readings

American Chronic Pain Association. (n.d.). *The family manual.* Rocklin, CA: Author.

Bates, M. C. (1996). *Biocultural dimensions of chronic pain: Implications for treatment of multi-ethnic populations.* Albany: State University of New York Press.

Eimer, B. N., & Freeman, A. (1998). *Pain management psychotherapy.* New York: Wiley.

Fordyce, W. E. (1995). *Back pain in the workplace: Management of disability in nonspecific conditions.* Seattle, WA: IASP Press.

Jamison, R. (1996). *Mastering chronic pain: A professional's guide.* Sarasota, FL: Professional Resource Press.
　　—A companion version for patients is also available.

Margoles, M. S., & Weiner, R. (Eds.). (1998). *Chronic pain: Assessment, diagnosis, and management.* Boca Raton, FL: CRC Press.

Melzack, R. (1989). *The challenge of pain* (rev. ed.). New York: Penguin.
　　—The classic book in the field.

Philips, H. C., & Rachman, S. (1996). *The psychological management of chronic pain: A treatment manual* (2nd ed.). New York: Springer.
　　—A patient's manual is also available.

Schwartz, M. S., & Andrasik, F. (1995). *Biofeedback: A practitioner's guide.* New York: Guilford Press.

Turk, D. C., & Gatchel, R. J. (Eds.). (2002). *Psychological approaches to pain management: A practitioner's handbook* (2nd ed.). New York: Guilford Press.

Free *Clinical Guides* are available for the management of back pain, cancer pain, headache pain and acute pain from the U.S. Department of Health and Human Services, Public Health Service, Agency for Health Care Policy and Research, AHCPR Publications Clearinghouse, P.O. Box 8547, Silver Spring, MD 20907; 800-358-9295. They are also available via the Internet from PainNet (see below).

Journals

Pain Research and Management
Headache: The Journal of Head and Face Pain
Journal of Pain and Symptom Management
Clinical Journal of Pain
Pediatric Pain Letter

Online Resources

The Arthritis Foundation
http://www.arthritis.org
—This site has resources on FMS, juvenile arthritis, and rheumatoid arthritis for professionals and clients.

Pain Research Center
http://painresearch.utah.edu
—Under "Pain Patients Resources" you will find over one hundred patient resources for all kinds of pain issues and diagnoses. A major resource.

Dick Chapman's Home Page
http://painresearch.utah.edu/crc
—An expert's selections. The "Introductory Information on Pain" offers a superb background in pain treatment and research.

Professional Organizations

American Academy of Pain Management
13947 Mono Way #A, Sonora, CA 95370; 209-533-9744
e-mail: aapm@aapainmanage.org   http://www.aapainmanage.org
—An interdisciplinary organization for pain professionals focusing on alternative medicine, which includes biopsychosocial approaches. More than 60% of the membership consists of physicians. It publishes the *American Journal of Pain Management*; provides information on accreditation; provides access to the National Pain Databank, an outcomes measurement system, which provides diagnosis-specific

treatment outcomes information; and publishes the *National Registry of Multidisciplinary Pain Practitioners*, which lists all credentialed practitioners and accredited pain programs.

American Chronic Pain Association
PO Box 850, Rocklin, CA 95677; 916-632-0922.
e-mail: ACPA@pacbell.net   http://www.theacpa.org
    —A very interesting site with some basic Q&As; very current downloads for professionals on pain medication, pain awareness, and clinical trials; and several focused publications for both professionals and patients.

American Society of Clinical Hypnosis
140 N. Bloomingdale Road, Bloomingdale, IL 60108-1017; 630-980-4740
e-mail: info@asch.net
    —Offers workshops and certification in clinical hypnosis.

American Academy of Pain Medicine
5700 Old Orchard Road, Skokie, IL 60077; 708-966-9510
http://www.painmed.org
    —A pain medicine organization for physicians. Excerpts from its publication *Pain Medicine Network* are available at the Web site. It also sells brochures on pain management for patients, a brochure on cancer pain, and one for insurers and referral sources that can be personalized and used in marketing. Available for downloading are "Writing and Defending Your Expert Report: The Step-by-Step Guides with Models" and "Forensic Opioid Bibliography."

International Association of Industrial Accident Boards and Commissions
    (IAIABC)
http://www.iaiabc.org/
    —A multidisciplinary organization for those interested in workers' compensation issues. This is probably the richest site on facts, procedures, regulations, training, and any other concerns and questions you might have regarding injured workers, for example, on Social Security, definitions and assessment of impairments, EDI (Electronic Data Interchange), and online training. Even HIPAA is fully addressed.

Patient Education Materials: Online Resources, Printed Resources, and Organizations

American Pain Foundation
201 N. Charles Street, Suite 710, Baltimore, MD 21201-4111
e-mail: info@painfoundation.org   http://www.painfoundation.org
    —Here you will find the Pain Management Bill of Rights, articles, and links to many specific resources.

National Foundation for the Treatment of Pain
1330 Skyline Drive, Suite 21, Monterey, CA 93940; 831-655-8812; fax 831-655-2823

e-mail: mgordon@mbay.net   http://www.paincare.org
  —Support and advocacy for pain patients and their families.

Caudill, M. A. (2002). *Managing pain before it manages you* (rev. ed.). New York: Guilford Press.
  —This book is the gold standard in this area. Empirically based on Caudill's treatment and research program, it is a workbook with handouts and is also available in Spanish.

Fransen, J., & Russell, I. J. (1996). *The fibromyalgia help book: Practical guide to living better with fibromyalgia.* St. Paul, MN: Smith House Press.

Starlanyl, D., & Copeland, M. E. (1996). *Fibromyalgia and chronic myofascial pain syndrome: A survival manual.* Oakland, CA: New Harbinger.

Treating Survivors of Motor Vehicle Accidents

OVERVIEW AND OPPORTUNITIES

We all know that motor vehicle accidents (MVAs) are damaging to our bodies, highly disruptive to our lives, and also quite common. Indeed, MVAs constitute the single most frequent trauma experienced by men and the second most frequent trauma experienced by women (Blanchard et al., 1996). Survivors of MVAs sometimes suffer multiple psychological and physiological sequelae, such as acute stress disorder (ASD), posttraumatic stress disorder (PTSD), pain disorders, mood disorders, and phobic reactions to accident-related stimuli (Koch & Taylor, 1995)—all of which can persist for years, creating considerable limitations in functioning. The development of specific interventions for survivors' psychological problems is recent and is still a work in progress. Nonetheless, these treatments show great promise for reducing the suffering and the psychosocial and economic limitations experienced by some survivors of MVAs.

Family members of survivors may likewise benefit from treatment. de Vries et al. (1999), for example, found a high level of PTSD not only among children who had been in MVAs but among their parents, particularly if the parents witnessed the accidents. Sprang (1997) recommends evaluating for PTSD among those who have lost a family member to an alcohol-related MVA. Grief interventions may also be needed if an accident has involved loss of life or serious injury to another, such as a family member or friend. Loss of one's own physical functions as a result of an accident may provoke grief reactions as well.

This area is still actively developing, and clinical work could focus on such aspects as the relationship between attribution of accident responsibility and the development of PTSD (Bulman & Wortman, 1977; Delahanty et al., 1997); the effect of premorbid functioning on the development of PTSD (Malta et al., 2002); and the role of physical injury and pain in the development of and recovery from PTSD (Blanchard et al., 1995).

YOUR POTENTIAL SATISFACTIONS

- You can be one of the first to specialize in this needed area.
- At least one well-formulated and effective treatment program is available for your implementation.
- Medical care (including psychotherapy) that may be required as a result of an MVA is not as micromanaged as care in other health/mental health areas.
- There is the opportunity for secondary prevention, in that early interventions are likely to reduce further deterioration (Blanchard et al., 1996; Bryant et al., 1999).

YOUR SKILL SET

Recycling Your Current Competencies

- Standard treatment skills for anxiety disorders and depression are the core of this therapy.
- There is no additional certification required for work in this area, but see below.

Retreading for Added Skills

- It is essential to have a thorough understanding of ASD, PTSD, and their treatments.
- Hypnosis and other pain management techniques can be useful for work with survivors of MVAs.
- Grief interventions, anger management, relaxation techniques, and substance abuse interventions may be useful adjuncts in many cases.
- You should understand the medico-legal context that survivors of MVAs are placed in and be able to work within this framework.
- Some understanding of the neuropsychology of mild brain injury and TBI.

NATURE OF THE WORK

Approaches and Techniques

The core treatment could be the implementation of the Direct Therapeutic Exposure program. This is a manualized approach described by Blanchard and Hickling (1997) and developed from their intensive clinical experience working with this population. It is a 10-session, exposure-based treatment approach, involving *in vivo* and imaginal flooding as well as cognitive restructuring, positive self-talk, imagery, and relaxation. It offers validated interventions that can be adapted for each client at the clinician's discretion. Shipherd et al. (2000) offer a brief description of a similar CBT model usable with individuals and small groups. *In vivo* desensitization of driving avoidance can be provided with audiotapes that incorporate cognitive and stress management methods; a survivor can listen to these while driving (see Sy Cohn, under "Patient Education Materials," below).

Cross-References to Related Specializations

Niche 1.4. Psychological Management of Chronic Pain
Niche 1.6. Collaborative Practice with Primary Care Physicians

Subspecialization

Prevention

Although the numbers are difficult to determine precisely, it is likely that a substantial number of accidents are related to driver impairments such as drowsiness (Young et al., 1997), to age-related declines in driving ability (Underwood, 1992), to aggressive driving (Lowenstein, 1997), and/or to substance use/abuse (Mancino et al., 1996). You might consider offering additional services for these, depending on your practice's setting.

Practice Models

Both independent practice and team treatment models are widely used. Using a multiple-intervention model, you can provide the kinds of direct treatment services described above.

Rehabilitation is usually a team function. You must know the roles, functions, the terminology, and procedures of all members of the team (including physiatrists; medical social workers; nurses; dietitians; recreational, occupational speech, and physical therapists; etc.).

You can work with survivors and their families, peers, or affected others.

Financial Considerations

Treatment for the psychological sequelae of MVAs is reimbursable under the medical benefits provided by automobile insurance; although it will vary by plan, generally psychological treatment is well covered. For example, such services are typically reimbursed at 110% of Medicare levels. If the automobile insurance limits are reached, the client's regular health insurance may become available.

Cautions, Ethical Dilemmas, Culture Clashes, and/or Managed Care Issues

Consideration must be given to premorbid and comorbid conditions. Blanchard and Hickling (1997) found a significantly greater probability of prior serious MVAs, prior traumatic events, and prior PTSD in survivors of MVAs than in controls without MVAs. Significant childhood trauma may complicate treatment and referral should be considered. PTSD was also more likely in survivors diagnosed with personality disorders (Malta et al., 2002).

As in any collaboration with medical professionals, you must be sensitive to the assignments of responsibilities (boundary or "turf" issues) and the expectations about communication.

To avoid the possibility of becoming entangled in role conflicts, make it very clear to your clients that your role is as a treater, not a forensic expert.

See "Financial Considerations," above, for some managed care issues.

PROSPECTS AND PROSPECTING

Where Is the Need?

Blanchard and Hickling (1997) found that of the survivors of MVAs seen at their clinic, 39% met full diagnostic criteria for PTSD (1 to 4 months after the accidents), and another 28% met criteria for subsyndromal PTSD. Although the rate of spontaneous remission of PTSD symptoms following MVAs is high, some survivors appear not to improve on their own and may suffer long-term limitations in functioning. A subset of this population may have a comorbid diagnosis (e.g., substance abuse) or other problems (e.g., regarding anger modulation) that may have contributed to their involvement in an accident, and these aspects may benefit from psychotherapy.

As public and physician awareness both of these problems and of the availability and effectiveness of treatments develops, increased demand for services can be expected. Clinicians with knowledge, skills, and experience in working with survivors of MVAs should be in demand.

Competition

No profession besides psychology has the combination of skills necessary, and none has entered this area.

Reaching Clients/Directions for Marketing

- Many survivors of MVAs immediately develop ASD, which you can evaluate and treat. To get to see these clients, you could make an effort to educate trauma teams, emergency medical technicians, emergency room personnel, and even PCPs in your area on how to identify those who may need evaluation and/or treatment for ASD.
- Lawyers who work with survivors of MVAs are a large potential referral source. Let them know that you specialize in treating these survivors and specify what services you offer (assessment, pain management, therapy for stress disorders, family interventions, grief interventions, etc.).
- In every community there are physical rehabilitation programs currently serving survivors of MVAs. Most of these are too small to have their own psychologist and might welcome your services.
- Efforts could include writing newsletter articles or delivering oral presentations to these rehabilitation groups, or to community groups like Mothers Against Drunk Driving.
- Companies that insure drivers may be interested in your expertise in evaluation as well as treatment, and so "independent medical examinations" may be a valuable service to offer.

INCREASING YOUR FORMAL KNOWLEDGE BASE

Core Readings

Blanchard, E. B., & Hickling, E. J. (1997). *After the crash: Assessment and treatment of motor vehicle accident survivors.* Washington, DC: American Psychological Association.
—This is *the* core reading and resource.
Hickling, E. J., & Blanchard, E. B. (Eds.). (2000). *International handbook of road traffic accidents and psychological trauma: Current understanding, treatment, and law.* New York: Elsevier.
Wilson, J. P., & Keane, T. M. (Eds.). (1997). *Assessing psychological trauma and PTSD.* New York: Guilford Press.

Online Resources

National Center for Post-Traumatic Stress Disorders
http://www.dartmouth.edu/dms/ptsd

—An excellent resource for further exploration on your own is the Published International Literature On Traumatic Stress (PILOTS) database.

Professional Organizations

Anxiety Disorders Association of America
11900 Parklawn Drive, Suite 100, Rockville, MD 20852; 301-231-8368
—You can purchase a pamphlet on PTSD from this group for $.60 each to distribute to patients, to mail out, or to have available in your waiting room.

Association for the Advancement of Automotive Medicine
2340 Des Plaines Avenue, Suite 106, Des Plaines, IL 60018; 708-390-8927; fax 708-390-9962

Patient Education Materials: Online Resources, Printed Resources, and Organizations

The Driving Therapist
http://www.phobiafreeway.com
—Sy Cohn (the "Driving Therapist") has created *Overcoming Driving Fears and Stress* tapes and CDs designed for use in the car to treat anxious avoidance and phobia. A driving kit that includes the tapes is for sale at the Web site.

Post-Traumatic Stress Disorder—What It Is and What It Means to You
http://www.aafp.org/afp/20000901/1046ph.html
—If you want to receive referrals from PCPs, you should consider creating a handout describing the PTSD symptoms, or request permission to use a published article such as this one, available from American Family Physician.

Allen, J. G. (1995). *Coping with trauma: A guide to self understanding.* Washington, DC: American Psychiatric Press.
Caudill, M. A. (2002). *Managing pain before it manages you* (rev. ed.). New York: Guilford Press.
Matsakis, A. (1992). *I can't get over it: A handbook for trauma survivors.* Oakland, CA: New Harbinger.
Rosenbloom, D., Williams, M. B., & Watkins, B. E. (1999). *Life after trauma: A workbook for healing.* New York: Guilford Press.
Saperstein, R., & Saperstein, D. (1994). *Surviving an auto accident: A guide to your physical, economic and emotional recovery.* Oxnard, CA: Pathfinder.
Smith, J. (1995). *Car accident: A practical recovery manual.* Cleveland, OH: StressPress.
—(Also available at http://cmd-epubs.com/sforms/sporder.html)
Smith, J. C. (1985). *Relaxation dynamics: Nine world approaches to self-relaxation.* Champaign, IL: Research Press.

Collaborative Practice with Primary Care Physicians

OVERVIEW AND OPPORTUNITIES

As noted at the beginning of this section, primary care patients who have psychological disorders utilize a disproportionate amount of medical services (Lechnyr, 1992; Katon, 1995). Olfson et al. (1996) found that even subthreshold symptoms of depression and anxiety carry with them significant disability. This situations represents an enormous financial burden to health insurers. Many studies have shown that providing mental health services reduces this overuse of medical services. An early but classic study of "at-risk" Medicaid patients in Hawaii (Cummings et al., 1993) discovered a substantial decrease in medical utilization among those who received mental health care that was integrated with their medical care. In keeping with findings such as these, the American Academy of Family Physicians (1995) has issued a position paper recommending the inclusion of mental health care in primary care, calling the savings thus achieved "impressive."

Since patients often don't describe their problems as depression or other psychological disorders, and there is no lab test for these, PCPs often don't diagnose them. Although PCPs often make some kind of psychological intervention during a visit (Pace et al., 1995), they are unlikely to make a referral to a mental health clinician (Jones et al., 1987; Regier et al., 1993; Zimmerman & Wienckowski, 1991). And without *adequate* treatment, many patients do not improve (Tiemens et al., 1996; McAleer, 1997). As a result, psychological disorders are both seriously underdiagnosed and sadly undertreated in primary care (e.g., Sartorius et al., 1993). Yet studies have repeatedly demonstrated that psychological interventions in primary care can improve patient satisfaction (Katon et al., 1997), in addition to reducing inappropriate use of medical services (and thus the total costs of care).

Results of collaborations between mental and physical health specialists have shown "win–win–win–win" outcomes, with patients, providers, caregivers, and payers all benefiting from more targeted, integrated, and informed care.

YOUR POTENTIAL SATISFACTIONS

- As McDaniel (1995) has observed, "While collaboration with physicians may result in many new referrals, it may also enliven our work. Crises involving medical illness are frequently intellectually stimulating, technically challenging, and emotionally and spiritually satisfying" (p. 120).
- Because most interventions are short-term and focused on symptoms, you can often see dramatic improvements because of your interventions.
- This is an opportunity to be involved at a relatively early point in what has been called the "linchpin" of our health care system, primary care (McDaniel, 1995).
- Linking mental health and primary care practice in a multidisciplinary collaboration takes physicians and patients alike one giant step closer to the ideal of the biopsychosocial perspective of treating the entire person–family unit.

YOUR SKILL SET

Recycling Your Current Competencies

Basic skills are those outlined in the introduction to this section, particularly crisis intervention, relaxation skills training, and family systems approaches.

Retreading for Added Skills

- Also important are pain management skills, including knowledge and training in hypnosis and biofeedback.
- You will need knowledge of the terms, dynamics, course, treatments, and symptoms of the medically presented disorders in whose treatment you wish to take part.
- Personal experience with extensive medical treatment or chronic conditions is an advantage here.

NATURE OF THE WORK

Areas of Practice

Below we present a sampling of some of the most commonly encountered psychosocial problems seen in primary care, and review some of the findings most suggestive of the benefits of collaborative care.

Depression and Anxiety

PCPs often do not fully recognize and therefore do not treat or refer patients with mood and anxiety disorders. In fact, Katzelnick et al. (2001) found that in a health maintenance organization cohort, only 0.5% of those with generalized social anxiety disorder were appropriately diagnosed or treated. Furthermore, PCPs misdiagnose two-thirds of patients with major depression and about three-quarters of those with any mood disorder (Coyne et al., 1995); even when they recognize mood disorders, PCPs are usually not effective treaters of these (Lin et al., 1997). Yet psychologists can make big differences. Katon et al. (1997) concluded that both psychiatrists and psychiatrist–psychologist teams were effective in improving outcomes with depressed primary care patients. Collaboration between PCPs and mental health clinicians can "dramatically improve adherence, satisfaction with treatment, and depressive outcomes" (Katon, 1995, p. 351).

Mood and anxiety disorders also often co-occur with medical disorders. For instance, panic disorder has been found to be highly associated with cardiac, respiratory, gastrointestinal, and neurological illnesses (Zaubler & Katon, 1996). Cardiac symptoms such as chest pain and palpitations, as well as disorders such as mitral valve prolapse, hypertension, and cardiomyopathy, share significant comorbidity with panic disorder. It seems logical and beneficial that physicians treating such disorders should evaluate and refer a significant number of these patients for treatment of the comorbid panic disorder.

Substance Abuse

Substance abuse (in the general sense of the term, which includes the specific DSM-IV diagnoses of both substance abuse and substance dependence) is also significantly underdiagnosed by PCPs (Milhorn, 1988)—perhaps by as much as 90% (Maly, 1993). In particular, according to Pursch (1978), 75% of physicians do not treat alcohol-related problems effectively.

Screening instruments such as the CAGE, the Michigan Alcohol Screening Test (MAST), and the Short MAST (SMAST) can discern approximately 80% of alcohol problems (Mayfield et al., 1974). Israel et al. (1996) report on the success of an unobtrusive and brief (four-item) questionnaire that identifies between 62% and 85% of alcohol problems in primary care practice. Those individuals who were detected by questionnaire and were then given a very brief (3-hour) CBT showed significant reductions in alcohol intake at a 1-year follow-up, improvement in psychosocial problems, and a reduction in physician visits. However, physicians do not appear to have the time for even such brief and effective interventions.

Somatization Disorder

Somatization is associated with increased medical usage of medical care, significant disability, and comorbidity with depression and anxiety. One study (Fink et al., 1999) found that between 22% and 58% of primary care patients met the standard criteria for somatoform disorder. However, despite calls by leading experts for compassionate care of the somatizing patient through collaboration with behavioral health specialists (Lipsitt, 1996) these patients are rarely seen by therapists. Why not?

Although physicians are eager to refer such patients for mental health services, the patients usually do not follow through on such referrals; they are convinced of the physical basis for their complaints. Only with a close collaborative relationship will they be enticed into appropriate treatment. And psychological treatment has been effective. McLeod et al. (1997) demonstrated a 6-week behavioral medicine intervention with somatizing patients in primary care that produced significant decreases in somatization, anxiety, and depression at a 6-month follow-up compared to controls. Lidbeck (1997) reported on a CBT group intervention for somatizing patients that led to symptom relief and medication use reduction at a 6-month follow-up.

Morse et al. (1997) interviewed a small sample of female patients with somatization disorder and found an association between childhood abuse and somatizing symptoms. After making the connection between their physical symptoms and their childhood abuse experiences, 70% of the women reported reductions in health care utilization. Hotopf et al. (1999) found a "powerful relationship" between unexplained symptoms in adulthood and a history of parental illnesses during childhood.

Childhood Disorders

The need for screening of pediatric patients is great: Bowman and Garralda (1993) found that 21% of children who visited a general practice were "frequent attenders," accounting for 50% of services provided. This group showed three times as much psychological disturbance as those who utilized the services less often, yet the psychosocial component of their illness was missed by their pediatricians.

Typical psychosocial interventions for children that can be implemented very effectively within a collaborative care model (Schroeder, 1997) include surgery preparation and the management of chronic diseases (e.g., asthma, recurrent abdominal pain, and other chronic pain). Pediatric obesity is another area where physicians feel undertrained (Pratt et al., 1997), frustrated, and lacking in referral sources for treatment (Alday et al., 1999). Psychological problems commonly brought to pediatricians include enuresis, encopresis, sleep disorders, childhood anxieties, attachment disorders, stressful life events, behavioral problems, sexual abuse, and learning disorders. Of course, this whole list can be effectively addressed by psychologists.

Cross-References to Related Specializations

Niche 1.2. Supporting Caregivers and Working with Chronic Illnesses
Niche 1.4. Psychological Management of Chronic Pain
Niche 5.1. Gerontology and Services to Aging Populations
Niche 5.2. Clinical Practice in a Rural Area
Niche 5.5. Wellness and Positive Psychology

Practice Models

The consensus of many who practice in this area is that collaborating with physicians works best in a shared physical location (Cummings, 1992; Kainz, 2002; McDaniel, 1995). Lesser forms of integration are probably not as effective, since they put the onus on patients to make the transition to your "specialist" care. Distance may raise those familiar resistances associated with mental health care and its attendant stigma. Furthermore, the opportunity to develop collegial relationships with physicians is greater when physicians and therapists are under the same roof. Follow-up and feedback on referred patients and mutual education are maximized in this arrangement.

Collaborative care may require some adjustments in the way you practice. McDaniel (1995) suggests these:

- Short-term models are predominant, and one-session interventions are not unheard of.
- Shorter sessions (less than 50 minutes) are common, with appointments made hours or a day or two, not weeks, ahead.
- Assessments are rapid, with immediate and concise feedback to physicians on diagnosis, prognosis, and treatment plans.
- Progress reports should be frequently updated.
- Call-in hours when physicians and patients can reach you are essential.
- Visiting patients at home, in a hospital, or at a rehabilitation center may be necessary.

See also Kainz (2002) and Bray and Rogers (1995) for more on what physicians expect from collaborating psychologists.

For PCPs, a distinct advantage of working with psychologists as opposed to psychiatrists is that the psychologists will not "steal patients" or "take over cases," but instead will work with the PCPs around medication issues and case management. The PCPs are happy to know that patients' mental health needs will be taken care of by competent professionals, and they will not have to spend their allotted 15 minutes with this kind of case or refer to someone who will simply write out a prescription.

Two illuminating descriptions of pediatric collaborative care are provided by Schroeder (1997) and Evers-Szostak (1998). Although their average number of sessions per patient is five, they find that for patients requiring long-term interventions for serious emotional problems, "neither the parents nor the pediatricians want us to refer these children out of the practice. They argue for continuity of care and working with people with whom they have come to trust. . . . In addition to new referrals, we have discovered that a number of children and parents return for help at different points in the children's development" (Schroeder, 1997, p. 113). Evers-Szostak (1998) reports that parents' feedback indicated a high satisfaction with the availability of psychological services within the context of the pediatric primary care practice. For ideas about possible collaboration modes and some of the social and financial issues, all from an MD's perspective, see Slomski (2000).

Financial Considerations

If you are interested in working in a PCP's office, you also need to think about what financial arrangements you will make. Options to consider range from paying rent for the time you use the office and doing your own billing to becoming an employee of the physician's practice.

Cautions, Ethical Dilemmas, Culture Clashes, and/or Managed Care Issues

As mentioned in the introduction to this section, you must pay careful attention to the boundaries of each profession and of your own areas of competency. Also, medical patients will most often be using their health insurance, and so this is not a managed-care-free area. However, since your interventions are likely to be brief, self-pay is more likely than in a traditional psychotherapy practice.

Fee splitting is still felt to be ethically questionable by most clinicians, although it is allowed by the APA's code of ethics (APA, 2002) if the patient is fully informed, so make very clear all your arrangements and relationships.

PROSPECTS AND PROSPECTING

Where Is the Need?

As more insurance companies strive to provide better services and recognize the benefits of cost offset, opportunities should expand. Physicians are becoming more aware of the importance of psychological and relationship factors in the practice of medicine (see, e.g., Novack et al., 1997).

Competition

The word is out, and you will find social workers (mainly) as well as all kinds of counselors, therapists, and consultants trying to partner with PCPs. However, as a psychologist you have many advantages (and no disadvantages), such as these:

- Having a doctoral degree and thus being able to be called "Doctor" by patients and staff. (Do not underestimate or discard the power of the ascribed social status to bring relief.)
- A comprehensive understanding of the various interactions involved in the biopsychosocial model.
- Skills in psychological assessment and diagnosis.
- Familiarity with the treatments shown to be effective.
- Eligibility for health insurance reimbursement.

Reaching Clients/Directions for Marketing

If you are interested in collaborating with PCPs—pediatricians, internists, family practitioners, or obstetricians/gynecologists—there are large opportunities simply because they tend to have very large practices and therefore many patients in need of psychological services.

- Writing about the opportunities for psychologist-physician collaboration, McDaniel (1995) notes: "Once good collaborative relationships are formed, psychosocially sensitive physicians will often refer a wide range of problems and a large number of patients so that the professional psychologist can build a full practice with these contacts alone" (p. 119).
- Divisions 29 and 42 of the APA have brochures for practitioners working with the psychosocial aspects of illness (e.g., coping with cancer, heart disease, or chronic illness), which you can personalize for use in your marketing efforts with physicians.
- In one model, staff members at Behavior Resources in Greenville, South Carolina, provide information to physicians at monthly hospi-

tal meetings on such topics as depression in children, suicide, and appropriate referrals to a mental health specialist ("Practice Building," 1995). They also offer information to pediatric residents. This gives them the opportunity to familiarize 15–20 physicians a month with the services they offer. Consider whether you could adopt a similar educational approach.

- Mori et al. (1999) present PRIMECARE, an innovative direct-contact model for working with primary care patients that does not depend on direct physician-generated referrals. A brief questionnaire is given to patients as part of a primary care visit. In addition to measuring symptomatology, the questionnaire asks about interest in such services as pain management, cardiac rehabilitation, cancer support, substance abuse treatment, chronic illness coping, smoking cessation, and so forth. (The questionnaire can be adapted to reflect the services you provide.) Follow-up by phone is initiated by mental health clinicians if a patient expresses any interest in services. This method was able to increase referrals almost fourfold over a 6-month period, compared with traditional physician-initiated referrals.

INCREASING YOUR FORMAL KNOWLEDGE BASE

Core Readings

Belar, C. D., & Deardorff, W. W. (1995). *Clinical health psychology in medical settings: A practitioner's guidebook*. Washington, DC: American Psychological Association.

Blount, A. (Ed.). (1998). *Integrated primary care: The future of medical and mental health collaboration*. New York: Norton.
   —This book offers case examples of such integration, as well as many perspectives.

Drotar, D. (1995). *Consulting with pediatricians: Psychological perspectives*. New York: Plenum Press.

Haley, W. E., McDaniel, S. H., Bray, J. H., Frank, R. G., Heldring, M., Johnson, S. B., Lu, E. G., Reed, G. M., & Wiggins, J. G. (1998). Psychological practice in primary care settings: Practical tips for clinicians. *Professional Psychology: Research and Practice, 29*(3), 237–244.
   —This article describes the culture of primary care medicine and offers 10 practical tips for the adaptation of psychological practice to primary care.

Hamberger, K. L., Ovide, C. R., & Weiner, E. L. (1999). *Making collaborative connections with medical providers*. New York: Springer.

Pollin, I. (1995). *Medical crisis counseling: Short-term therapy for long-term illness*. New York: Norton.

Schroeder, C. S., & Gordon, B. N. (2002). *Assessment and treatment of childhood problems: A clinician's guide* (2nd ed.). New York: Guilford Press.

You may find books and articles of relevance under "liaison psychiatry" or "psychiatric consultation."

Journals

Families, Systems and Health
Journal of Interprofessional Care
Journal of Health Psychology

Online Resources

Center for the Advancement of Health (CFAH)
2000 Florida Ave. N.W., Suite 210, Washington, DC 20009-1231; 202-387-2829;
     202-387-2857
e-mail: cfah@cfah.org   http://www.cfah.org
—Dedicated to the advancement of behavioral medicine, the center "sponsors and participates in symposia that explore the intersections of physical and mental health and their implications for research, policy and practice." Many free articles are available at the Web site.

Academy of Psychosomatic Medicine
http://www.apm.org
—There is much of value at this consultation psychiatry organization's Web site, including current and back issues (full text) of its journal *Psychosomatics* and its newsletter.

Counseling in Primary Care Trust
http://www.cpct.co.uk/
—This site's database, Counsel.lit, is searchable online on such topics as collaborative team work, research methods, systems theory, somatization, physician stress, patient satisfaction, and health psychology as they relate to primary care.

Pediatric Development and Behavior
http://www.dbpeds.org
—This is a good place to learn about issues regarding how pediatricians deal with psychosocial problems in their day-to-day practice.

Health Psychology and Rehabilitation
http://www.healthpsych.com
—Many useful articles and practical suggestions about practicing psychology in medical and rehabilitation settings can be found here.

Professional Organizations

Society of Behavioral Medicine
http://www.sbm.org

American Psychological Association divisions:

Division 29 (Psychotherapy)
http://www.apa.org/divisions/div29

Division 38 (Health Psychology)
e-mail: apadiv38@erols.com   http://www.apa.org/divisions/div38
—Membership entitles you to the Division's newsletter, the *Health Psychologist*, as well as its journal, *Health Psychology*.

Division 42 (Independent Practice)
http://www.division42.org
—The largest division of APA, Division 42 offers many resources for practitioners interested in working with physicians.

Section 2

Couples, Families, Children, and Schools

Introduction, Overview, and Commonalities

Years ago, adults were considered either single or married. Today, couple relationships can be widely varied and complex. They can include long-term unmarried couples, recently engaged couples, newlyweds still in the "honeymoon stage," existing distressed marriages, abusive marriages, actively divorcing couples, separated but not yet divorced couples, "newly single" former spouses—and, of course, couples where the partners are of different races, ethnicities, or religions; same-sex couples; "marriages of convenience"; and so on (and on). Many additional complexities arise when children are added (or not added) to relationships. Couples may be childless by choice, or may be undergoing fertility treatments, infertility, fetal loss, or adoption proceedings. Then there are families of special-needs children; parents of twins, triplets, or other multiples; single-parent families; stepfamilies and blended families; gay, lesbian, and bisexual parents; parents (and siblings) who have lost a child; parents with an "empty nest"; and families caring for frail or ill elderly relatives. No doubt, dozens more types of couples and families could be listed.

Besides the changed landscape of relationships, there have been significant changes among our youth as well. The American Academy of Pediatrics Committee on Psychosocial Aspects of Child and Family Health (2001) has stated:

> The mortality of meningococcemia is appreciated by all pediatricians, but the morbidity of depression and the mortality of adolescent suicide are more appreciable. In other words, after infancy, children in the United States are more likely to die from injuries or violence than from infectious diseases. (p. 1228)

The committee identifies many "newer morbidities" that have transformed pediatric practice. These include school problems, such as learning disabilities and attention difficulties; child and adolescent mood and anxiety disorders; adolescent suicide and homicide, and other violence both at school and at home; drug and alcohol abuse; HIV+ syndrome; eating disorders and obesity; and early sexual activity. Changes such as these create opportunities for psychologists to establish linkages with physicians in order to develop methods of prevention, enhance resilience, smooth transitions, serve special needs, and address the issues raised by heightened multicultural awareness.

OUR INCREASED KNOWLEDGE

Recent research has underscored the importance of the family as both a protective factor and a force in recovery from mental illness and substance abuse. Studies of risk and resiliency have developed ways of identifying couples at risk for various dysfunctions and of marshaling protective factors, allowing more efficient focus for prevention and early secondary intervention. Examples of other important advances that can be utilized in our interventions with children and families include the following:

- Fundamental shifts have occurred in our understanding of the relationships between family functioning and the onset, course, comorbidity, outcome, and relapse of certain psychological disorders. Interventions that focus on parents, families, and couples have produced positive results for at-risk children and "identified patients" in families (e.g., Patterson et al., 2000; Mari & Streiner, 1996; Cordova & Gee, 2001; Morrison et al., 2000).
- As research has accumulated about the importance of ethnicity, a need has been created for clinicians who can craft specific clinical interventions for ethnically diverse groups. Applied to the niches discussed in this section, this knowledge could be used to create subniches according to a diversity perspective. (See Niche 5.3 for more on culturally informed interventions.)
- Our growing understanding of gender differences and gender-specific issues has led to greater specificity of our interventions in this area as well. You will see an example of this in Niche 2.4.
- Recent research has suggested the efficacy of combining couple or family interventions with other approaches to augment outcomes. For example, behavioral couple treatment for alcohol and drug use disorders (e.g., Epstein & McCrady, 1998) and relapse prevention via couple therapy sessions (e.g., O'Farrell et al., 1998) are promising developments; they suggest that including significant others in substance abuse treatment improves outcomes.

As a result of such developments, couple and family therapy interventions can now be thought of as a panoply of finely tuned and targeted approaches for each of these populations. The niches in this section are often overlooked areas of family and relationship functioning that are likely to benefit from a greater specificity of approach. These niches may not be the only or even the very best areas for specializing your family/relationship practice; they are meant simply as examples, ideas, and starting points. (Be sure to check under niches' "subspecializations" headings for additional ideas.)

RECYCLING YOUR CURRENT COMPETENCIES

If you are a couple and/or family therapist, you probably already have the following skills, experiences, and attitudes that will stand you in good stead for work with the niches in this section:

- A core understanding of couple and familial factors that affect individual functioning, and knowledge of how to communicate that understanding to aid individual psychological development as it is rooted in the couple or family.
- A respect for the complexity of, and a comprehensive grasp of, life-span, cognitive, interpersonal, and systems theory approaches to relationships, families, and parenting.
- Skills in using techniques of proven efficacy to ameliorate dysfunctional patterns and augment the healing and nurturing properties of couples and families.
- Familiarity with consultation and group interventions that will be useful for networking with agencies, school systems, and parent groups.

ATTENDING TO THE TRENDS

Developments in such fields as genetics, health care, and communications have created new demands and adaptive challenges for families.

- The field of genetic counseling for parents, for example, has been extended by the improved ability to identify genetic predispositions to breast cancer and other serious diseases.
- Developments in health care have created new choices and new conundrums for families, ranging from assisted reproduction to assisted suicide. In particular, the ability to prolong life has produced a "sandwich generation" of caregivers.

- Families are also coping with increased demands on wage earners' time, since the number of hours that Americans work has been increasing, shrinking the time parents and children spend together. As one result, children may come to kindergarten without the social and emotional skills that have been shown to be early predictors of success or failure in school.
- Developments in telecommunications have an impact upon families by blurring the boundaries of work and family life, thus creating new demands and stresses on working parents and children.
- Finally, the Internet has, for better or worse, opened new vistas of influence for families, new sources of connection and community, and new anxieties for parents, with the prefix "cyber" defining new genres of relationships (even sexual relationships).

REACHING CLIENTS/DIRECTIONS FOR MARKETING

Services to Couples and Families

- Create linkages with attorneys, courts, and agencies that specialize in matrimonial or family law (prenuptial, custody, divorce).
- Collaborate or network with medical specialists who may be gatekeepers and case finders, such as gynecologists (for women), urologists (for men), and primary care physicians (PCPs).
- Clergy can provide access to distressed couples and families, and they may be happy to refer their more challenging cases. Psychoeducational offerings to parishioners can serve as an entry point for collaboration with clergy. See Weaver et al. (1997), Edwards et al. (1999), and McMinn et al. (2001) for more on this topic.
- Valentine's Day is an opportunity to reach out to couples. Other holidays (e.g., Thanksgiving or Christmas) can be stressful events for families in transition, especially for families with newly single or never-married parents.

School-Related Services

- Collaborate with other professionals who work with students (e.g., pediatricians, adolescent health specialists, learning disability specialists, college counselors, or coaches for the SAT and similar examinations) by forming a group practice or through sharing office space.
- Offer seminars to parents, PTAs/PTOs, schools, Scout groups, and clubs for children and families. These will make them better able to recognize problems, and thus more likely to seek services for these problems.

- Help your school system improve detection of students' emotional problems, and make school personnel aware of the services you can provide. Explore synergistic relationships with guidance counselors and others in your local school district who deal with student behavior and disciplinary problems. Tell them you are available for consultations, presentations to teacher in-service sessions, or whatever formats they have available. Offer to provide prevention or early intervention programs in local public agencies.
- Locate your office close to schools. Make certain your signage is prominent and clear. Offer descriptive brochures in commonly accessed locations.
- Link your marketing efforts with upcoming events—for instance, Children's Mental Health Week, Childhood Depression Awareness Day, Learning Disabilities Awareness day/week/month, or various Education Days (e.g., math or science appreciation events). Go to http://www.healthieryou.com/advocacy/observe.htm to find information by month and year for national observances. The first day of school (for school refusal issues) and the end of the semester (for test anxiety) are other opportunities to highlight your services.

THIRD-PARTY PAYER ISSUES

Each specialization in this section has some non-managed-care aspects, which are discussed where relevant.

OPPORTUNITIES

The phrase "an embarrassment of riches" might describe the many opportunities for offering needed and effective psychological services to couples and families today. As noted earlier, in this section we present only a few examples of the many possibilities for niching your services as a couple and/or family therapist. Other potential niches—to name a few—include premarital counseling, sex therapy, interventions for divorcing families, adoption or infertility counseling, "empty nest" counseling, and so on. Still other opportunities for family and relationship therapists exist in working with older adults (see Niche 5.1), working with caregivers (see Niche 1.2), helping families cope with death and dying (see Niche 1.3), and consulting to family-owned businesses (see Niche 3.2).

Relationship Enrichment Programs

OVERVIEW AND OPPORTUNITIES

No one has ever said that being part of a couple is easy, and for many people a "functional" relationship is "good enough." However, many souls long for more intimacy, communication, romance, commitment, sex, or some more personal definition of a "better" relationship.

Adding a relationship enrichment program to your practice may be of value both to those who do not need couple therapy and to those who have made significant progress in such therapy and want to make more. Although enrichment may be provided in many formats and from any orientation, several researchers and clinicians have developed programs to improve the quality of relationships and have empirically demonstrated their value. We present here only well-developed, time-limited, brand-named, psychoeducational-model programs. The programs are structured but not rigid, and their authors often suggest modifications to suit your setting and audience while retaining their essential aspects and benefits.

YOUR POTENTIAL SATISFACTIONS

- You will be working with generally solid relationships, and that is less stressful. Enrichment programs come under the heading of "wellness" rather than "curing illness."
- Clients will be expanding and exploring new territory for them, which is exciting and satisfying work for both them and you.
- These programs are quite complete, comprehensive, and easily adopted.

- The programs are time- or session-limited, and the content and schedule are largely prepared and tested for you.
- Enrichment will never be covered by managed care, as it is not, by definition, "medically necessary."

YOUR SKILL SET

Recycling Your Current Competencies

- You must, of course, have skills, experience, knowledge, and training for working with committed relationships. Core skills might include the ability to assess relationships so that you can identify and refer those inappropriate for these programs; group therapy skills to manage the interactions of the member couples; educational skills because of the contents of the programs; the ability to evaluate the outcomes of your programs; and an acceptance and tolerance of a variety of relationship styles and arrangements.
- In our opinion, you must be in a rich couple relationship yourself.

Retreading for Added Skills

We recommend learning one of the packaged programs described below, as these have some demonstrated validity, and their structure is comforting to both clients and therapists. Each of the programs has a structured training and supervision path to skill and expertise. You will find their materials clear and highly polished. Training costs range from a few hundred to a few thousand dollars in money and time.

Since there is no body of research to show significant differential benefit of one program over another in all areas explore several before choosing to get training in or to implement one.

NATURE OF THE WORK

In setting up the treatment groups, the first issue is to exclude clients with severe conflicts, who are unlikely to benefit from enrichment programs but who may benefit from individual treatment or couple therapy. Of course, you will use your interview and history taking to help make this distinction, and there are dozens of relationship assessment instruments to support your decision making and for documenting pre–post changes due to enrichment services. See Corcoran and Fischer (2000) for a variety of measures.

Another aspect of the selection process could involve John Gottman's work. His two books (Gottman, 1994; Gottman with Silver, 1994) offer an amazing package. The measures he has developed and validated for married couples can predict who will divorce with surprising accuracy. These are presented in one book (Gottman, 1994), while the other (Gottman with Silver, 1994) describes how they were developed and offers lots of ideas about the trajectories of marriages. Providing this kind of feedback to couples might be a very valuable premarital counseling service.

Cross-References to Related Specializations

Niche 2.2. Assisting Stepfamilies and Blended Families
Niche 3.2. Consulting to Family-Owned Businesses

Subspecializations

Enrichment program skills can be extended into niches that have significant growth potential. Here are some examples:

- Kushnir et al. (1996) have combined couple enrichment with cognitive stress management and behavioral treatment components to reduce the conflicts of relationships with two employed partners.
- Accordino and Guerney (1998) have extended the well-researched Relationship Enhancement program (described below) to prisoners and their wives.
- Filial therapy is a version of the Relationship Enhancement program. It has been very widely implemented to teach parents to work therapeutically with their disturbed children. See, for example, VanFleet (1994, 2000), Harris and Landreth (1997), and Costas and Landreth (1999).

Practice Models

Most of these programs are provided in groups, and so you will need group space.

An issue common to all group work is securing sufficient clients to create groups that will be large enough to allow the mutual support among members and make the time profitable to you. No one likes to wait for treatment, but couples seeking enrichment are more patient than most. If you advertise your groups far in advance, scheduling them to start each 3 months, and are willing to run a group for a small number on occasion, you should succeed.

However, offering enrichment in a dyadic format answers a need by giving those who are not comfortable with sharing in a group the benefits of these methods. Practitioners who offer both formats may do best.

Financial Considerations

- These are structured programs and so have a set fee for a set number of sessions.
- Since group presentations are the norm for efficiency and social learning, fees can be low enough to attract numbers of couples and yet high enough to be profitable.
- Each couple should pay the whole program fee in advance, and it may be advantageous for motivation to advertise a "no-refunds" policy, although you could then make some exceptions in very unusual circumstances.

Cautions, Ethical Dilemmas, Culture Clashes, and/or Managed Care Issues

Although doing "enrichment," not "therapy" or "counseling," does not technically require a license, be aware that couples may not make this distinction—nor may licensing bodies or courts, if there is a complaint or lawsuit.

Because these programs are not "medically necessary," they are managed care-free. Resist making inaccurate, illegal, and unethical overdiagnosis of one partner so that insurance can be used.

PROSPECTS AND PROSPECTING

Where Is the Need?

- Except for married couples committed to divorcing, and couples who have settled into stable but unhappy relationships and have no wish to upset these, all intimate relationships are potential candidates for relationship enrichment programs. The market is therefore enormous and bottomless.
- With more people staying together and more concern for relationships' quality, there should be a growing market for these services. The "baby boomers" now have the time and money to invest in their relationships.

Competition

Unfortunately, almost anyone can get training in using these methods, so difficulty of entry is not a barrier to competition. Worse is that all kinds of "relationship counselors" consider that they can do enrichment just because they have experience with counseling.

Reaching Clients/Directions for Marketing

- A substantial percentage of unhappily yoked folks will not accept the "patient" or "sick" role required to seek couple *therapy* or even *counseling*. However, they can be attracted to programs labeled "enrichment." Even if they find these insufficient to alter their situation, they will have become educated and socialized into a therapy analogue and so will be more accepting of couple therapy, which you could then provide.
- Although few people will brag to their friends about their couple therapy, many will be happy to tell others of your enrichment program's value because it allows them to praise themselves and their partners, the efforts they have made, and the benefits they have gained. Generally, to make these referrals work, you must ask participants specifically to talk to their friends and relatives, describe exactly what they might say and how to say it, and give them literature to pass on. Some of this can be done during a late-phase evaluation-of-progress session.
- Most religious and social organizations will be happy to publicize your work. Advertisements in local publications for families and children may be very productive. As for all advertising, you should plan your campaign to last at least a year.
- Some of these programs offer ready-made advertising materials and trademarked names. Several are already well established in the public's mind.
- Offering a brand-named product distinguishes you from other providers rest and so can allow you to flourish.
- You might choose to offer several of the programs described below—not only to enlarge the number of clients, but to allow your graduates to try a different approach later to work for even better relationships.

INCREASING YOUR FORMAL KNOWLEDGE BASE

Core Readings

Berger, R., & Hannah, M. T. (1999). *Preventive approaches in couples therapy*. New York: Brunner/Mazel.
  —Many relationship enrichment programs are described here, along with the research supporting their efficacy.

Ginsberg, B. G. (1997). *Relationship Enhancement family therapy*. New York: Wiley.
  —Ginsberg extends the work of Bernard and Louise Guerney from the 1950s. Solidly researched and comprehensive, with many practical ideas.

L'Abate, L., & Weinstein, S.E. (1987). *Structured enrichment programs for couples and families.* New York: Brunner/Mazel.

—This book is replete with exercises and homework for enrichment and prevention. Topics include parenting, in-laws, sex, expressing anger constructively, conflict resolution, being direct, communicating feelings, self-assertion, intimacy, openness, and finances. They also include transitions, such as becoming a parent, midlife, retirement, and widowhood.

L'Abate, L., & Young, L. (1987). *Casebook: Structured enrichment programs for couples and families.* New York: Brunner/Mazel.

—A companion to the L'Abate and Weinstein book.

Philpot, C. L., Brooks, G. R., & Lusterman, D.-D. (1997). *Bridging separate gender worlds: Why men and women clash and how therapists can bring them together.* Washington, DC: American Psychological Association.

—The book's jacket copy states that this "provides therapists with gender-sensitive techniques and interventions to help clients understand the challenges of today's confused gender expectations." Like fish that can't discover water, most of us barely pay attention to these issues, but we need "top-of-mind awareness" to do therapy on male–female relationships. An antidote to John Gray's astrology.

Schnarch, D. (1997). *Passionate marriage: Keeping love and intimacy alive in committed relationships.* New York: Holt.

—Schnarch's is by no means a packaged program, but an intense and wise exploration of love and marriage.

Packaged Programs and/or Franchises

Quite logically, the major researchers in the marriage area have developed programs and/or written popular books (see "Patient Education Materials," below) to reduce the stresses or increase the pleasures of marriage. Here are some of the better-known ones to explore and evaluate. You can get current information from their Web sites.

Couple Communication

Interpersonal Communications Programs, Inc.
7201 S. Broadway, Littleton, CO 80122; 800-328-5099; fax 303-798-3392
http://www.couplecommunication.com

—Developed by Sherod Miller, Couple Communication teaches communication and conflict resolution skills in four 2-hour groups or a couple format (six 50-minute sessions). Training consists of a 1-day workshop, homework, a written test, and treating 20 couples with supervision feedback.

The following two programs (EFMT and Imago) are designed as couple therapies, but can be used for enrichment programs and are included here because of their advanced development.

Emotionally Focused Marital Therapy

Susan M. Johnson has developed Emotionally Focused Marital Therapy (EFMT) from attachment theory, a psychodynamic orientation. Spouses explore the feelings, thoughts, and needs that are believed to underlie their current distress. The aims are greater empathy and understanding, which then free the couple to interact in different ways. For more information on EFMT, see Greenberg and Johnson (1988), Johnson and Greenberg (1994), and Johnson (1996).

Imago Relationship Therapy

Institute for Imago Relationship Therapy
335 North Knowles Avenue, Winter Park, FL 32789; 406-644-3537, 800-729-1121
e-mail: info@imagotherapy.com   http://www.imagotherapy.com
    —Developed and taught by Harville Hendrix for many years, Imago focuses on the unconscious influences on mate selection and in one's adult relationships, and the potential for personal and spiritual growth. Publications include a brief overview by Zeilinski (1999), a casebook by Luquet and Hannah (1998), and Luquet (1996)'s manual for a six-session version.

GROW: Relationship Counseling

Couples take a shortened version of the Adult Personality Inventory, which is then used to generate data for a four-session/8-week counseling program (with a workbook). The Introductory Kit ($25) offers a manual, two test booklets, test processing, and the four lessons. The reference publication is Henry et al. (1984).

Worldwide Marriage Encounter

Worldwide Marriage Encounter
909-863-9963   http://www.wwme.org
    —The oldest and most widely presented program, Worldwide Marriage Encounter uses a structured discussion format, lasting a weekend. It is most frequently offered in mainline (especially Roman Catholic) churches, as well as synagogues. Typically the charge is small. There is also an Engaged Encounter. Though not hostile to therapists, the leaders are not professionals. You might consider approaching this group in your community to see whether there might be referrals for those who do not benefit from these brief, primarily educational programs.

Practical Application of Intimate Relationship Skills

PAIRS Foundation, Ltd.
1056 Creekford Dr., Weston, FL 33326; 888-PAIRS-4U, 954-389-9596
e-mail: info@pairs.org   http://www.pairs.com
    —Lori Gordon designed the Practical Application of Intimate Relationship Skills (PAIRS)—a 4- to 5-month, 100- to 120-hour ("Semester") program that emphasizes

developing self-knowledge as well as relationship skills. Shorter (1-day and week-end) program formats are now also available. PAIRS uses paired teachers, who can be certified in a 4-day intensive program, and it is not inexpensive (several thousand dollars).

Prevention and Relationship Enhancement Program

PREP Inc.
P.O. Box 102530, Denver, CO 80250-2530; 303-759-9931, ext. 932; fax 303-759-4212
e-mail: prepinc@aol.com   http://www.prepinc.com
—Howard Markman and his associates, founders of the Prevention and Relationship Enhancement Program (PREP), are well-respected researchers and clinicians in this area. They offer video- and audiotapes, and professional materials such as "Concept Sheets," a package of research publications. Their books include Notarius and Markman (1994), Markman et al. (1996), and Stanley et al. (1998), which offer PREP as well as research findings on communication, skills training, commitment, forgiveness, friendship, fun, and physical intimacy.

PREPARE/ENRICH

Life Innovations, Inc.
P.O. Box 190, Minneapolis, MN 55440-0190; 800-331-1661
http://www.prepare-enrich.com
—The four PREPARE/ENRICH programs are aimed at premarital, premarital with children, married, and over-age-50 married couples. In the first meeting, couples complete a questionnaire about issues they struggle with. This questionnaire has excellent research support. It is sent for scoring, and in the next meeting each couple is given a 15-page computerized report designed to create a meaningful dialogue between the couple and the counselor. Couples return for three to six feedback sessions. The Web site describes 3-hour training workshops or a self-training manual.

Relationship Enhancement

National Institute of Relationship Enhancement
4400 East–West Highway, Suite 28, Bethesda, MD 20814-4501; 800-4-FAMILIES, 301-986-1479; fax 301-680-3756
e-mail: info@nire.org   http://www.nire.org
—Relationship Enhancement is the best researched and most widely used method in this area. Originally designed to improve communication with active listening, it has been extended over the years with additional foci. Developed originally by Bernard and Louise Guerney, it has been successfully applied to hundreds of populations and settings. The Web site offers training, books, and professional materials. The best up-to-date survey and introduction are provided by Ginsberg (1997) and the original book by Guerney (1977) is still highly relevant.

Training in Marriage Enrichment

Don Dinkmeyer, Sr., and Jon Carlson developed Training in Marriage Enrichment (TIME), a group educational program, some years ago. It is distributed by American Guidance Service (800-328-2560). The package ($150) includes a Leader's Guide, Participant's Handbooks, six audiotapes, and other materials. TIME can be presented as 10 sessions of individual or group therapy or as a weekend retreat.

Patient Education Materials: Online Resources, Printed Resources, and Organizations

Beck, A. T. (1988). *Love is never enough: How couples can overcome misunderstandings, resolve conflicts, and solve relationship problems through cognitive therapy*. New York: Harper & Row.
> —Beck applies cognitive therapy and its ideas to couple relationships.

Gottman, J. G. M., with Silver, N. (1995). *Why marriages succeed or fail: What you can learn from the breakthrough research to make your marriage last*. New York: Simon & Schuster.
> —Solidly based on his many years of research, John Gottman's models and advice are trustworthy. In brief, he believes that marriages cope with conflicts in one of these three styles: validating, conflict-avoiding, and volatile. Couples are in trouble if they interact with criticism, contempt, defensiveness, or withdrawal. Stable and happy marriages have a 5:1 ratio of positive-to-negative interactions.

Gottman, J. M. (1999). *The marriage clinic: A scientifically-based marital therapy*. New York: Norton.
> —A popular version of Gottman's findings and techniques.

McKay, M., & Fanning, P. (1994). *Couple skills: Making your relationship work*. Oakland, CA: New Harbinger.
> —This is a collection of descriptions of the skills seen as essential for marriage, mainly communication and negotiation. Clients will like the book for its simplicity and clarity, but are unlikely to be able to implement these skills without professional support.

Scarf, M. (1996). *Intimate partners: Patterns in love and marriage* (reissued ed.). New York: Ballantine Books.
> —Scarf presents the stages of relationship development (idealization, disenchantment, child rearing, career building) through many cases. She attends to multiple generations to show how the past is repeated and unconscious needs shape current behaviors.

Assisting Stepfamilies and Blended Families

OVERVIEW AND OPPORTUNITIES

Making a family work is one of the hardest jobs in the world. How much harder then is making two families work as one? The research indicates that it is a great deal harder, and this is why our skills are needed.

- Stepfamilies are very common. More than 40% of children will live in a stepfamily at some point in their lives, according to Bray (1999). When children from one or both parents are brought into a stepfamily, and the parents have additional children in the new marriage, the result is often called a "blended family."
- Stepfamilies experience a high degree of stress, especially during the early years after remarriage. Research confirms that stepfamilies are characterized by less positive relationships, less cohesion, and more conflict (Bray & Berger, 1993; Waldren et al., 1990; Ganong & Coleman, 1993). Fine and Kurdek (1995) report that problems in the stepparent–stepchild relationship are correlated with less marital satisfaction for the stepparents.
- A wide range of studies have found children of stepfamilies to be at increased risk for emotional, behavioral, learning, and health-related problems (see Bray & Harvey, 1995, for a review). One particular trouble spot is the relationship between parents (both biological parents and stepparents) and children during the first 2 years following stepfamily formation (Hetherington, 1989). Solomon (1995) found that mother–daughter relationships seem to be especially vulnerable to difficulties inherent in stepfamily formation. Girls also have more negative interactions with stepfathers (Vuchinich et al., 1991) and such negative interactions may be related to lower self-esteem in girls (Haberstroh et al., 1998).

The steps of divorce, single parenthood, and remarriage combine in various ways to produce stress and even trauma—through multiple losses, relocations, conflict with former spouses, visitation and support issues, and relationship challenges among stepsiblings. Outcome research has already shown that family therapy interventions improve outcomes for stepfamilies (see, e.g., Bray & Kelly, 1998). Given all the stresses and vulnerabilities of individuals in stepfamilies, preventive interventions could also have utility.

Coping with a stepfamily is, for many, a struggle for psychic survival. Parents do not want to go through, or put their children through, another marital dissolution. Many spouses who are highly motivated to succeed simply lack the tools to make it happen, and we psychologists can provide these.

YOUR POTENTIAL SATISFACTIONS

As with any therapy directed at a relationship, the satisfactions are complex. However, they might include reducing the pain of no longer necessary conflict, seeing others blossom with support, helping generations interact appropriately, and guiding people toward productive levels of closeness and distance.

YOUR SKILL SET

Recycling Your Current Competencies

- The basic skills include knowledge of family systems theory; familiarity with family therapy, couple therapy, and parenting interventions; and knowledge of child/adolescent development. If you have been doing family and couple work, and have an understanding of child development issues, you already have many of the skills necessary to provide stepfamily interventions.
- Ancillary skills that you may already possess include knowledge of substance abuse assessment and treatment, anger management interventions, and multicultural sensitivities and skills.
- If you have been personally affected by divorce and remarriage, you will bring particular insights to bear on the struggles of stepfamilies.

Retreading for Added Skills

- A thorough understanding of the special dynamics of stepfamilies and blended families, and of what makes these families unique, is essential. Some issues that commonly arise are the involvement of the noncustodial parent (child support payments, visitation rules, shared decision making, etc.); diffusion of authority between parents; consistency of rules and discipline; children's relations with stepsiblings; and children's allegiances to various adults.

- You should also have a working knowledge of your state's child custody laws and regulations.
- Understanding gender issues is a pertinent proficiency.

NATURE OF THE WORK

Bray (1995, 1996) has identified five areas for intervening with stepfamilies: planning for remarriage, marital relationships, parenting in stepfamilies, stepparent–stepchild relationships, and nonresidential-parent issues.

Children are a great stressor to these families. Lawton and Sanders (1994) offer an integrated model of the development and maintenance of child behavior problems in stepfamilies that addresses skill deficits. Nicholson and Sanders (1999) provide an effective way of working with child behavior problems in a stepfamily context. Kelley (1996) notes the limitations of traditional behavioral and systemic models of intervention for working with stepfamilies, and presents a model that integrates narrative and educational approaches in ways that can be customized to each family's unique needs.

Building a strong marital relationship can be a neglected focus in stepfamilies because the demands and issues related to parenting often take precedence over the new spouses' needs, resulting in weaknesses in their own relationship. In terms of interventions, Khehgi-Genovese and Genovese (1997) focus on the parental dyad, aim to reduce stressors, and work from a strengths orientation with remarried spouses.

Cross-Reference to Related Specialization

Niche 2.4. Competent and Resilient Girls

Subspecializations

Preparation for Remarriage

If you can reach those considering remarriage, Lyster (1995) reported a high level of satisfaction with a marriage preparation program tailored to those about to remarry. Aspects of the program rated highly for remarrying couples were family-of-origin issues, finances, and spirituality.

Other Possible Subspecializations

- Work with adolescents in stepfamilies.
- Interventions with immigrant stepfamilies (Berger, 1997).
- Counseling minority stepfamilies.
- Work with issues involving noncustodial parents.
- Interventions for stepsibling relationships.
- Counseling culturally diverse stepfamilies (i.e., stepfamilies with members of different ethnicities).

Practice Models

The format of intervention should be tailored to each family's needs, and indeed many formats are utilized. Family and couple therapy and the use of groups are the most common modalities. This work is usually done in the clinician's office although some groups (e.g., the Stepfamily Foundation; see "Patient Education Materials," below) offer home and telephone consultation, as well as intensive sessions (2- or 3-day programs).

Financial Considerations

The usual methods of reimbursement for family therapy and educational presentations apply here.

Cautions, Ethical Dilemmas, Culture Clashes, and/or Managed Care Issues

Be sure you are familiar with your state's laws in terms of requirements for parental consent for treating children when there has been a separation, divorce, or adoption. Ask to see the legal arrangements if you have any doubts. You should know whose consents are needed for your kind of intervention, and how to keep and release records in these circumstances. Your brochure for clients should make clear your position on clinical and legal issues. All the usual family therapy concerns apply here. Make clear your role (e.g., therapist to the family), roles you will not assume (e.g., custody evaluator), and other boundary issues.

PROSPECTS AND PROSPECTING

Where Is the Need?

- The statistics cited above clearly indicate that large numbers of individuals are personally affected by remarriage—either their own, their spouses', their ex-spouses', their parents', their children's, or some combination of these.

- The number of stepfamilies is growing, according to Barry Miller, PhD, who forecasts that businesses will soon be providing services for employees who are affected by remarriage and stepfamilies (cited in Fisher, 1999). Miller contends that stepfamily problems cost businesses $6.8 billion annually in lost productivity.
- The popularity of books on topics related to resolving difficulties and coping in blended families can be taken as another indicator of need. We found 355 books in a December 2001 search for "stepfamilies" at Amazon.com (about half of these were for children, and 90 were on parenting and families).

There is a surprising dearth of practitioners who specialize in this area, and there is great need. Whether you want to run psychoeducational groups for parents and/or children; conduct family therapy; or provide counseling on relational, developmental, or educational issues, there is ample opportunity to build a full practice.

Competition

Of course, many family and couple therapists can work with stepfamilies, but few advertise this, and so a specialization can be very productive. Rochelle Rogers, a therapist on Long Island, New York, who is marketing stepfamily services to individuals and payers, has said: "What I can't figure out is why there aren't more people specializing in this. The demand is definitely there" (quoted in "Stepfamilies," 1998, p. 8).

Reaching Clients

- Since troubled stepfamilies often involve troubled stepparent–adolescent relationships, networking with parents of teens through PTOs/PTAs can be productive.
- Speaking at or forming a local chapter of a stepfamily organization, such as the Stepfamily Association of America (see "Patient Education Materials," below), could be a good way to reach potential clients. The Stepfamily Foundation (again, see below) will list your practice if you pursue certification with this group.
- Parents Without Partners may seem an unlikely source of referrals, but since many who attend will remarry, there will be interest in such topics as "Should you remarry?" or "Transitioning into stepfamilies."
- Holidays can be particularly stressful times for stepfamilies and thus

present opportunities for you to reach out (with free seminars, newspaper articles, etc.).

DIRECTIONS FOR MARKETING

- Brochures and educational materials that can be given to lawyers, clergy, and school counselors can be productive. In particular, attorneys who deal with family law (divorce, custody and support, estate planning, etc.) meet many stepfamilies.
- You may want to offer materials or presentations to businesses, since, as noted above, employers may be developing an interest in providing help for employees undergoing stepfamily transition or experiencing stepfamily problems. Other topics of potential interest to stepfamilies include family-owned businesses affected by remarriage and the loss of family pets due to divorce and remarriage.

INCREASING YOUR FORMAL KNOWLEDGE BASE

A survey of clients' satisfaction with therapy for stepfamily issues (Pasley et al., 1996) found that therapists' unfamiliarity with stepfamily issues was the most frequent complaint. Obviously, then, learning all you can about these issues in a major skill goal.

There is no special certification required for work in this area at present.

Core Readings

Bray, J. H. (2001). Therapy with stepfamilies: A developmental systems approach. In S. McDaniel, H. Philpot, & D.-D. Lusterman (Eds.) *Casebook for integrating family therapy: An ecosystemic approach* (pp. 127–140). Washington, DC: American Psychological Association.

Bray, J. H., & Kelly, J. (1998). *Stepfamilies: Love, marriage, and parenting in the first decade.* New York: Broadway Books.
    —Based on a large longitudinal study of stepfamilies, the book includes vignettes from the lives of real families to illustrate the findings. Topics include the natural life cycle of stepfamilies, the process of developing a stepfamily into a family unit, the types of stepfamilies, the four basic tasks stepfamilies need to accomplish in order to succeed, and how a stepfamily can help heal the scars of divorce.

Einstein, E. A. (1994). *The stepfamily: Living, loving, and learning* (2nd ed.). Ithaca, NY: Author.
    —This won an American Psychological Association National Media Award.

Hetherington, E. M. (Ed.). (1999). *Coping with divorce, single parenting and remarriage: A risk and resiliency perspective.* Mahwah, NJ: Erlbaum.

—This volume presents a comprehensive array of research on varied topics (e.g., children of divorced parents as adults; single parents; stages of development in stepfamilies, multigenerational families; diverse stepfamilies; risk and protective factors; and interventions).

Kaslow, F. W. (1996). Understanding and treating the remarried family. In Hatherleigh Editorial Board (Ed.), *The Hatherleigh guide to marriage and family therapy.* New York: Hatherleigh Press.

Pasley, K., Dollahite, D. C., & Huntley, D. K. (1995). The nine Rs of step-parenting adolescents: Research-based recommendations for clinicians. In D. K. Huntley (Ed.), *Understanding stepfamilies: Implications for assessment and treatment* (pp. 87–98). Alexandria, VA: American Counseling Association.

Visher, E. B., & Visher, J. S. (1996). *Therapy with stepfamilies.* New York: Brunner/Mazel.

—The authors are a psychologist and a psychiatrist who are stepparents themselves. Their book is helpful for learning how to work with the various roles and relationships that make up stepfamilies; it also considers children's reactions based on their developmental level.

Journals

Journal of Divorce and Remarriage
Journal of Family Psychology
Journal of Marital and Family Therapy
Families in Society

Professional Organizations

American Association for Marriage and Family Therapy (AAMFT)
1133 15th Street N.W., Suite 300, Washington, DC 20005-2710; 202-452-0109; fax 202-223-2329
e-mail: Central@aamft.org   http://www.aamft.org
—The AAMFT offers tapes of seminars on stepfamilies.

Clinical Tools

Einstein, E., & Albert, L. (1986). *Strengthening stepfamilies.* Champaign, IL: Research Press.

—This kit consists of three audio cassettes, leader's guide, manual, charts, and other materials.

Visher, E. B., & Visher, J. S. (1988). *Stepping together program—Creating strong stepfamilies.* Lincoln, NE: Stepfamily Association of America.

—This package includes the *Stepfamily Workshop Manual.* It covers 12 hours of group meetings, and includes leader and participant workbooks, as well as the text *Therapy with Stepfamilies.* These authors have also written other books in this area.

Patient Education Materials: Online Resources, Printed Resources, and Organizations

Bray, J. M., & Kelly, J. (1998). *Stepfamilies: Love, marriage, and parenting in the first decade.* New York: Broadway Books.

Lofas, J., & Sova, D. B. (1997). *Stepparenting.* New York: MJF Books.
    —The book describes the first author's approach to stepfamilies. (Lofas is the president of the Stepfamily Foundation.)

Newman, M. (1994). *Stepfamily realities: How to overcome difficulties and have a happy family.* Oakland, CA: New Harbinger.
    —This book covers topics such as communication skills, intimacy and sexuality, and coparenting issues; it takes a family systems view of achieving balance within stepfamilies.

Norwood, P. K., & Wingender, T. (1999). *The enlightened stepmother: Revolutionizing the role.* New York: Avon.

Pickhardt, C. E. (1997). *Keys to successful stepfathering.* Hauppauge, NY: Barrons Educational Series.
    —This book takes a look at the stepfamily from the perspective of the stepfather. It emphasizes the importance of the coparenting team, communication and conflict resolution.

Visher, E. B., & Visher, J. (1991). *How to win as a stepfamily* (2nd ed.). New York: Brunner/Mazel.

Wisdom, S., & Green, J. (2002). *Stepcoupling: Creating and sustaining a strong marriage in today's blended family.* New York: Three Rivers Press.

The Step Family Foundation
333 West End Avenue, New York, NY 10023; 212-877-3244
http://www.stepfamily.org
    —The Web site provides many resources, patient materials, patient and professional message boards, membership, and information on the group's own training and certification and audio and video seminars for professionals.

Stepfamily Association of America (SAA)
650 J Street, Suite 205, Lincoln, NE 68508; 402-477-7837, 800-735-0329
e-mail: stepfamfs@aol.com   http://www.saafamilies.org
    —SAA publishes books and other materials on divorce and stepfamilies written for adults and children in stepfamilies and for professionals; provides a directory of mental health professionals, who specialize in stepfamily life; and sponsors professional conferences.

Stepfamily Network
http://www.stepfamily.net
    —The Web site provides a listing of organizations that offer various counseling services, from online member-to-member support to local professional resources.

Stepmothers International, Inc.
222 West Las Colinas Blvd, Suite 1750, Irving, TX 75039; 972-501-1491
http://www.stepmothers.org

Gifted Children

MEETING THEIR EMOTIONAL NEEDS

OVERVIEW AND OPPORTUNITIES

By convention, intellectually gifted individuals comprise the top 2% of the IQ range—a small percentage, but a significant number (about 5 million Americans, of whom 1.5 million are children). In addition, individuals can be considered "gifted" in realms other than the intellectual, such as artistic and music talents or interpersonal sensitivity and skills; broadening the definition in this way will expand the possible client base many-fold.[1] Moreover, many children with gifts, talents, or creativity (GTC) also exhibit particular problems such as attention-deficit/hyperactivity disorder (ADHD) or learning disabilities (LDs). They can thus be subdivided in terms of both their special assets and their problems, as well as by gender and age. Different subgroups may benefit from different services.

Children with GTC constitute one of society's most valuable resources, yet it is a sad fact that few of these children go on to be eminent adults in their particular domains of giftedness. All such children can suffer the same social stressors, and so may benefit from similar supportive services to flourish as adults (Winner, 1996). Very few clinicians practice with gifted individuals, and few specific clinical interventions have been developed for work with this group (Moon & Hall, 1998). Research and clinical attention to this group have been curiously lacking (Sternberg, 1996a, 1996b; Sternberg & Lubart, 1996). Gifted students receive less than 1% of all funding for special education, yet their potential to contribute to society is enormous (Sternberg, 1996b). This neglect is "a quiet crisis," according to a U.S. Department

---

[1]In fact, we address gifted (academically), talented (in other areas), and creative children together in this niche.

of Education report (Ross, 1993), with resultant boredom, lack of challenge, and underachievement (Winner, 2000).

YOUR POTENTIAL SATISFACTIONS

- Individuals with GTC are stimulating to work with.
- Helping individuals who have exceptional abilities and/or talents unlock or augment their potential is personally gratifying and of enormous value to society.
- Gifted students often feel different and are vulnerable to feelings of isolation, social awkwardness, and depression, particularly during adolescence. Common psychosocial interventions that address such problems could help these children reach their full potential.
- Because this population receives very few psychological services, providing services can be rewarding.

YOUR SKILL SET

Recycling Your Current Competencies

- Assessment is a core skill. You should be able to administer, score, and interpret the standard tests and batteries for intelligence, LDs, and ADHD.
- Children with GTC can benefit from all kinds of family interventions, so family therapy skills are useful.
- If you or members of your family have been identified as gifted, creative, or talented, you may come to this area with special insights and experiences.

Retreading for Added Skills

- You should have some sophistication in the assessment of multiple intelligences (e.g., Gardner, 1983; Sternberg, 1997) and the many manifestations of GTC because traditional IQ tests are less useful in evaluating this population, due to ceiling effects and narrowness of focus.
- The assessment of coexisting ADHD and LDs is a growing area of practice, and so a solid background in these areas is valuable.
- Clinicians serving this population should be knowledgeable about and sensitive to the unique psychosocial stressors, identity issues, developmental asynchronies, psychosocial vulnerabilities, and intellectual challenges faced by gifted children.

NATURE OF THE WORK

As noted earlier, most gifted children and adolescents do not fulfill their potential (Winner, 1996). Many could benefit from expert help with motivation, planning, follow-through, and personal and family issues that might interfere with fulfillment of their potential. Gifted children who are academically underachieving report greater family issues and/or poorer self-concept (Freeman, 1994). The lack of support for children with GTC in the public school system is a major stressor for these children and their families. School and educational issues include helping children to adjust either to academic acceleration or to boredom caused by insufficiently challenging materials, and working to change inadequately grounded educational policies regarding these students' unique needs (Benbow & Stanley, 1996; Reis et al., 1998).

Clinical issues can include being perceived as "different," the trauma of accelerated development and asynchronies in development (Roedell, 1984), and the effects of real or perceived multipotentiality (Frederickson, 1979; Kerr & Erb, 1991). According to Silverman (1986), the majority of gifted children are introverted, and the proportion of introversion increases with IQ. Although data are not consistent, some authors (e.g., Silverman, 1983; Orange, 1997) suggest that a relationship exists between perfectionism and giftedness—an effect that may be mediated by parental expectations (Ablard & Parker, 1997). Finally, children may underachieve in order to fit in with peers. All of these issues are suitably addressed in psychotherapy.

Research suggests that emotional intensity is a characteristic of many gifted children (Piechowski, 1991). Although this intensity can motivate greater achievement and creativity, family members and teachers do not always react positively to the intensity of some highly gifted children. "Emotional overexcitability" (Dabrowski & Piechowski, 1977) can combine with other sensitivities and abilities to magnify stress in children with GTC (Freeman, 1994).

Areas of Practice

Moon et al. (1997) found that parents of gifted students who responded to a survey expressed the need for specialized counseling services for those students. Parents of children with GTC report stresses related to the challenge of raising their exceptional children. These families have unique concerns that can be addressed by informed family therapy interventions. Although family background and encouragement influence high achievement (Albert & Runco, 1986; Bloom, 1985; Freeman, 1995), some family systems are emotionally stressed by the presence of gifted children, and interventions that provide coping strategies for parents and siblings of these children is an area of need (Moon & Hall, 1998).

Sternberg (1996b) and Sternberg and Lubart (1996) describe society's prejudices and stereotypes regarding persons with GTC, particularly with respect to how these translate into the marginalization of such individuals. In particular, Alsop (1997) cited "negative and unsupportive behaviors" on the part of educators, community, and even friends and family networks, concluding that "With few exceptions parents in this study were subjected to a repertoire of characteristically negative responses across socially important contexts" (p. 32).

Support groups for gifted individuals and their families, parenting groups, sibling groups, and group therapy for socialization skills or for depressed adolescents are some services you might consider offering.

Cross-References to Related Specializations

Niche 2.4. Competent and Resilient Girls
Niche 2.5. Clinical Interventions for Students and Schools
Niche 5.5. Wellness and Positive Psychology

Subspecializations

Career Counseling

The unstated societal assumption that gifted individuals will find optimal career paths on their own seems simple-minded. Career counseling for this population has not been fully tried.

Helping Gifted Students with LDs or ADHD

How significant a problem is the co-occurrence of GTC with LDs or ADHD? According to a Department of Education report (Ross, 1993), over half of the top 1% of U.S. students are underachieving, and a subset of these are likely to have LDs and/or ADHD (Reis & McCoach, 2000). Mendaglio (1993) found that gifted students with LDs experienced a great deal of frustration, anger, and resentment, which affected their behavior and their peer and family relationships. There is significant comorbidity with psychological disturbance: In a high-IQ, young adult sample with LDs, Holliday et al. (1999) found that 30% had sufficient emotional or behavioral problems to qualify for a formal psychiatric diagnosis. Professional psychology should not miss this important opportunity, according to Pfeiffer (2001), who states that "the gifted have many unmet social, emotional, and psychoeducational needs and are arguably one of America's most valuable resources" (p. 175).

Good introductions to this area are an article by Baum et al. (1998) and a handbook by Baum et al. (1991).

Assessments

You might consider offering assessment services to help identify multiple exceptionalities among gifted students. According to Pfeiffer (2001), assessment of gifted students for LDs or ADHD is complex, requiring "psychological testing at the hands of skilled clinicians equipped to make difficult differential diagnoses" (p. 177).

Vocational testing is another area where professional psychology can fill a need for specialized services (Pfeiffer, 2001). You might also consider helping gifted students with LDs choose a college, fill out applications, and develop "survival skills." Bramer (1996) can guide counseling those with ADHD about college. Kravets and Wax (2000) is a guide to college programs for those with LDs, as is a Web site (http://www.ldpride.net/ldlinks.htm). *The PostSecondary LD Report* is a guide to college choice, published four times a year by Block Educational Consulting, Columbus, OH 43214.

Examples of interventions that focus on talents rather than on deficits are provided by Baum (1988) and Whitmore and Maker (1985).

Other Possible Subspecializations

- Helping gifted minority children (Plucker, 1996).
- Identifying individuals with unrecognized GTC (Azpeitia & Rocamora, 1994).
- Creativity enhancement in gifted children (Csikszentmihalyi et al., 1993; Sternberg & Lubart, 1996).
- Helping gifted girls (Frey, 1998; Klein & Zhems, 1996; Kerr, 1997) and women (Kerr, 1997).

Practice Models

- Specialization in this area could augment a more general practice in one of several areas (work with children and adolescents, family therapy, testing and assessment, or pediatric neuropsychology).
- You might create a network with pediatricians or other child and adolescent medical specialists; educators; school counselors; art, dance, and music teachers; and academic coaches. You can also explore networking with school systems—particularly, of course, schools for gifted children, but also with extracurricular programs for such children, private schools, and summer camp personnel. Let them know that you have a specialization in the unique issues related to gifted

children. If you plan to network with schools, be sure to take the time to become knowledgeable regarding both which system currently provides services to these students and what the political realities of that system are. Be careful not to step on the toes of those from whom you would like to receive referrals. This will help you to emphasize areas of need and offer interventions that augment existing services, rather than duplicating them.

- Consider forming a multidisciplinary group practice consisting of those who do assessment and treatment; educators who provide mentoring, create intellectual challenges, and combat boredom; counselors specializing in career guidance; and psychotherapists who provide targeted psychosocial interventions and support for children and their families.
- Some interventions—for example, creativity enhancement—are easily adapted to a group format, and as such will produce some economic advantages in terms of pricing your services.

Financial Considerations

Although managed care issues may apply to some work in this area, parenting interventions, evaluation/assessment, and coaching will be mainly managed-care-free areas of practice. Also, managed care contracts generally exclude evaluations for GTC and LDs as educational concerns, not behavioral health.

Cautions, Ethical Dilemmas, Culture Clashes, and/or Managed Care Issues

Therapists who are not familiar with giftedness can misdiagnose certain traits associated with giftedness as pathology (Azpeitia & Rocamora, 1994).

PROSPECTS AND PROSPECTING

Where Is the Need?

There are many indications of need for specialized clinical services for children with GTC and their families. Needs have been noted in the literature (e.g., Mahoney, 1998; Moon et al., 1997; Azpeitia & Rocamora, 1994; Moon & Hall, 1998; Winner, 1996), and by parents and teachers of these children (Moon et al., 1997).

- Critical needs exist for clinicians who understand the unique emotional development of gifted children; who can identify the stressors related to giftedness, as well as family and educational issues; and who can provide differential diagnosis for gifted children with ADHD or LDs.

- Those who work with gifted children have maintained that specialized counseling services are needed for this population, and that practitioners have generally failed to provide these needed services (Colangelo, 1988; Moon et al., 1997).
- At-risk subpopulations appear to be those with extreme GTC, gifted girls, gifted adolescents, and gifted individuals of lower socioeconomic status.
- To get an estimate of the percentage of students with identified GTC in your state as of the mid-1990s, see National Center for Education Statistics (1996, Table 53).

Competition

School psychologists and school counselors serve this market.

Reaching Clients

- Parents of gifted children have formed support and advocacy organizations (see "Patient Education Materials," below), providing additional evidence that this population perceives unmet needs. Your community may already have such an organization. If not, you might look into starting one.
- Presentations at GTC-related events can bring many referrals, because those attending are already focused and motivated.

Directions for Marketing

- Pediatricians, other child health specialists, teachers, and tutors, as well as preschools and specialized camps for gifted children, can be prodigious case finders. Presentations and brochures aimed at these audiences can be highly productive.
- Consider Mensa for your marketing activities. Mensa U.S.A. (47,000 members) has over 100 special interest groups. Use the Web site (http://us.mensa.org/local_groups/overview.php3) to find a group in your locale.
- The ERIC Clearinghouse (see "Online Resources," below) has a listing of resources for gifted students that you might explore for your marketing efforts. See the Web site's listings for state departments of education, state directors of special education, and other resources by state.

INCREASING YOUR FORMAL KNOWLEDGE BASE

Core Readings

Csikszentmihalyi, M., Rathunde, K. R., Whalen, S., & Wong, M. (1993). *Talented teenagers: The roots of success and failure.* New York: Cambridge University Press.

Gardner, H. (2001). *Intelligence reframed: Multiple intelligences for the 21st century.* New York: Basic Books.

Silverman, L. K. (Ed.). (2001). *Counseling the gifted and talented.* Denver, CO: Love.

Sternberg, R. J., & Lubart, T. I. (1995). *Defying the crowd: Cultivating creativity in a culture of conformity.* New York: Free Press.

Willard-Holt, C., & Holt, D. (1998). *Applying multiple intelligences to gifted education: I'm not just an IQ score!* Manassas, VA: Gifted Education Press.

Winner, E. (1996). *Gifted children: Myths and realities.* New York: Basic Books.

—This is arguably the best book in the area, and certainly a fine place to start.

Journals

Journal for the Education of the Gifted
Gifted Child Quarterly
Advanced Development

Online Resources

Educational Resources Information Center (ERIC) Clearinghouse on Disabilities and Gifted Education (ERIC EC), 800-328-0272; TTY 703-264-9449
e-mail: ericec@cec.sped.org   http://ericec.org
—The Web site is a huge resource for information on LDs and giftedness, including focused minibibliographies and reviews.

Hoagies' Gifted Education Web Page
http://www.hoagiesgifted.org
—Here are many useful materials on the topics of gifted children; gifted children with LDs or ADHD; and parenting gifted children. There are also links to research articles, bibliographies, educational resources, support groups, and parent/family organizations at the state and national levels.

Professional Organizations

Organizations for gifted children have educational conventions you could attend to obtain continuing education credit, familiarize yourself with current issues and formulations, discover what materials are available for therapy, and do networking.

American Association for Gifted Children
1121 West Main Street, Suite 100, Durham, NC 27701; 919-783-6152
http://www.aagc.org

National Association for Gifted Children
707 L Street N.W., Suite 550, Washington, DC 20036; 202-785-4268
http://www.nagc.org

National Foundation for Gifted and Creative Children
395 Diamond Hill Road, Warwick, RI 02886; 401-738-0937
http://www.nfgcc.org

Division 16 (School Psychology) of the American Psychological Association
750 First Street N.E., Washington, DC 20002-4242; 202-336-6013; fax 202-218-3599
http://www.indiana.edu/~div16/

Supporting the Emotional Needs of the Gifted, Inc. (SENG)
c/o Dr. James Delisle, College of Education, 405 White Hall, Kent State
    University, Kent, OH 44242; 216-672-2294
http://www.sengifted.org/mis_diag.htm

Patient Education Materials: Online Resources, Printed Resources, and Organizations

For parents of gifted children with LDs, Smart Kids with LD (http://smartkidswithld.org) has a newsletter and online resources that may be of interest.

GT World (http://www.gtworld.org) provides sign-on capability for five e-mail lists—GT-Families, GT-Special and GT-Spec-Home (for those with GTC and disabilities), GT-Adult, and GT-Talk—as well as other resources for persons with GTC and their families.

The Hollingworth Center for Highly Gifted Children (http://www.hollingworth.org), named for Dr. Leta Hollingsworth, is a clearinghouse for information on gifted children. It publishes a newsletter (several articles are online), sponsors regional support groups and workshops, holds an annual national convention, can provide tapes of prior conferences, and posts event information on the Web site.

Baum, S. M., Owen, S. V., Dixon, J. P. (1991). *To be gifted and learning disabled: From identification to practical intervention strategies.* Mansfield Center, CT: Creative Learning Press.

Kerr, B. A. (1994). *Smart girls two: A new psychology of girls, women and giftedness.* Dayton, OH: Ohio Psychology Press.

Kerr, B. A., Cohn, S. J., Webb, J. T., & Anderson, T. (2001). *Smart boys: Talent, manhood, and the search for meaning.* Scottsadale, AZ: Great Potential.

Kiesa, K. *Uniquely gifted: Identifying and meeting the needs of the twice exceptional student.* Gilsum, NH: Avocus.

Walker, S. Y. (1991). *The survival guide for parents of gifted kids: How to understand, live with and stick up for your gifted child.* Minneapolis: Free Spirit.

Competent and Resilient Girls

GUIDING THEIR PERILOUS JOURNEY THROUGH ADOLESCENCE

OVERVIEW AND OPPORTUNITIES

Any adolescent is likely to tell you what a recent poll revealed: It's tough being a teenager today (Shell Oil Company, 1999). The further finding that more girls than boys agree with this statement is consistent with the research that adolescence truly is a time of stress, danger, and crisis for many girls. For example, Schoen et al. (1997) found high levels of physical and sexual abuse, eating disorders, and depression among girls, and also found that girls were more likely than boys to say that they had no one to turn to for support. Adolescent girls are more likely than boys to have decreased self-esteem, to worry, to be dissatisfied with their appearance, and to have suicidal thoughts and attempts. Even their substance abuse and tobacco use are on par with boys' (Schoen et al., 1997).

Although some assert that girls' distress is more likely to be overlooked because they present "a portrait of quiet disturbance" (Harris et al., 1991), parents and others involved in the lives of girls often do perceive girls' distress (or can be made aware of it through our educational efforts) and will be motivated to help them. As clinicians trained in assessment, child and adolescent development, gender issues, and family and group dynamics, we are singularly, relevantly, and fully qualified to help girls emerge from this life passage stronger, healthier, and more self-assured. We can help by mobilizing and reinforcing personal, family, and community strengths; supporting healthy attitudes and beliefs; identifying risks and vulnerabilities at a still changeable early point; and maximizing family functioning. All these efforts can fortify girls for confronting the many challenges that await them.

YOUR POTENTIAL SATISFACTIONS

- This is an opportunity to make a significant, lifelong difference in the lives of girls.
- Your practice can be quite varied: It can include both preventative and treatment interventions; can utilize individual, group, and family modalities; and can include consulting with schools and other organizations concerned with girls.
- Organizations already advocating for girls (see below) provide a wide range of materials and handouts, which you could use in reaching this population.

YOUR SKILL SET

Recycling Your Current Competencies

- This is a natural specialization for those already in a child/adolescent practice.
- Knowledge of child and adolescent development, of gender roles, and of parenting approaches and techniques forms the base of any work in this area.
- There is no special formal certification needed at present in this area.

Retreading for Added Skills

A proficiency in assessing the need for treatment in more specialized areas such as substance abuse, eating disorders, LD, and ADHD would be of great benefit to clients.

NATURE OF THE WORK

Your services can be very diverse and adapted to your resources and style.

- Interventions can prepare girls for the hazards of the transition to adulthood by promoting assertiveness, resiliency, and self-efficacy.
- Clinical interventions have been shown to be effective with adolescent girls for many anxiety and depressive disorders, somatic com-

plaints, suicidal behavior, and drug and alcohol problems (cf. Kazdin & Weisz, 1998; Reinecke et al., 1998).

- Anxiety over performance in math reduces working memory and produces poorer achievement (Ashcraft & Kirk, 2001). Interventions for math anxiety (see, e.g., Anton & Klisch, 1995) can help girls to improve performance, reduce avoidance, and resolve ambivalence about achievement; they can thus support the pursuit of a wider range of career choices with higher incomes.
- Clinicians can maximize parental support and help parents appreciate their importance in the development of their daughters' self-esteem. Therapists can reinforce known protective factors, such as an empathic relationship with parents and family (Chandy et al., 1996) and positive gender role identity.
- Through consultation and seminars, teachers can be encouraged to devise gender-fair classrooms that support girls' learning and social development.

Areas of Practice

Anxiety, Depression, Substance Abuse, and Eating Disorders

According to the National Center for Health Statistics (1999), 31% of girls in grades 9 through 12 believe they are overweight and 60% are trying to lose weight. In a population of dieting teens, Rosen et al. (1987) found high levels of social anxiety, depression, and low self-esteem present only in the girls, not in the boys. Whether these symptoms caused recurrent dieting or were results of it is unknown, but clearly they are all linked. Sadker and Sadker (1994) found a disturbing correlation: Body image dissatisfaction that causes compulsive dieting lowers a young woman's ability to concentrate, potentially decreasing her academic achievement. Interventions aimed at increasing protective factors such as self-esteem, according to Striegel-Moore and Cachelin (1999), "would not only decrease the likelihood of disordered eating, but would also promote general mental health in this population" (p. 102). Fortunately, clinical interventions have been effective for adolescent anxiety, depression, disordered eating, somatic complaints, suicidal behaviors, and drug and alcohol problems (see Kazdin & Weisz, 1998; Reinecke et al., 1998).

Undetected LDs and Math and Science Anxiety

To be competitive in math and science at the college level (and beyond), young women must avail themselves of the same learning opportunities that their male peers choose. However, at the high school level, young women are underrepresented in advanced placement classes in math, physics, and other sciences (data cited in Campbell, 1999). The fact that more girls than boys are opting out of these opportunities seems to reflect not talent but self-esteem issues, "math anxiety," less parental encouragement of girls, and/or fewer female role models in these courses. Overall, girls tend to rate their own abilities more negatively, have lower expectations, and are more likely to attribute failure to low ability compared to boys (Stipek & Gralinski, 1991). Also, according to Shaywitz et al. (1990), girls are under-diagnosed for LDs, and thus are much less likely to receive remedial services for LDs than are boys.

Clinicians can be of great help to teenage girls by treating math and science anxieties. Also needed are interventions for identifying and building on the strengths and coping skills of gifted girls and/or girls with LDs. Assertiveness and leadership interventions can help girls become more effective in presenting their ideas in class and school settings. Lastly, psychoeducational programs for parents can help them encourage, motivate, and model their daughter's achievements.

Career Development, College Counseling, and Test Anxiety

Research indicates that girls often start to limit their career options in early adolescence (Gottfredson & Lapan, 1997). Factors that constrict girls' perceptions of their career options include poor self-concept and sex-typing of occupations (Stitt-Gohdes, 1997). The quality of the mother–daughter relationship has been found to be influential in a girl's career development (Blustein et al., 1991). Rainey and Borders (1997) found that mothers' educational levels, work experience, personality characteristics, and gender role attitudes were all influential in middle school girls' career aspirations. See Gottfredson and Lapan (1997) for suggestions regarding gender-neutral career counseling.

Services you could provide might include combining your efforts with that of an SAT coach to help girls with SAT (or other test) anxiety; offering guidance, coaching, and mentoring for adolescent girls working on career issues; and providing family interventions centered around girls' career issues and family attitudes and assumptions.

Parenting Girls Effectively

A positive relationship with parents has been found to be a crucial protective factor for girls (Humphrey, 1988; Miller, 1998; Simantov et al., 2000). Parents may need to become aware of their importance both as role models and as the primary social support for their daughters. These could be carried out through parenting interventions (see examples below) and psychoeducational programs.

Confronting Sexual Harassment and Abuse

Sexual harassment in the schools begins early and takes an unremitting course, according to a survey from the American Association of University Women (AAUW). *Hostile Hallways II* (AAUW, 2001) found that 80% of girls reported having experienced sexual harassment. According to Rowell et al. (1996), sexually harassed girls report "feelings of confusion, depression, embarrassment, shame, and self-blame," for which individual counseling can be beneficial; interventions at the system level, and the teaching and supporting of assertiveness in girls, can also be very productive.

According to a national study, half of rapes occurred when the victim was 17 or younger (Kilpatrick, 1992). Nagy et al. (1994) surveyed 3,000 students in grades 8–10 and found that 13% of girls and 7% of boys reported sexual abuse (defined in this study as forced intercourse). Evidence is mounting that child sexual abuse has a variety of emotional and behavioral sequelae, including suicidal behaviors and ideation, disordered eating, unwanted pregnancies, chemical use, anxiety and mood disorders, and conduct disorder (Fergusson et al., 1996; Nagy et al., 1994; Davidson et al., 1996; Briere & Runtz, 1993; Briere et al., 1997; Tebbutt et al., 1997). Clinical interventions can address the spectrum of abuse, from prevention to resolution of the emotional aftermath, and can treat perpetrators as well as the victims.

Healthy Mind, Healthy Body

Writing at the beginning of the last decade, Robinson (1991) observed:

> Adolescents are the only age group in this country whose mortality rate has increased over the last thirty years. Increases in adolescent mortality rates have been accompanied by a shift in the causes of mortality from those due to disease to those related to social, environmental, and behavioral factors. (p. 243)

Girls are much more vulnerable to sexually transmitted diseases, unintended pregnancy, physical and sexual abuse, and increased substance use and abuse (including tobacco use)—all of which have behavioral components and for which our skills are needed. The Girl Power! Web site (see "Online Resources," below) provides a summary of these statistics.

Expertise in health and wellness interventions (e.g., smoking cessation, substance abuse interventions, and exercise and sport interventions), combined with a sensitivity to developmental and gender issues, can be invaluable to girls and the problems they face. Addressing the affects and cognitions shaping or supporting risky behaviors would be an almost unique contribution you could make as a psychologist. Your practice can focus on consulting to schools or collaborating with pediatricians or adolescent health practitioners. (See Niche 1.6 for ideas on how to collaborate with PCPs.) You could combine your skills with those of nutritionists and offer weight management interventions. Working with chronically ill adolescents is another possible focus (see Kibby et al., 1998, for a review of the many effective interventions for this population).

Cross-References to Related Specializations

Niche 1.6. Collaborative Practice with Primary Care Physicians
Niche 2.2. Assisting Stepfamilies and Blended Families
Niche 2.5. Clinical Interventions for Students and Schools
Niche 3.2. Consulting to Family-Owned Businesses
Niche 5.5. Wellness and Positive Psychology

Subspecializations

- Counseling ethnic minority girls.
- Counseling girls with physical disabilities or chronic illness.

Practice Models

A private practice model that includes collaboration with other professionals (e.g., pediatricians, adolescent health specialists, LD specialists, college counselors, SAT coaches) is recommended. In addition, clinicians should explore networking opportunities with the school system and other community organizations that have a stake in and concern about girls' futures.

Financial Considerations

- Although some of this work will be paid for as psychotherapy (treating eating disorders, depression, etc.) much of it is public education, consultation, or staff training (paid for by contracts), or private practice (as for LDs).
- You will probably find that few others are offering these services in your locale.
- Work that is not related to formal medical or psychiatric diagnoses—such as parenting training, consulting, and leadership interventions—is managed-care-free.

PROSPECTS AND PROSPECTING

Where Is the Need?

Callan (1999) notes that various social and cultural developments—such as increased sexual freedom, changes in family structure, heightened violence and unsafe environments, increased rates of families with both parents working, increased rates of girls' employment, and technological changes—have converged to expose girls to more environmental stressors. Increased levels of emotional distress may be expected to continue as girls try to cope with the societal consequences of these changes, such as exposure to sexually transmitted diseases, substance use and abuse, and increased levels of physical and sexual abuse. Surveying the new landscape of adolescence, Callan (1999) concludes that the problems of adolescent girls are "pervasive" and "complex." Moreover, "The sheer range of problems is challenging and the number of adolescents needing mental health treatment plus those who require support in their journey through 'normal' adolescence is great" (Callan, 1999, p. 363).

This increased need has produced responses from policy makers and professionals who work with girls. The field of adolescent medicine was recently launched; the Girl Power! Web site was created by the U.S. Department of Health and Human Services; and the American Psychological Association (APA) has formed a Presidential Task Force on Adolescent Girls (Dougherty, 1999). These developments augur well for a continued specialized focus on this population. "With increased policy attention to health care for children and adolescents, now is a good time for more researchers and providers to turn their attention to these populations" (Dougherty, 1999, p. 318).

Competition

There is at present very little competition in this specialty. Adolescence has been an overlooked specialization in mental health, perhaps because teenagers are considered too difficult or uncooperative to treat, or because clinicians' stereotypes of adolescent pathology excludes nonclinical interventions.

Reaching Clients

You can base your strategy for reaching this population on research on how adolescents seek help. Girls are significantly more likely to seek help with their problems both from informal social support networks (such as friends and parents) and from professionals than are boys (Dubow et al., 1990; Schonert-Reichl & Muller, 1996). Since girls tend to turn to family members and friends when distressed, networking with community and parent groups will let the girls and their families know about your services.

Directions for Marketing

In addition to the marketing ideas for reaching students presented in the introduction to this section, try approaching women's business and professional groups via ads, newsletters, and presentations. Professionally developed marketing materials are available from Girl Power!

You might also consider subscribing to several of the popular publications aimed at girls and young women and displaying these titles in your waiting room, to get the word out to your adult clients that you specialize in this area.

Consult a calendar of upcoming events (see the introduction to this section) to "piggyback" with national recognition days and draw attention to the services that you offer.

INCREASING YOUR FORMAL KNOWLEDGE BASE

Core Readings

Bem, S. L. (1993). *The lenses of gender: Transforming the debate on sexual inequality.* New Haven, CT: Yale University Press.
    —An eminent authority on gender roles, Sandra Bem will help you to see our concepts of "masculine" and "feminine" with new eyes.

Gilligan, C. (1993). *In a different voice: Psychological theory and women's development.* Cambridge, MA: Harvard University Press. (Original work published 1982)
    —Beautifully and convincingly rendered, this book changed rules and assumptions in psychology, in medical research, and among teachers and other professionals about male–female distinctions.

Gilligan, C., Rogers, A., & Tolman, D. (Eds.). (1991). *Women, girls and psychotherapy: Reframing resistance.* Binghampton, NY: Harrington Park Press.
    —A feminist reinterpretation of the psychotherapeutic process.

Johnson, N. G., Roberts, M. C., & Worell, J. (Eds.). (1999). *Beyond appearance: A new look at adolescent girls.* Washington, DC: American Psychological Association.
    —This wide-ranging volume includes contributions on self-esteem, body image, ethnicity and racial factors, relationships, sexuality, school, health care, dating violence, and treatment.

Kerr, B. A. (1997). *Smart girls: A new psychology of girls, women, and giftedness.* Scottsdale, AZ: Gifted Psychology Press.
    —Kerr summarizes research on gifted girls, presents biographies, discusses gender-specific issues, and makes suggestions for helping girls realize their potential.

Pipher, M. (1994). *Reviving Ophelia: Saving the selves of adolescent girls.* New York: Putnam.
  —This is the book that raised public awareness of the costs borne by girls and what can be done.
Risman, B. (1998). *Gender vertigo: American families in transition.* New Haven, CT: Yale University Press.
  —Utilizing qualitative and quantitative data, this book provides evidence that gender equality in families is an attainable goal.
Silverstein, B., & Perlick, D. (1995). *The cost of competence.* New York: Oxford University Press.
  —Using historical analysis, these authors posit the existence of a new syndrome that is the outgrowth of the conflict between girls' achievement goals and society's expectations and prejudices. Original and thought-provoking, this book could change how you think about disordered eating.
Smolak, L., Levine, M. P., & Striegel-Moore, R. (Eds.). (1996). *The developmental psychopathology of eating disorders: Implications for research, prevention, and treatment.* Mahwah, NJ: Erlbaum.
  —A comprehensive assessment of the role of biopsychosocial factors in the development of eating disorders.

Journals

Psychology of Women Quarterly
Sex Roles
Journal of Adolescent Health

Online Resources

Girl Power!
e-mail: gpower@health.org   http://www.girlpower.gov
  —This Web site is sponsored by the U.S. Department of Health and Human Services to "encourage and empower 9- to 14-year-old girls to make the most of their lives." The "Parents" section contains links to summaries of research on girls' health, substance use, and physical fitness. Girl Power! provides a large, varied, and free media kit to raise awareness and advance issues. You can personalize the materials with your practice name and logo.

The Society for Adolescent Health has a multidisciplinary listserv. To subscribe, send a message to listserv@uconnvm.uconn.edu with "subscribe SAM-L" (and your name).

Professional Organizations

Division 35 (Society for the Psychology of Women) of the American Psychological Association
750 First Street N.E., Washington, DC 20002-4242; 602-246-6615
e-mail: div35apa@aol.com   http://www.apa.org/divisions/div35

—An e-mail list, POWR-L, is cosponsored with the Association for Women in Psychology. Other APA divisions, such as Health Psychology and Counseling Psychology, also have special-interest groups for women's issues.

Patient Education Materials: Online Resources, Printed Resources, and Organizations

Preventing Substance Abuse among Children and Adolescents: Family-centered approaches—evidence-based guidelines. Available as a book-length guideline, a practitioner's guide, and as a brochure from the National Clearinghouse for Alcohol and Drug Information at 800-729-6686 or at a Web site (http://www.samhsa.gov).

Girl Tech
P.O. Box 4062, San Rafael, CA 94913-4062; 415-256-1510
http://www.girltech.com
—This Web site encourages girls use of technology through products and services developed for girls. A parent/mentor section has a great deal of research-based information on girls' learning styles and gender equity in the classroom.

Melpomene Institute
1010 University Avenue, St. Paul, MN 55104; 612-642-1951
http://www.melpomene.org
—Melpomene is a nonprofit organization that helps girls and women link physical activity and health through research, education, and publications. Pamphlets are available on topics such as eating disorders, body image, sports, and self-esteem.

Girls Incorporated, National Resource Center
441 West Michigan Street, Indianapolis, IN 46202-3233; 317-634-7546
e-mail: hn3580@handsnet.org   http://www.girlsinc.org
—This group serves 350,000 young people ages 6–18 at over 1,000 sites nationwide. It provides a variety of publications on topics relevant to girls and achievement.

Advocates for Women in Science, Engineering and Mathematics (AWSEM)
P.O. Box 91000, Portland, OR 97291-1000; 503-690-1261
e-mail info@awsem.com   http://www.ogi.edu/satacad/awsem.html
—AWSEM provides listings of resources and products to help women in pursuing science careers.

Mann, J. (1994). *The difference: Growing up female in America.* New York: Warner Books.

Clinical Interventions for Students and Schools

OVERVIEW AND OPPORTUNITIES

Psychological interventions are often the treatments of choice for a wide array of problems that affect students, including youth drug and alcohol use, school violence, truancy, bullying, sexual harassment, LDs, ADHD, and of course behavioral and emotional problems.

The integration of mental health services with the medical side in "school health clinics" should lead to expanded opportunities for psychologists (Carlson et al., 1996). If the school system in your community is taking this tack, you might look into how you might become part of this system, either on a consultant basis or by providing direct services. According to an article in *Communiqué*, the National Association of School Psychologists (NASP) newsletter (Crespi & Nissen, 1998), some school systems are moving toward reducing school psychologist staff. This may well lead to more "outsourcing" (i.e., contracting with nonstaff providers—maybe you) for mental health services.

Surveying recent developments in the educational reform movement and looking to the future, Tharinger et al. (1996) describe the potential opportunities for psychologists to work with schools as "vast." These go well beyond the traditional school psychologist role of assessment, and beyond contemporary practices as well. The opportunities listed by Tharinger et al. (1996, p. 30, with our additions in brackets) include the development of new and creative methods for the following:

- Performance assessment and portfolio review [beyond current grades and statistical measures].
- Health and education outcomes measurement [beyond academic skills and abilities].

149

- Program and systems evaluation [including program development and management].
- Systems consultation, not just to teachers, but to parents, student support staff, and administration.
- Prevention and early intervention for at-risk behaviors and health promotion [by providing direct services, staff training and supervision, and program development].

The discussion that follows concerns services that psychologists who are *not* school psychologists could provide. In other words, we consider here those kinds of problems and responses that a generally trained clinician might explore.

YOUR POTENTIAL SATISFACTIONS

What could be more meaningful than preventing or ameliorating the life-long consequences that can result from failure to address children's psychosocial problems? Our knowledge base of the psychosocial risk factors that predispose children to the development of psychological problems is rapidly growing, providing for effective early identification and intervention with children.

Since family problems and parenting issues have frequently been identified as related to the development of behavioral problems in school children, those who enjoy working with family interventions will find much good work to do in this population.

YOUR SKILL SET

Recycling Your Current Competencies

If you have training and experience in working with children and their families, you have some of the basics to provide interventions for school children. The core clinical skills involve child, developmental, and educational psychology; family systems theory; and child and family therapy.

Retreading for Additional Skills

Important additional knowledge bases can include the following:

- Familiarity with the substance abuse literature, concepts, and interventions.
- Training in multicultural skills.

- Awareness of how gender issues, sexuality, and sexual orientation issues affect adolescents.
- Experience with anger management interventions.
- Crisis intervention techniques.
- Interventions appropriate for posttraumatic stress disorder (PTSD) in children.
- Treatments for school refusal and social phobia.
- Interventions for childhood depression and anxiety, including test anxiety.
- Parent training methods.
- Various psychoeducational approaches.

Knowledge of consultation models for working with school systems can be invaluable. To this end, you might want to learn about consultation through continuing education seminars or readings and/or consider developing a collaborative arrangement with others who already provide school consultation services. The resulting synergism would be likely to benefit all. (Edens [1998] provides a useful and generalizable guide to school-based consultation for children with externalizing problems.)

Although this book is about specialized practices, you might also consider becoming a generalist and an employee. You might make the effort to become certified as a school psychologist or as a school counselor and to take a job inside the system. For those still in training, consider that the entry-level credentials are typically a masters degree and a year of paid internship, and entry-level salaries are typically around $40,000 per school year (about 200 workdays with paid holiday, sick leave, and often summers off). Salaries for those with doctorates and experience are typically in the $45,000 to $60,000 range (see http://www.nasponline.org/publications/cq282sp2000.html). See Crespi and Fieldman (2001) for one clinician's experience in respecializing as a school psychologist.

NATURE OF THE WORK

Areas of Practice

Treating Students with Work and Study Inhibitions

Many kinds of professionals can coach or train students in study and test-taking skills, but clinicians can bring more powerful therapeutic methods to bear on these areas, and such interventions will be even more appreciated when simple reteaching methods have failed to improve performance. Typical clinical issues include faulty and self-defeating attributions, fears of failure or success, low self-esteem, excessive perfectionism, depression, defective self-direction, and low frustration tolerance.

In particular, poor time management and procrastination can be crippling, especially among college and graduate students (Muszynski & Akamatsu, 1991). A prospective study by Britton and Tesser (1991) found that time management skills were in fact better predictors of college achievement than SAT scores, so you can see that addressing the psychological roots of poor time management is a worthy clinical endeavor. As for resources, Ferarri et al. (1995) discuss treatment approaches to procrastination; Zimmerman et al. (1994) present a method for teaching college students to systematically improve their use of study time; and Sapadin (1999) is useful to clinicians, parents, and students. (See also Learning Commons, 2002).

Treating School Refusal

Depending on the criteria used, school refusal (formerly referred to as "school phobia") affects between 1% and 2% of the school population (Paige, 1993); milder forms affect upwards of 10%, most frequently in the earliest grades and then again around adolescence (Murray, 1997). Situational factors (e.g., home relocation or school transitions) can trigger school refusal, as can social factors at school (e.g., bullying, teasing, and similar abuse). Being the youngest child or having a mother who also had school refusal will increase a child's risk. School refusal can often be indicative of psychological problems, such as generalized anxiety and depression (perhaps masked by somatic complaints), social phobia, public speaking anxiety, and, less often, separation anxiety. Of course, all of these can be effectively addressed by appropriately trained psychologists.

In treating school refusal, besides the general interventions for anxiety disorders and depression, some specific interventions have been devised (see, e.g., Blagg, 1992: Last & Strauss, 1990; Kearney & Silverman, 1995). A comprehensive volume by King et al. (1995) is aimed at school and clinical psychologists and presents many specific cognitive and behavioral interventions for school refusal, using a team approach. Kearney (2001) offers an empirically based assessment and systemic interventions, based on functional analysis of school refusal behaviors.

Interventions for Bullying and Aggression

The severity, extent, and consequences of bullying have only recently been recognized, and responses to it are still needed in most communities. About 30% of 6th- and 10th-grade students report being involved in bullying (Nansel et al., 2001). Student fears of assault can contribute to school refusal and/or have damaging long-term effects on self-esteem (Banks, 1997;

Leitman et al., 1995). According to Banks (1997) studies have established that approximately 15% of children are affected by bullying, as either bullies or victims. Victims of bullying behavior describe lifelong emotional consequences (Batsche & Knoff, 1994).

Early identification of bullying behaviors can assist in prevention, because such behaviors may be early markers of serious pathology in adulthood (Amminger et al., 1999). Bullies are more likely to experience problems with the law and problems in maintaining positive adult relationships (Oliver et al., 1994). For example, Tobin and Sugai (1999) were able to predict later discipline problems, violence, and school failure in students by analyzing records from the sixth grade. When evaluating students who have demonstrated aggressive, noncompliant, bullying, or violent behaviors, clinicians should be guided by the research, which shows that such children are often themselves prior victims of violence and/or witnesses to violence (e.g., Brown et al., 1999; Espleage et al., 1996; Eckenrode et al., 1990 cited in James, 1994), as well as the awareness that a substantial proportion of child witnesses and victims may also be suffering from PTSD (Durant et al., 1994).

Practitioners can provide effective psychoeducational and behavioral interventions for students identified as aggressive or violent, or for teachers or parents of these students. Larson (1994) offers a review of primary, secondary, and tertiary violence prevention programs. Empirical support has been found for programs such as Second Step (Grossman et al., 1997), Think First (Larson, 1992), Peacebuilders (Embry et al., 1996) and the Rethink Anger Management Program (see below). Deffenbacher et al. (1996) combined cognitive approaches, relaxation skills training, and social skills training into an effective program, and Aber (1999) and colleagues were able to reduce violence in New York schools by providing children with opportunities to learn how to deal constructively with conflict. Finally, Snook et al.'s (1999) description of "student alienation syndrome" suggests that school atmosphere and teachers' attitudes can overtly or covertly promote violence and educator-induced PTSD. You may be able to interest schools in an assessment of schools' climates as a basis for your subsequent preventative interventions.

Clinicians can also assist the victims of bullying with programs and consultations to instill pride, teach assertiveness and reporting of bullying, model coping skills and appropriate behaviors, and reinforce changes.

Treating Test Anxiety

Because test anxiety is common, can be crippling, and is treatable, this might become a focused clinical specialization as well as a point of entry into the schools. Every student suffers from some test anxiety, and for most, low to moderate levels of it promote better performance. However, a significant number suffer more distress, lower grades, and narrowed life choices.

After some triage, providing psychoeducational efforts in a group format can be both economical and profitable. A combination of relaxation and other anxiety reduction methods with training in test-taking skills (e.g., strategies for multiple-choice tests) and some study and memory techniques appears to be the best. Although purely educational approaches do exist, helping students to deal with generalized anxiety or fears of being judged, and to change their pathological self-perceptions, requires psychotherapeutic techniques. Vagg and Papsdorf (1995) describe and compare the use of cognitive therapy, study skills training, and biofeedback in reducing test anxiety. Gonzalez (1995) describes systematic desensitization, study skills counseling, and anxiety-coping training in the treatment of test anxiety. Older students with LDs improved on measures of self-esteem and test anxiety following cognitive-behavioral therapy (Wachelka & Katz, 1999). Johnson (1997) is a self-help guide; Newman (1996) is widely used; and Zeidner (1998) is very comprehensive.

School systems usually cannot provide these kinds of programs directly, and so they can serve as points of entry as you consult with teachers, counselors, and vice-principals. In addition, college and graduate students intimidated by oral examinations may constitute a small number, but are fairly easily located through advertising or inquiring at local colleges and universities.

Cross-References to Related Specializations

Niche 2.3. Gifted Children
Niche 2.4. Competent and Resilient Girls
Niche 5.3. Culturally Informed, Diversity-Sensitive Practice

Practice Models

A private practice model can be combined with consultation to the school system, and networking with other professionals and organizations working with school children (e.g., pediatricians, adolescent health specialists, school counselors, learning disability specialists, college counselors, SAT coaches, PTAs/PTOs) is recommended.

Financial Considerations

Although some of this work can be paid for as psychotherapy (e.g., work with children who have formal diagnoses of social phobia or conduct disorder), much of it is public education, consultation, or staff training (paid for by contracts), or private practice (as for LDs). As we have noted earlier, work that is not related to formal medical or psychiatric diagnoses (e.g., parenting training, prevention interventions, staff training, and consulting) is managed-care-free.

PROSPECTS AND PROSPECTING

Where Is the Need?

The U.S. Center for Mental Health Services (1997, cited by the American Academy of Child and Adolescent Psychiatry, 1999) estimated that 9–13% of children aged 9–16 suffer from serious mental disorder, yet only one in five of these children receives any treatment. Many who do receive treatment get only medication (Goleman, 1993), the effectiveness of which has been questioned (e.g., Malone et al., 1997; Ambrosini et al., 1999; Antonuccio et al., 1995). Many more school children have issues that do not meet formal criteria for frank mental illness. These are called "subclinical" cases and can benefit greatly from the services we can provide or support in the schools. Generally, psychological interventions with children have been shown to be effective, and many clients prefer them to pharmacological solutions for most disorders (Antonuccio et al., 1995). The general effectiveness of therapy for children has been demonstrated by meta-analysis (Weisz et al., 1995). And, lastly, there is a shortage of clinicians who can work effectively with children (Culbertson, 1993).

In addition, in 1996 NASP predicted, on the basis of population trends, that 3,000 additional school psychologists will be required in the United States by the year 2006 just to maintain the current ratios (Ejime, 1996). Although the American Counseling Association recommends a ratio of 1 counselor for every 250 students, current levels across the United States are 1:561 and decreasing ("A Dearth of School Counselors," 1999). These ratios range from 1:300 to 1:1,171 across states, and so there may be significant opportunities almost everywhere for specialized services to be provided by outside psychologists.

Competition

Of course, school psychologists and school counselors both serve this population, but their services are likely to be more traditional or more generic because of regulations, their training, or their preferences. Therefore, specializations like the ones described above can give you significant market advantages.

Reaching Clients/Directions for Marketing

An important step in becoming more involved in your local school system will be learning about the political realities affecting that system. Knowledge of funding levels, staffing realities, demand for services versus supply, quality of services provided, accessibility, and level of satisfaction with the services provided are all areas that may reveal unmet needs. Since each school system is unique, you will need to locate key resources for understanding the trends in your particular school system. One such resource—your state professional organization—can provide information about regulations, as well as predictions about how any upcoming changes might affect practices interfacing with school systems.

How can you learn more about your school system's unique needs? One approach would be to ask school staff members about what kinds of topics they would be interested in for presentations. Meeting with members of the instructional support team, guidance counselors, or others at the schools who are knowledgeable about needs could be helpful. You may gain entry by approaching a peer currently providing services to the schools. Consult a calendar of upcoming events (see the introduction to this section) to "piggyback" with national recognition days and draw attention to the services you offer.

INCREASING YOUR FORMAL KNOWLEDGE BASE

Core Readings

Consultation

Caplan, G., & Caplan, R. B. (1993). *Mental health consultation and collaboration.* San Francisco: Jossey-Bass.
    —An authoritative guide and update of the original *Theory and Practice of Mental Health Consultation.* Harvard psychiatrist Gerald Caplan is the originator of much of the theory and practice of mental health consultation.
Edens, J. F. (1998). School-based consultation services for children with externalizing behavior problems. In L. VandeCreek, S. Knapp, & T. L. Jackson (Eds.), *Innovations in clinical practice: A source book* (Vol. 16, pp. 337–353). Sarasota, FL: Professional Resource Press.
Marks, E. S. (1995). *Entry strategies for school consultation.* New York: Guilford Press.
    —Written for a school psychologist consultant audience by a school psychologist consultant, this book provides many insights and contains useful information and suggestions for effectively interfacing with schools through relationship building and understanding how schools function.
Sherman, R., Shumsky, A., & Rountree, Y. B. (1994). *Enlarging the therapeutic circle: The therapist's guide to collaborative therapy with families and schools.* New York: Brunner/Mazel.
    —The authors have worked extensively with schools and families. The book describes five successful models of family- and school-based collaboration. Many case studies make the material accessible.

Bullying

Elliott, D. S., Hamburg, B. A., & Williams, K. R. (Eds.). (1998). *Violence in American schools: A new perspective.* New York: Cambridge University Press.

—These authors believe that the best approaches to youth violence intervention are comprehensive and multidisciplinary, and take into account such variables as developmental level, social context, peer and family relationships, and community.

Hazler, R. J. (1996). *Breaking the cycle of violence: Interventions for bullying and victimization.* Washington, DC: Accelerated Development.

—This book presents a step-by-step model for working with bullying in the schools.

Juvonen, J., & Graham, S. (Eds.). (2001). *Peer harassment in school: The plight of the vulnerable and victimized.* New York: Guilford Press.

—This volume addresses who is likely to become a victim, responses to victimization, health effects, and peer variables, and discusses school-based prevention and intervention approaches.

Larson, J., & Lochman, J. E. (2002). *Helping schoolchildren cope with anger: A cognitive-behavioral intervention.* New York: Guilford Press.

Newman, D. A., Horne, A. M., & Bartolomucci, C. L. (2000). *Bully busters: A teacher's manual for helping bullies, victims, and bystanders.* Champaign, IL: Research Press.

—This is a manual in seven modules, designed to raise awareness and teach skills for upper elementary and middle school teachers. It includes very complete and practical exercises.

Test Anxiety

Johnson, S. (2000). *Taking the anxiety out of taking tests: A step-by-step guide.* Oakland, CA: New Harbinger.

Spielberger, C. D., & Vagg, P. R. (Eds.). (1995). *Test anxiety: Theory, assessment, and treatment.* Washington, DC: Taylor & Francis.

Zeidner, M. (1998). *Test anxiety: The state of the art.* New York: Plenum Press.

Journals

School Psychology Review
Psychology in the Schools
Journal of Clinical Child Psychology
Behavioral Disorders
Journal of Emotional and Behavioral Disorders

Online Resources

Bullying in Schools
http://www.ericps.ed.crc.uiuc.edu/eece/pubs/digests/1997/banks97.html

—Discusses prevalence, causes, consequences, and interventions for bullying in schools.

Bullying in Schools and What to Do About It
http://www.education.unisa.edu.au/bullying
—This is the Web site of Ken Rigby, PhD, a social psychologist, and offers many
materials of practical value.

Partnerships Against Violence Network (PAVNET)
http://www.pavnet.org
—PAVNET is a "virtual library" of information about violence and youth at risk,
representing data from seven different Federal agencies.

Early Warning, Timely Response: A Guide to Safe Schools
http://cecp.air.org/guide/guidetext.htm
—This guide identifies early warning signs of violence and other troubling behaviors, and recommends intervention and prevention strategies for students who are at
risk for behavioral problems.

Professional Organizations

National Association of School Psychologists (NASP)
4340 East–West Highway, Suite 402, Bethesda, MD 20814; 301-657-0270; fax
    301-657-0275
e-mail: nasp8455@aol.com   http://www.nasponline.org/index2.html
—NASP publishes a newsletter, *Communiqué*, and hosts a convention, a national
certification program, meetings, training institutes, and self-study programs.

Division 16 (School Psychology) of the American Psychological Association
750 First Street, Washington, DC 20002-4242; 202-336-6013; fax 202-218-3599
e-mail: kcooke@apa.org   http://www.indiana.edu/~div16
—The division offers a book series, "Applying Psychology to the Schools," with
detailed, empirically supported intervention recommendations. Titles include *Collaborative Family–Provider Partnerships in Early Intervention: Intervention and Systems Change; Responding to the Needs of Aggressive Children and Their Parents: A
Practitioner's Guide to Parent Training; Relationship-Based Interventions between
Teachers and Children: Developmental Systems Perspectives on the Practice of School
Psychology*; and *Psychology in Schools and Communities*.

Center for the Prevention of School Violence
Dept. of Juvenile Justice, 1801 Mail Service Center, Raleigh, NC 27699-1801;
    800-299-6054
http://www.juvjus.state.nc.us/cpsv/

Institute for Mental Health Initiatives (IMHI)
4545 42nd Street N.W., Suite 311, Washington, DC 20016; 202-364-7111; fax 202-
    363-3891
e-mail: info@imhi.org   http://www.imhi.org
—IMHI offers advanced training seminars for practitioners. The goal of these
workshops is to bring the Rethink Anger Management Program and similar programs into the community.

Patient Education Materials: Online Resources, Printed Resources, and Organizations

Bullying: A Survival Guide
http://www.bbc.co.uk
—Enter "Bullying" into the search box. A collection of about half a dozen articles.

Centre for Children and Families in the Justice System, London [Ontario] Family Court Clinic
http://www.lfcc.on.ca
—This Canadian site offers several publications for parents and teachers on youth violence, aggression, and bullying.

Scottish Council for Research in Education
http://www.scre.ac.uk
—Click on "Bullying at School Info" for many pages and articles on this topic.

How to Study
http://www.howtostudy.org
—Provides links to many useful articles on overcoming procrastination and test anxiety. Complements of Chemeketa Community College.

Campus Blues
http://www.campusblues.com/test.shtml
—A comprehensive article on test anxiety, aimed at college students.

Stop Bullying Now
http://www.stopbullyingnow.com
—Support for targets, help for bullies, interventions, training for teachers, articles, bibliography, links. Very comprehensive.

TeensHealth: Dealing with Bullying
http://www.kidshealth.org/teen/school_jobs/bullying/bullies.html
—Sound advice for teens.

Casbarro, J. (2003). *Test anxiety and what you can do about it.* Port Chester, NY: National Professional Resources.
—For students from the elementary grades through high school.
Emmett, R. (2002). *The procrastinating child: A handbook for adults to help children stop putting things off.* New York: Walker.
—Sound advice for parents.
Evans, E. (1996). *No more test anxiety: Effective steps for taking tests and achieving better grades.* Los Angeles: Learning Skills.
—This book and accompanying CD provide a step-by-step approach to overcoming test anxiety.
Knaus, W. J., & Ellis, A. (2002). *The procrastination workbook: Your personalized program for breaking free from the patterns that hold you back.* Oakland, CA: New Harbinger.
—A step-by-step guide written for a general audience.

Levinson, S., & Greider, P. C. (1998). *Following through: A revolutionary new model for finishing whatever you start.* New York: Kensington.

   —While not strictly focused on academics, this is guide to overcoming procrastination in all areas of life.

McEwan, E. K. (1998). *When kids say no to school: Helping children at risk of failure, refusal, or dropping out.* Wheaton, IL: Harold Shaw.

NASP offers brochures for parents on a variety of topics including school refusal, teaching self-control, and ADHD (see "Professional Organizations").

Section 3

The World of Work

Introduction, Overview, and Commonalities

Work is integral to sustaining life and identity. Those who suffer impediments in their productivity or their "people skills" can be at a huge disadvantage—a disadvantage that can translate into lost income and low self-esteem. In addition, workplaces are in themselves sources of stress, often with conflicting demands and resulting burnout—a human factor that affects the "bottom line," and so is of concern to employers. Finally, recent history has witnessed massive corporate restructurings that have eroded employees' trust, loyalty, and commitment, and this breach is only now being addressed by corporate management. As a result, a remarkable confluence has begun to develop between those calling for improved work environments for psychological and humanistic reasons, and those calling for such environments as fuel for the engine of corporate success. This confluence provides a fine opportunity for behavioral science to utilize its sophisticated interventions for the benefit of business.

THE VALUE AND NEED FOR CLINICAL PSYCHOLOGY IN THE BUSINESS WORLD

Businesses' comfort level with psychological interventions is increasing. This is especially true when these skills are packaged as training, feedback about personality strengths and weaknesses, executive coaching, interventions to enhance productivity, and/or assistance with employees' career development.

Corporate America is increasingly turning to psychology to help solve some of its most vexing problems. By some thoughtful analysts, massive losses in productivity are attributed to "the people factor." In the current

163

highly competitive business environment, such suboptimal functioning places corporations at risk of not surviving.

How massive are the costs and losses? Wiesendanger (1995) has estimated that U.S. companies lose $200 billion every year because of the following factors: reduced productivity; preventable accidents and workers' compensation claims; employee absenteeism, turnover, and the costs of training replacements; health insurance and medical expenses related to low-quality workplaces; and worker dissatisfaction and burnout. In 1993, employers reportedly spent $22 billion on employee counseling and therapy alone—a figure that was a 57% increase from 5 years earlier (Wiesendanger, 1995). Many of the remedies that have been applied have been developed or adapted from the interventions we use in everyday clinical practice.

According to Martin (1996), the application of psychology to the workplace is viewed by executives "not as a clinical science but as a technology of understanding and accelerating growth; transforming perceptions and belief systems; unlocking creativity, motivation and commitment; healing the organization's grief from change and loss; and most importantly, predicting the future behavior of individuals and groups based upon their past" (p. 37).

Some of the ways psychological knowledge is routinely incorporated into business settings are as follows: conflict management, leadership training, enhancing productivity, creativity training, and change management. The American Psychological Association (APA) Task Force on Envisioning, Identifying, and Accessing New Professional Roles (Levant et al., 2001) describes other functions clinically trained psychologists could legitimately offer:

> Psychologists who are skilled and creative may be able to offer businesses a broad array of services within the scope of their training and expertise. These services might include (a) programs aimed at stress in the workplace; (b) workplace violence prevention and intervention (e.g., critical incident stress debriefing); (c) training programs for managers to facilitate early identification and referral of employees in need; (d) prevention, screening, and early intervention programs; (e) training related to sexual harassment, diversity, and gender issues; and (f) team-building and communication development programs (see Katz & Miller, 1996; Quick, 1999; Resnick & Kausch, 1995, for specific examples). In addition, the emerging area of career and job coaching to assist people in developing their careers and managing difficulties in their work environments is receiving considerable attention in the business community (e.g., Saporito, 1996). (Levant et al., 2001, p. 82)

Depending on your interests, training, and experience, still other opportunities include reducing work dysfunctions; aiding in selection, evaluation, and promotion of employees at all levels; crisis management; and interventions for employee wellness and drug and alcohol problems.

Even the activities we and Levant et al. (2001) have listed do not encompass all of the uses to which behavioral science knowledge has been and can be put in business settings. Organizations that might avail themselves of such services range in size and type from "Mom-and-Pop" businesses to international corporations. They include professional groups and associations; privately owned companies (including family-owned businesses—see Niche 3.2) and public companies; and nonprofit and/or community service organizations.

YOUR SKILL SET

Because it is both risky and unethical to practice beyond your knowledge, you must bear in mind the boundaries of other professionals practicing in this area. Industrial/organizational psychologists, financial consultants, lawyers, and others have skills and legitimized abilities that you may lack and should not compete with. Moreover, a business setting involves complexities and interactions of factors that may not be apparent to a person without business training. For example, when you are working from a clinical perspective with individuals in their workplace, knowledge of the workplace's norms, motivations, and "culture" is valuable. But changing these factors requires organizational consultation, not clinical work. That said, there are nonetheless areas where your clinical training and experience make you highly qualified to provide services to businesses.

For all but the first of the niches in this section, your knowledge base should include organizational theory and development, consultation approaches, and process facilitation (Perrott, 1999). Although you do not need an MBA to be competent in these niches, an understanding of business law, finance, and management provides perspectives on the complex rules and procedures under which businesses operate. In addition to formal coursework, supervision and/or mentoring opportunities are pathways to competency and can also provide networking opportunities.

For work in these niches, adapt your practices to the culture of business. Everything—your attire, your vocabulary, your title, your business card, and your practices—should convey that you are a businessperson, not simply a clinician. An active, collegial approach is what is expected. Be aware that boundaries differ considerably from those in traditional clinical work (e.g., socializing with clients is often expected and clearly not taboo). Change is still your work product, but "changes in observable behavior rather than changes in subjective experience" are the goals, as are "efficiency, productivity, and profit" (Hilburt-Davis, 1996). In addition, "The consultant takes a leadership position—the role of change agent. You are paid to have an opinion, to give advice. . . . The expectations are that the consultant takes more responsibility for making changes happen than in the clinical setting" (Hilburt-Davis, 1996).

Finally, embrace and confront timelines, deadlines, and bottom lines (both yours and businesses') up front, in the form of a written contract for your services.

DIRECTIONS FOR MARKETING

Marketing is of major importance when you are working with businesses, and so you will need to put aside several hours per week to develop and execute your marketing strategy.

- Start with the most accessible part of the local business community: Join, attend, and give presentations at Rotary Clubs, Chambers of Commerce, and similar organizations. Nurture contacts with people who are well connected in your community. These could be other professionals, community leaders, "power brokers" (Martin, 1996), or "angels" (Grodzki, 1999) who can send multiple referrals, provide endorsements, and make business introductions for you. In addition to this core of networking activities, the following are important perspectives.
- Businesspeople usually do not know how to evaluate your skills and experience, so you must convey to them how your particular knowledge and skills can be helpful to them. Look for your natural advantages over any competition. Distinguish your services from the "dark side" of consultancies, especially "poor ethics and lack of confidentiality, simplistic analysis methods, poor implementation skills, and being unable to provide and measure results. By contrast, the ethics and boundaries that regulate the psychotherapy disciplines are viewed as a welcome relief" (Martin, 1996, p. 52).
- Be cognizant of the culture of business, as noted above. In particular, bear in mind that informality, sloppiness, and tardiness will cause rejection.
- Detailed marketing strategies for breaking into the world of business can be found in Perrott (1999), Martin (1996), Heller (1997), Weiss (1992), and Ackley (1997). They cover the essentials that will need your attention: consultancy models, delineating and distinguishing your services, identifying your target audience, conducting a needs assessment, developing promotional letters and brochures, "cold calling," following up, rehearsing for interviews, writing proposals, setting fees, closing a deal, and so on.
- An approach that involves only a small commitment of time and al-

most no expense is described by Dean (1999). He uses a free e-mail newsletter to market his "virtual coaching" practice nationally to thousands of subscribers (he calls this "permission marketing," because recipients must request the newsletter). As in most other marketing strategies, the key is to regularly provide relevant content that, over time, creates positive perceptions of you as a trustworthy source of information and services.

- Several years ago, I (RLL) participated in the Business Committee of the New Jersey Psychological Association, which was seeking ways to approach businesses to raise their awareness of the value of psychology in the workplace. We decided on an annual award for psychologically healthy workplaces, which turned out to be a very exciting and productive way for psychologists to make personal connections with businesses. As media chair, I contacted a reporter for *The New York Times*, who wrote a feature article on the award (Sommers, 1999). The *APA Monitor* also did an article on New Jersey's and other states' awards, and noted:

> The awards have also put psychologists into some forums they might not otherwise be in. Associations have advertised the award in business publications. Some of the winners have asked that the award be presented to them a second time during the conferences where they meet with their peers. (Foxhall, 2001)

- Harry Beckwith (1997) has written a remarkable and valuable book, *Selling the Invisible: A Field Guide to Modern Marketing*, in which he extols the importance of cultivating trust and developing relationships with clients in order to sell one's services. "Giving psychology away" will take on whole new meanings for you after reading his analysis of how to overcome clients' fears.

Many practitioners have already perceived these confluences and seized opportunities to provide services to business, but we believe that there are still great opportunities for competent, business-oriented practitioners in this area. Almost all of the opportunities are managed-care-free. Furthermore, a business-oriented practice can evolve from an initial commitment of just a few hours a week (plus time for personal and practice development, of course) to a majority of your practice, depending upon your level of interest and need. Whether you would like to work with business as a solo practitioner or have an interest in group practice (multidisciplinary or interdisciplinary), there are many creative examples. What is important is that you acquire a good sense of the needs of businesses and of how your skills and experience can help meet these needs.

Become a reader of business newspapers, magazines, and books, so that you can stay abreast of developing trends that present opportunities to create new services. Don't forget to follow local business developments as well. If you have not read *Forbes, Business Week, Fortune*, or even *The Wall Street Journal* in years, you may be surprised at the liveliness of the writing, the creativity of the innovations described, and the psychological perspectives on the individuals and issues described.

The APA Task Force quoted earlier (Levant et al., 2001) has suggested that many services could be easily provided to smaller businesses:

> Industrial psychologists currently assume critical roles in large companies, particularly in employment screening, testing, and certification programs. Organizational, consulting, and a variety of other psychologists provide a range of in-house and external consulting services. In addition to these roles, there are a variety of services reasonably within the scope of practice of more generally trained psychologists that can be offered to businesses (e.g., see Maddi, 1997; Somerville, 1998). This may particularly be an opportunity in smaller communities or with smaller businesses, where there are less likely to be specialized resources available. (Levant et al., 2001, p. 82)

The niches in this section provide examples of specializations that offer benefits both to businesses and to individual employees, as they seek to adapt, succeed, and prosper in the context of the many challenges and trends affecting them. We hope that this sampling of possibilities will inspire you to explore how you might find effective, creative, and synergistic ways to get into business with businesses.

Treating Public Speaking Anxiety for Work Success

OVERVIEW AND OPPORTUNITIES

Developing a specialty practice in treating public speaking anxiety (PSA) is based on three simple facts:

1. PSA is the most common form of social anxiety. Indeed, it is listed as the leading type of fear among Americans, according to the Bruskin Report (cited in Whitworth & Cochran, 1996).
2. PSA is vocationally and socially costly, because so many business settings require personnel to address small or even large groups. Those with PSA have severe inhibitions across these situations.
3. Clinicians have training and experience in effective therapies for various types of anxiety, including PSA.

YOUR POTENTIAL SATISFACTIONS

- Most of those coming for treatment are higher-functioning, hopeful, and ready to work on their problem. Working with these clients usually comes under the heading of "making well people weller," which can be a welcome balance to the more usual focus of clinical attention—namely, psychopathology. It may balance some of the burnout potential of working with more seriously disordered individuals.
- The methods available are familiar, are effective, and do not require enormous efforts on the part of the client or therapist.
- Because PSA is only one of several kinds of performance anxieties, it

is quite possible to build upon success in this area and use it to enter business consulting.

YOUR SKILL SET

Recycling Your Current Competencies

If you already know many methods for treating anxiety and avoidance, you are likely to need few new skills to treat PSA. Knowledge of and experience with cognitive-behavioral therapy (CBT), exposure, and social skills training for anxiety disorders will all be useful. See Bourne (1995) for a nuts-and-bolts collection of many methods besides those discussed below under "Approaches and Techniques."

Your training should include the skills to assess, differentially diagnose, and recommend appropriate treatments. Group skills are important if you use a group treatment format. You should not have significant personal problems with PSA, but some reluctance to speak in public may be useful. There is no additional formal certification needed at present for work in this area.

NATURE OF THE WORK

Approaches and Techniques

Clinical expertise is required for intelligent and valid triage, because those who present with PSA may include those with depression, more generalized or intense social phobia, specific phobias, and personality disorders (avoidant and paranoid, most likely). Lewin et al. (1996) indicate that those with just "circumscribed speech fear [constitute] a meaningful subtype and can be independent of generalized social anxiety" (p. 387).

There are many assessment instruments to choose from. The following are the most widely used:

- The Personal Report of Communication Apprehension—24 (PRCA-24; McCroskey et al., 1985).
- The Speaker Anxiety Scale (SAS; Clevenger et al., 1992), derived from the PRCA-24 and consisting of 32 factorially derived items measuring nine factors, including "positive anxiety."
- The Personal Report of Confidence as a Speaker (Phillips et al., 1997).
- The Timed Behavioral Checklist for Performance Anxiety (Paul, 1966).

Evidence suggests that offering a combination of treatment components is most effective (Allen et al., 1989; Heimberg et al., 1985). The three most common and most effective treatments are skills training; systematic desensitization (SD) with exposure *in vitro* or *in vivo*; and cognitive modification (Whitworth & Cochran, 1996). Zemore (1975) is an early but clear demonstration of SD with progressive muscle relaxation training, and Hekmat et al. (1985) used what they called "instructional desensitization." Although unpleasant for clients and demanding of the therapist, flooding has been shown to be a highly effective and brief treatment for PSA, often more effective than SD (Marshall et al., 1982). Only a psychologist who understands the principles behind it can use flooding appropriately and safely. Cognitive methods that have been demonstrated to be effective in PSA include CBT (Woody et al., 1997), rational–emotive therapy (Straatmeyer & Watkins, 1974), stress inoculation training (Jaremko, 1980; Altmaier et al., 1982) and visualization (Hopf et al., 1994). Other methods include hypnosis (Schoenberger et al., 1997), video feedback of performance, and a self-help program of readings (Motley & Molloy, 1994). Note, however, that paradoxical intention (Worthington et al., 1984) and neurolinguistic programming (Krugman et al., 1985) have not been shown to be of value.

Cross-References to Related Specializations

Niche 2.5. Clinical Interventions for Students and Schools
Niche 3.3. Improving Work Performance

Subspecializations

Treating Performance Anxieties

Many artists suffer from "stage fright," which is a variant of PSA. Not only actors, but musicians, radio and television performers, and many others who must give public presentations are afflicted. Students and professionals alike in the performing arts must attend tryouts and casting calls that involve repeated "failures." The anxieties have similar dynamics and so are highly responsive to our techniques. To explore this area, you might look at Desberg and Marsh (1999), which is a self-help book about stage fright. Ashley (1997) offers an 8-week program based on a Jungian approach.

Treating Extreme Shyness

People who are painfully shy hold negative expectations about the outcome of social situations and underestimate their ability to deal with social situations. They remember negative feedback better than people who are not shy, and are overly sensitive to the negative reactions of others. Shyness, according to Henderson and Zimbardo (1998), "becomes a self-handicapping strategy—a reason or excuse for anticipated social failure that over time becomes a crutch." Assertiveness (especially with strangers) is inhibited, and interpersonal conflict is avoided, with sadly negative consequences for job performance and career development (Hamer & Bruch, 1997). Shy people may feel that they are treated unfairly at work because others who are less diligent workers receive promotions and they do not. Shy employees may be viewed as lacking "people skills" and leadership qualities, and thus may be denied opportunities in the workplace. Furthermore, anxious self-preoccupation (Melchior & Cheek, 1990) may reduce performance in evaluation situations. A hidden consequence of shyness includes greater health problems (Bell et al., 1993), due perhaps to the combined effects of a subpar social support network and discomfort discussing health problems with medical personnel.

The treatments available for this population are easy to administer and highly effective, yet constitute a neglected area of practice for researchers and clinicians (Judd, 1994). Like treatments for social phobia, interventions for shyness employ a comprehensive approach that includes exposure and behavioral practice in feared situations, social skills training, cognitive restructuring for negative thoughts, communication exercises both for getting acquainted and for deepening relationships, and assertiveness training.

Zimbardo pioneered research and then treatment in this area. His popular book (Zimbardo, 1990) introduced the ideas. He has worked with Henderson, and an article by Henderson (1992) is a brief but detailed guide to the groups they run. Heimburg et al. (1995) provide comprehensive coverage of social anxiety and social phobia. Beidel and Turner's (1997) book is solidly based on their longitudinal research and long practice. Rapee and Sanderson (1998) offer both guidance to treatment and a client workbook. Hope et al. (2000) provide a fully developed treatment manual with workbook. For the lay reader, Schneier and Welkowitz's (1996) book is surprisingly comprehensive.

Prevention of PSA

PSA may possibly be prevented by interventions in the schools (or other childhood settings such as churches and civic organizations) consisting of short-term groups for "psychological immunization" (graded preliminary exposure to potentially threatening stimuli), although the content of this approach requires additional development (Hiebert et al., 1989; Cradock et al., 1978).

Consulting about PSA

It is possible to present workshops to the public or any kind of social group or business groups on many aspects of conversation, presentations, meetings, and business relationships.

Other Potential Populations for Subspecializations

Depending on your local situation as regards service providers and population needs, consider developing services for related populations, such as the following:

- Those who have lost jobs and whose PSA cripples their job searching.
- Salespeople who may suffer from rejection anxiety.
- Workers from other cultures, who need to adapt to the American social expectations for assertion, public speaking, and demonstrations of confidence.
- Workers with substance abuse. Many people with social phobia cope with their anxiety by using alcohol and can benefit from addressing the anxiety component.

Practice Models

Structured individual and group treatments are common and may range from a few hours to about 14 weekly sessions. Although group treatment has been used very successfully, many clients will be so vulnerable to debilitating embarrassment that they will require or just prefer individual treatment. For an exceptionally distressed individual, SD as a supplement to the group program may be clinically helpful.

There are many self-help and informal approaches (see above and "Patient Education Materials," below), but even with the use of self-administered treatments (such as a take-home manual), therapist supervision and contacts will reduce the dropout rate and thus improve outcome (Marshall et al., 1976).

Organizations may hire therapists on a contractual basis to run groups for reducing their members' PSA.

Financial Considerations

Current and local fees for individual and group therapies would apply to this area. Most business clients will pay "out of pocket," but some may use health insurance for either individual or group treatment if the severity of their PSA rises to diagnosable levels of social phobia, or if they have comorbid diagnoses. Additional services could include intake diagnostic workups, telephone consultations, and long-term maintenance or "booster" sessions.

Cautions, Ethical Dilemmas, Culture Clashes, and/or Managed Care Issues

Treating PSA or shyness is a managed-care-free practice area, because neither of these is a formal psychiatric diagnosis. However, the client may have a related anxiety disorder or other diagnosis, and this might be covered under health insurance. Therefore, you should do a thorough assessment for other comorbid conditions.

PROSPECTS AND PROSPECTING

Where Is the Need?

The market is enormous. A community sample survey found that one-third of people have substantial fears of public speaking, and 20% of these people reported that these fears had an adverse impact on at least one aspect of their lives (Stein et al., 1996). Therefore, the minimum potential market is about 6% of the population, or 15 million Americans.

Surveys of adults indicate that almost half consider themselves to be chronically shy, 78% believe it can be overcome, and 87% are willing to do something about their shyness (Carducci, 2000). Ironically, perhaps, sufferers often delay treatment because the very dynamics of shyness make accessing care difficult.

Competition

For PSA, there are a number of competitors: college speech teachers, some speech therapists, generic counselors, organizations like Toastmasters and the Dale Carnegie Institute, and medications. Your professional advantages lie in possible health insurance coverage, guaranteed privacy and confidentiality, and your clinical skills. Only a clinician can do the following:

- Make a careful, complete, and accurate differential diagnosis
- Evaluate a client in all relevant dimensions.
- Consider all the treatments and match the treatment(s) to the client's needs.
- Understand and use *any and all* of the treatments available.
- Rationally choose a backup treatment when one disappoints or fails.
- Select and properly administer the most appropriate evaluation methods before, during, and at the end of treatment.

College speech instructors use a variety of techniques to deal with PSA, which they label "communication apprehension" (CA). Robinson (1997) reports that they "teach the necessary speaking skills," create "a supportive and positive classroom environment," relabel students' CA as normal, and teach "techniques that help students handle feelings of apprehension." The traditional method of dealing with CA in the regular classroom is "progressive oral communication performances designed to teach skills and increase self-confidence" (Stacks & Stone, 1984, p. 318). However, this method may hurt rather than help those with high PSA (Stacks & Stone, 1984). It appears that the typical CA treatment, which consists of simply rehearsing positive self-statements, is less therapeutic than exploring and countering the typical unproductive and irrational self-statements (Thorpe et al., 1976). Because those with high PSA minimize their preparation efforts (Daly et al., 1995), offering training in rhetorical skills before reducing their anxiety is not likely to be effective. For a better understanding of how university speech and communication teachers address these issues, have a look at a common textbook's (Richmonds & McCroskey, 1998) contents and perspective.

Reaching Clients/Directions for Marketing

- Because PSA is so common, it is easily understood by the public, as is shyness. Potential clients are well aware of the problem and the costs to their lives. Whereas those with PSA seek treatment on their own, shy people may require outreach efforts that are tailored to their social apprehensions, with particular attention to keeping these efforts warm, sensitive, low-threat, and nonpathologizing.
- Simple ads and announcements of services can be placed in newspapers and the newsletters of many organizations.
- A brochure for practice promotion and patient education, entitled *Painful Shyness in Children and Adults*, is available from APA Division 42 as of Spring 2002 (Henderson et al., 2001).

INCREASING YOUR FORMAL KNOWLEDGE BASE

Psychologists have generally considered PSA a variety of social phobia, and so the most useful literature can be found under that heading.

Core Readings

Beidel, D. C., & Turner, S. M. (1997). *Shy children, phobic adults: Nature and treatment of social phobia.* Washington, DC: American Psychological Association.
—A comprehensive overview of what we know about social phobia and its treatments.

Greist, J. H. (1995). The diagnosis of social phobia. *Journal of Clinical Psychiatry*, 56(Suppl. 5), 5–12.
—A quick overview.
Heimberg, R. G., Liebowitz, M. R., Hope, D. A., & Schneier, F. R. (Eds.). (1995). *Social phobia: Diagnosis, assessment, and treatment*. New York: Guilford Press.
—A very comprehensive review of all aspects of social phobia.
Stein, M. B. (Ed.). (1995). *Social phobia: Clinical and research perspectives*. Washington, DC: American Psychiatric Press.
—Good for deep background information from all perspectives: clinical, epidemiological, psychodynamic, and genetic. Treatments are also reviewed.

Online Resources

Public Speaking Anxiety: The Basics, Symptoms and Effects, Resources, Getting Help
http://www.nutrition-health-online.com/dir/speaking_and_anxiety/index.shtml
—Though very commercial, this site has many booklets and articles easily usable as patient education handouts.

Communication Studies Department, Hamline University
http://www.hamline.edu/depts/commdept/prca-2.html
—Discussion of the uses of the PRCA-24 and how to get more information. The test itself is available online at http://www.usm.maine.edu/com/prca.htm.

The Shyness Institute
http://www.shyness.com
—This site serves as an excellent example of marketing to this population, and also contains considerable information on shyness including questionnaires, support groups, and a list of professional treatment centers.

Clinical Tools

Babior, S. (1996). *Overcoming panic, anxiety, and phobias: New strategies to free yourself from worry and fear*. Duluth, MN: Whole Person Associates.
—This highly structured book is aimed at a lay audience, but includes worksheets that clinicians can use. It offers CBT strategies for specific fears and phobias, information for family members, and 14 successful case studies.
Babior, S., & Goldman, C. (1996). *Working with groups to overcome panic, anxiety, and phobias*. Duluth, MN: Whole Person Associates.
—A treatment manual for all kinds of anxieties, with activities, treatment plans, and so forth.
Heimberg, R. G., & Becker, R. E. (2002). *Cognitive-behavioral group therapy for social phobia: Basic mechanisms and clinical strategies*. New York: Guilford Press.
—An empirically supported treatment manual.
Hope, D. A., Heimberg, R. G., Juster, H. R., & Turk, C. L. (2000). *Managing social anxiety: A cognitive-behavioral therapy approach*. San Antonio, TX: Psychological Corporation.

—Expert clinical researchers describe their interventions and provide the relevant homework, exercises, and handouts. Highly recommended.

Patient Education Materials: Online Resources, Printed Resources, and Organizations

Anxiety and Public Speaking
http://www.brad.ac.uk/acad/civeng/skills/pubspeak.htm
—Provides a brief overview and materials useful for a public information handout.

Background Information on the PRCA: The Personal Report of Communication Apprehension
http://www.hamline.edu/depts/commdept/prca-2.html
—A very brief explanation of the role of anxiety for PSA.

How to Conquer Public Speaking Fear, Morton C. Orman
http://www.stresscure.com/jobstress/speak.html
—A six-page essay on reducing the stress of public speaking by using 10 principles.

Antony, M. M., & Swinson, R. P. (2000). *The shyness and social anxiety workbook: Proven techniques for overcoming your fears.* Oakland, CA: New Harbinger.
—A well-structured workbook with CBT techniques for thought-changing and exposure. One of the best self-help books.
Dayhoff, S. A. (2000). *Diagonally-parked in a parallel universe: Working through social anxiety.* Placitas, NM: Effectivness-Plus.
—Solutions for shyness in the form of step-by-step CBT interventions.
Desberg, P. (1996). *No more butterflies: Overcoming stagefright, shyness, interview anxiety, and fear of public speaking.* Oakland, CA: New Harbinger.
—The author, a professor, offers a self-help guide based on his many workshops.
Greist, J. H., Jefferson, J. W., & Katzelnick, D. J (1997). *Social phobia: A guide.* Madison, WI: Dean Foundation.
—A very good introduction in 61 pages, suitable for the educated patient or family member. Includes a discussion of drug treatment.
Markway, B. G., Carmin, C. N., Pollard, C. A., & Flynn, T. (1992). *Dying of embarrassment: Help for social anxiety and phobia.* Oakland, CA: New Harbinger.
—The publisher says, "This book provides clear and supportive instruction for assessing your fears, practicing relaxation and deep breathing, and improving or developing new social skills."
Markway, B. G., & Markway, G. (2001). *Painfully shy: How to overcome social anxiety and reclaim your life.* New York: St. Martin's Press.
—An excellent overview with cases, ideal for patient education.

Consulting to Family-Owned Businesses

OVERVIEW AND OPPORTUNITIES

When you picture a family-owned business (FOB), do you see Mom, Pop, and the kids working together harmoniously and effectively in the corner store, pursuing their shared goals? Or do you envision family member stakeholders battling for control, profligate siblings engaged in ruinous rivalries, and rampant dysfunctionality? The reality of most FOBs lies somewhere between these extremes. The abilities of the family members to resolve conflict, negotiate transitions, and communicate effectively will determine whether a family firm survives or perishes.

Until recently, families needing expert help with process issues such as these had nowhere to turn, because their usual advisors (friends, relatives, accountants, attorneys, and business management consultants) lacked the skills to help them deal with family issues or the family firm as a unique type of business entity (Gersick et al., 1997). McKimmy (1996) found that 30% of family business owners reported having no trusted business advisor outside the family; of those who had outside advisors, accountants were relied on most frequently. We can provide independent opinions, utter confidentiality, and, most importantly, research-based advice on issues that no other profession can address with authority.

Like all businesses, FOBs are concerned with profitability, personnel productivity, job satisfaction, and the "fit" of individuals to their jobs. But in an FOB, in addition to experience and ability, decisions must consider familial ties, affection, primogeniture, and gender. Multiple and changing boundaries make for role confusion and role conflict. Families often have to resolve conflicts between what is in the best interests of the business on the one hand, and what would further an individual or relationship, provide leadership training to a successor, resolve long-standing sibling and parental issues, or reformulate the firm and the family after a divorce on the other. Examples of other areas in which FOBs may benefit from psychological advisors include grieving for the loss of the family firm's leader/parent, teaching siblings to colead the company, dealing with reorganization and emotions when a family member separates from the business, or helping the members of an entrepreneurial couple to improve their relationship where it limits the business. It's easy to understand why issues such as these have begun to attract the interest and talents of therapists (particularly family therapists) and clinicians who also have business training or experience.

YOUR POTENTIAL SATISFACTIONS

- Consulting to FOBs is a fresh opportunity to utilize your skills, particularly the sophisticated knowledge base of family and couple dynamics.
- Unlike publicly owned businesses, many FOBs are not exclusively bottom-line-driven.
- Although this niche may require effort to develop and market, it can be durable, lucrative, and personally rewarding, because FOBs will realize that your services have both personal and economic value.
- You will be one of the few offering these specialized services.
- This is a managed-care-free area of practice.

YOUR SKILL SET

Recycling Your Current Competencies

As with most new areas, no single theory or body of knowledge is required for work with FOBs. Rather, it requires competencies drawn from a number of other areas.

- A thorough understanding of and experience with family and couple dynamics and systems principles are the core skills. Couple and family methods are important modalities (Rosenblatt et al., 1985), and psychodynamic models (Kets de Vries, 1996) have been used. Sirkin (1996) has utilized multigenerational genograms with family businesses. Therapists trained in family treatment using these approaches already possess powerful methods for understanding and effecting change in FOBs.
- Organizational development, leadership training, team-building ap-

proaches, and executive coaching are also helpful skills and perspectives. In addition, training and experience with group dynamics (especially leadership and followership) and with being a change agent can be helpful.

- A family firm consultant must be comfortable dealing with business topics. Familiarity, training, and/or experience with legal and financial issues affecting FOBs, and the ability to interact effectively with lawyers and accountants, are important assets.
- Understanding and knowledge that you have developed from personal experience with an FOB would be an advantage.
- Being able to step outside of customary roles and assume an active, action-oriented approach is best.

Retreading for Added Skills

- Additional training on such topics as succession planning, organizational development, leadership training, and team development may widen your perspective, improve your ability to speak the language of business, and so expand your armamentarium of interventions for helping FOBs.
- The Family Firm Institute (FFI) offers a certificate in consultation to family firms. More information is available from its website (see "Professional Organizations," below). The FFI also offers mentoring and training at its annual conference.

NATURE OF THE WORK

FOBs vary widely in terms of size and complexity. Whereas 40% involve two spouses (and perhaps unrelated others) working together in day-to-day business operations (Massachusetts Mutual Life Insurance Company, 1994), other formats—such as sibling and cousin partnerships, intergenerational arrangements, and various other combinations—are also common.

Despite the fact that diagnosable disorders may exist among the members of a family firm, this work is consultation, not treatment. Most of those working with FOBs stress that the firm (and, to a lesser extent, the family system) is the client, not individual family members (Sirkin, 1996). As Hilburt-Davis (1997) points out, the relationship between the consultant and the family members is collegial, with a vocabulary that is nonpathological: " 'assessment' instead of 'diagnosis'; 'issue', 'problem' or 'concern' instead of symptom'; 'old baggage' instead of 'transference.' " Hilburt-Davis (1997) continues:

The work is not only with the family and business systems but with the interaction between the two. It involves helping the family to clarify roles, agreements, boundaries, assumptions, and expectations. It can include family retreats, strategic planning sessions, team building, conflict management, and role clarification. It is about helping the family [members] define what they want for themselves, in the family and in the business and, then, helping them to align their actions with their vision and values.

Areas of Practice

The pressure points of FOBs are most often in these areas:

- Succession—planning and arranging for passing on the leader's position.
- Conflicts over issues or personalities.
- Other issues (e.g., substance abuse in younger family members, gender and sibling issues, etc.).

Succession

Significantly, two-thirds of FOBs do not survive past the first generation, and only one-quarter of the remaining one-third survive the second generation (Kets de Vries, 1996). This fragile existence is understandably the focus of intense concern on the part of FOBs. There is much that can go amiss, and when this happens, families will be motivated to find solution-oriented expertise to get back on course. Succession planning is one of the most troubling issues for families that own businesses because it evokes the panoply of family dynamics, often in multigenerational relief.

In a recent survey of FOBs conducted for the MassMutual Financial Group (*American Family Business Survey*, 2002), almost 40% of family businesses expected their chief executive officers (CEOs) to retire or semiretire within the next 5 years, and 56% expected this to happen within 10 years. Since the tenure of the average FOB's CEO is as much as six times longer than that of the CEO of the typical public company, this level of turnover is described as "unparalleled." Management transition is difficult for most companies, but it can be especially painful and even catastrophic in a family business.

Interestingly, although surveys indicate that the great majority of family business owners want to pass the business on to another family member, many have not yet chosen a successor. Of those who have, only a small minority have actually written a succession plan. Clearly, there is much to be done in moving this process along by addressing the family issues that interfere.

Conflicts and Hostilities

Not every FOB is a hotbed of contention, but among those that are the financial and personal consequences of dysfunction can be staggering (Liebowitz, 1998). Results of a recent survey by Northeastern University's Center for Family Business ("Comprehensive Study Focuses . . . ," n.d.) indicate that conflict among family members in FOBs is fairly regular (weekly) for about 20% of FOBs, and at least monthly for another 20%. Of particular relevance for consultants is the finding that 40% of FOBs experiencing conflict had not discussed the issues prior to a crisis taking place. A 1998 survey by ReGeneration Partners found that "communication among family members" was the third most frequent issue mentioned as affecting FOBs ("Key Issues as Viewed . . . ," 1999).

In addition to family therapy and systems interventions, conflict resolution skills, goal-setting strategies, leadership interventions, communication skills, and many of the intervention strategies described in Niche 3.3, can be usefully adapted to work with FOBs.

Other Issues

Another area of great concern, according to Bork et al. (1996), is an increasing risk of substance abuse among younger members of FOBs. Approaches for training work teams to comanage in family firms (Fischetti, 1999), and for understanding the impact of sibling issues (Caroll, 1988), and gender issues (Salganicoff, 1990) have been developed. Approaches have included developmental (Gersick et al., 1997), relational (Flemons & Cole, 1994), and role-clarifying (Freudenberger et al., 1989) ones.

Cross-References to Related Specializations

Niche 1.3. Working with Dying and Grieving People
Niche 2.1. Relationship Enrichment Programs
Niche 3.3. Improving Work Performance
Niche 3.4. Consulting on Workplace Stressors

Subspecializations

- Working with gender issues in FOBs (Salganicoff, 1990).
- Consultation to lawyers and other FOB professionals.

Practice Models

Practice models are quite varied and flexible:

- The traditional approach of having the entire family appear at the clinician's office for a series of sessions is somewhat less often utilized because of the costs and disruption to the business.
- Practitioners may see clients at their place of work; they may even spend time sitting in on business meetings or witnessing business operations. In addition, the family business consultant may interview others in the business, including people outside the family who are key players in the FOB.
- Some consultants schedule family retreats.
- Consultation to lawyers and accountants who deal with FOBs may be quite beneficial to them for understanding stalemated or neglected issues in families.
- Mediation with family members who have been unable to settle their conflicts among themselves can save time, money, and the future of the business itself.
- The "full-service team" or multidisciplinary model is exemplified by the California Family Business Institute, which uses an investment banker, an attorney, a marketing specialist, and a business psychologist to simultaneously evaluate an FOB's current situation and develop a strategy to navigate the succession process ("Multi-Disciplinary Business Team . . . ," 1997).

Financial Considerations

- Consultation to FOBs is a managed-care-free realm of practice, as noted earlier.
- Business owners are accustomed to paying for consultants; they know that consultants have expertise that can save them time, money, and problems. Hourly fees have been reported to be in the $200 to $300 range, but certainly these will depend upon such factors as the skill and reputation of the consultant, as well as the company's resources, perceived need, level of concern, time involvement, and even geography ("Consulting to Family Businesses," 1998).
- Being seen in a company as an expert may lead to referrals to your private therapy practice. According to an article in *Clinical Psychiatry News*, "every expert we talked to stressed the increased flow of patients that will begin to show up once they've seen you around their offices. 'All of my private practice clients are now people I've picked up in my consultative practice,' Dr. Van Lew said" ("Business Tension Can Spur Consultations," 1999, p. 50).

Cautions, Ethical Dilemmas, Culture Clashes, and/or Managed Care Issues

The conflicting interests and multiple stakeholders in FOBs make it essential to communicate clear policies regarding who is your client, what your goals are, and what the nature of your role is (consultant vs. therapist).

Payment arrangements should be spelled out in advance, so that responsibility for your fees is not misperceived. Confidentiality's limits must be clarified with all family members and any other participants. Be sensitive to and examine any conflicts of interest. Also, acknowledge the limits of your knowledge, and do not hesitate to consult with or refer clients to other professionals (e.g., lawyers and accountants).

PROSPECTS AND PROSPECTING

Where Is the Need?

- According to Galagan (1985), more than 90% of American businesses are family-controlled, accounting for approximately 40% of the gross national product—and yet until recently, no field of advisors was dedicated to working with the needs of this group.
- Hilburt-Davis (1997) notes that "For qualified professionals there are many opportunities." A growing sensitivity to the "human side of change" (Kanter, 1985), and a "growing frustration with content experts" (Hilburt-Davis & Senturia, 1995) are among the developments fueling this trend. Family business consultation is an expanding area of opportunity for clinicians, according to Florence Kaslow, herself a family therapist and FOB consultant (Kaslow 1993).
- The unprecedented level of change in FOBs resulting from retirement or transitions will produce considerable turbulence and difficulty for these firms, and our skills can help smooth the transition for many.
- *Practice Strategies* ("Family Therapy Transfers to Corporate Setting," 1999), *Family Therapy Networker* (Sirkin, 1996), *Clinical Psychiatry News* ("Business Tension Can Spur Consultations," 1999), and *Psychotherapy Finances* ("Consulting to Family Businesses," 1998) have all featured FOB consultation as a new area of opportunity for therapists.
- The recent growth in interest in consulting to family firms is demonstrated by the fact that more than 60 universities have developed programs dealing with FOBs (Vinturella et al., 1994). These programs, many in centers for entrepreneurship, focus on enhancing the skills of consultants from a variety of fields such as law, accounting,

and psychology who can deal with the special circumstances of FOBs, including "the human side of change" in them.

Competition

There is likely to be competition with others who work with family firms (Sirkin, 1996) but are not trained in psychological approaches (e.g., accountants, lawyers, and financial planners). Although they may lack the particular skills that we possess, they are the ones to whom business traditionally turn for problem solving. You may find a formal alliance a viable option.

Reaching Clients

Networking with other professionals, such as lawyers and accountants, who can provide referrals or who may seek consultation for help in dealing with their difficult cases is a good place to start. According to Hilburt-Davis (1997, p. 34), "referrals can come from other professionals who have been stumped by the family dynamics. Some referrals come from therapists who cannot deal with the family business issues a client is raising in therapy."

Directions for Marketing

- The major avenues of access to FOBs are local business organizations such as Rotary Clubs and Chambers of Commerce, which are often dominated by family business owners. By joining, you will come to understand the needs of businesses in general for guidance and consultation in behavioral health areas and in work and family issues. Up to half of the topics addressed in their meetings concern family dynamics, work stress, and conflict management. You may begin to feel confident enough to provide some presentations on these topics. Such presentations will both educate and reach potential clients.
- Newsletters sent to lawyers and accountants can be helpful in educating these other professionals about the kinds of interventions and problem solving that can be accomplished by clinicians working with FOBs.
- Business schools' centers for entrepreneurship, and family business centers, often host seminars and functions to discuss business dynamics and healthy work environments. Depending on your location and knowledge, you could attend or present at these meetings. The FFI Web site (again, see "Professional Organizations," below) provides a listing by state of family business education programs, forums, and centers

INCREASING YOUR FORMAL KNOWLEDGE BASE

Core Readings

Bork, D., Jaffe, D. T., Lane, S. H., Dashew, L., & Heisler, Q. G. (1996). *Working with family businesses: A guide for professionals.* San Francisco: Jossey-Bass.
—Written from a family systems perspective it is aimed at all professions who advise family business but has much to offer therapists in providing a basic framework for process consultation.

Buchholz, B., Crane, M., & Nager, R. W. (1999). *The family business answer book.* Paramus, NJ: Prentice-Hall.
—An easy to read introduction to the issues from a business consulting point of view.

Cohn, M. (1992). *Passing the torch: Succession, retirement and estate planning in family-owned businesses.* New York: McGraw-Hill.
—A good orientation to the title's issues with a family-systems orientation.

Fischetti, M. (1999). *Building strong family teams.* Philadelphia: Family Business.
—It covers the issues faced by FOBs, provides strategies for family members working together as teams, and provides specific tools and approaches for working with FOBs.

Gersick, K. E., Davis, J. A., Hampton, M. M., & Lansberg, I. (1997). *Generation to generation: Life cycles of the family business.* Boston: Harvard Business School Press.
—This book presents a developmental model, based on 10 years of research with hundreds of FOBs, for helping family firms work effectively with change

Hilburt-Davis, J., & Dyer, W. G. (2003). *Consulting to family businesses: A practical guide to contracting, assessment, and implementation.* San Francisco: Jossey-Bass.
—Two recognized authorities in the field of FOBs take you step by step through the consultation process.

Ibrahim, A. B., & Ellis, W. H. (1994). *Family business management: Concepts and practice.* Dubuque, IA: Kendall/Hunt.
—A good basic text presenting the major methods and models for making the family business work.

Journals

Family Business Review

Journal of the Family Firm Institute

Family Business (Family Business Publishing Company, P.O. Box 41966, Philadelphia, PA 19101; http://www.familybusinessmagazine.com) provides a window into the current concerns and issues of FOBs. There are forums where individuals discuss problems and seek advice on FOB-related issues. There is a listing of consultants by state, so you might find other professionals in your area with whom to partner or for seeking referrals. You might keep a copy in your waiting room as a marketing opportunity.

In addition, relevant journals include those in the areas of family therapy (e.g., *American Journal of Family Therapy, Journal of Marital and Family Therapy, Family Relations: Interdisciplinary Journal of Applied Family Studies, Family Journal— Counseling and Therapy for Couples and Families*) and journals in business and management psychology.

Online Resources

Family Business NetCenter (http://www.fambiz.com) is an Internet hub catering to owners of family-controlled companies, with perhaps a thousand articles written by professionals in the field of family business consulting.

FAMLYBIZ is an e-mail list for researchers, academics, and professionals providing services to family businesses. Subscribe by sending an e-mail to listproc@ sandiego.edu with this message: "Subscribe famlybiz [your name]."

Professional Organizations

Family Firm Institute (FFI)
12 Harris Street, Brookline, MA 02146; 617-738-1591
e-mail: ffi@internetmci.com.   http://www.ffi.org
    —FFI offers a Directory of Consultants and Speakers, a yearly annotated Family Business Bibliography, the Family Business Case Series, proceedings of its annual conference, and other resources.

Patient Education Materials: Online Resources, Printed Resources, and Organizations

Family Enterprise Publishers
http://www.efamilybusiness.com/fep_home.php
    —Basically an online catalog of books and other materials for "business-owning families and the professionals who serve them."

A series of workbooks for use by FOBs is available from the Austin Family Business Program at Oregon State University (http://www.familybusinessonline.org) and could be helpful for your consulting. These include *Succession Survival Kit* (the financial and emotional aspects of succession planning); *Preparing . . . Just in Case* (preparing—financially, legally, and emotionally—for the death or incapacitation of a family's leader); *Passing on Strategic Smarts* (framework for leadership development within the FOB); and *Financial Smarts* (explanation of the interrelationship between the finances of the business and the family).

Improving Work Performance

OVERVIEW AND OPPORTUNITIES

We clinicians have much to offer to those who experience mild impediments in their daily work functioning, or who would like to function at a higher level, learn new skills, and feel more content and in control of their lives. Improved functionality and satisfaction in the workplace constitute an area where clinicians can make important contributions.

YOUR POTENTIAL SATISFACTIONS

- Working with managers and executives can be pleasant and stimulating.
- Working with complex organizations can be satisfying, in that it provides opportunities to apply your skills to true prevention and early intervention (for mild or developing conditions).
- Consulting gives you a stimulating window into how managers think about their work and challenges.
- Many of the improvements you can help employees make in work performance are win–win–win situations (for the employers, the employees, and you), in that your efforts can reduce stress on workers, improve morale and productivity, and benefit the larger community.

YOUR SKILL SET

Recycling Your Current Competencies

The basic skills for many of these interventions are likely to be in your repertoire already, although you will need to fine-tune the interventions for each particular corporate setting. For those interventions that are not already part of your clinical skills, guidance in the form of workbooks and brief training seminars is often available (see below). You should also be familiar with the culture of business.

Martin (1996) provides a lively and informative account of how she refocused her clinical practice on executive coaching and corporate consultation. She points out that "In providing corporate therapy there are as many approaches as there are to conducting psychotherapy in one's office" (p. 97).

- If your interests and abilities lie in diagnostics, you might focus on helping corporations make personality assessments in executive hiring and promotion decisions.
- If you have experience working with people from other cultures, offering acculturation counseling for newly transferred executives might be of interest to you.
- If you have experience working with women on career advancement or "glass ceiling" issues, you could help companies interested in facilitating retention and advancement for their women employees.
- Group therapy skills may be relevant to work teams. For example, teams may become stale, so interventions aiming to enhance communication and interactions will increase their productivity. Encouraging and rewarding risk taking, enhancing social support, communicating appreciation, and valuing honesty are all tasks with which experienced group therapists are quite comfortable. Other tasks for group therapists might involve helping groups resolve the "culture clash" issues that occur when two businesses merge or a company is reengineered.

Retreading for Added Skills

In addition to the general suggestions for retreading mentioned in the introduction to this section, specific suggestions for each area of practice are provided.

NATURE OF THE WORK

Areas of Practice

Psychologists have developed many ways of consulting with business leaders, but we present information on these three likely areas of practice:

- Coaching executives.
- Consulting with employers on accommodating to psychological disabilities.
- Implementing the drug-free workplace.

Coaching Executives

We use "coaching" here to mean helping an individual client overcome personal limitations or deficits that hamper job performance. The philosophy of coaching focuses on positive qualities as opposed to symptoms; on the future rather than the past; on unrealized potentials rather than deficits; and on such topics as problem solving, decision making, clarifying and achieving goals, finding and utilizing opportunities, and balancing work with home and play. A coach adopts roles described by such terms as "mentor," "consultant," "guide," "sounding board," and also "success partner" (with whom the client can share important news about promotions, breakthroughs, important developments, etc.).

Levinson (1996), a very early practitioner of coaching, distinguishes it from psychotherapy in this way: Coaching is short-term and issue-focused, and includes suggestions, information giving, and other forms of guidance. Another pioneer in this area, Sperry (1993), makes important points that need to be borne in mind when he offers profiles of healthy, distressed, and impaired executives, and distinguishes three types of services: executive consulting, executive counseling, and executive coaching.

A survey conducted by the International Coach Federation (1998) found that clients tended to utilize coaches for a variety of behavioral and psychological issues. These results give a good sense of how coaches present themselves and the kinds of issues they address. Specifically, 85% of respondents said that the main role of their coaches was to be sounding boards—to listen to them and give honest feedback. Seventy-eight percent called their coaches motivators, 56% mentors, 47% business consultants, and 41% teachers. Eighty-one percent of respondents said that they turned to their coaches for help with time management, 74% for career guidance, 74% for business advice, 59% for help with relationship/family issues, 52% for guidance on physical/wellness issues, 45% for assistance with personal issues, 39% for goal setting, 38% for financial guidance, and 11% for improving creativity. Other interesting facts revealed by this survey included that only one-third of coaches had master's degrees or higher, and that half of the respondents confided in their coaches as much as their spouses or therapists; 12% said that they confided in their coaches more than anyone else. The survey reported that 70% of respondents said their investment in their coaches was "very valuable."

Consulting with Employers on Accommodating to Psychological Disabilities

The Americans with Disabilities Act (ADA) of 1990 was designed to protect people with physical and psychiatric disabilities from workplace discrimination. Guidelines to ADA issued by the Equal Employment Opportunity Commission define these disabilities as including mood disorders, attention-deficit/hyperactivity disorder, schizophrenia, mental retardation, and personality disorders. Such accommodations as changes in work hours, leaves of absence for treatment, and appropriate adjustments of job duties for those suffering from these disabilities are considered to be reasonable changes on the part of employers.

According to an article in the *APA Monitor* ("Mental Disabilities No Barrier . . . ," 1998), psychologist and lawyer Peter David Blanck, director of the University of Iowa's Law, Health Policy and Disability Center, describes the cost to employers for such accommodations as minimal. But without an understanding of the particular needs and limitations faced by employees with mental and emotional problems, employers are unable to fashion such accommodations and may have exaggerated estimates of their costs. The same *Monitor* article quotes Yolanda Brooks a psychologist who advises attorneys dealing with work-and-disability cases: " . . . there's a wealth of opportunity when it comes to the ADA." It can range from reviewing individual cases as an objective third party, to helping employers figure out what would be a reasonable accommodation for a worker with a disability."

To work in this area, you must familiarize yourself with the ADA. Bruyere and O'Keeffe (1994) provide a guide to the ways psychologists can help implement the ADA fairly and effectively. Foote (2000), L. L. Hall (1997), and Houlihan and Reynolds (2001) offer additional perspectives, and Stefan (2000) gives a critique of disability law in practice with suggestions for change.

Implementing the Drug-Free Workplace

As a broadly trained mental health professional, you will often be able to tailor and implement comprehensive drug free workplace (DFW) programs, evaluate them, and provide follow-up clinical and consulting services to business and industry. If you are seeking a relatively simple and ethical way to enter the general realm of consulting to businesses, this could be it.

For legal reasons (federal agencies require that workplaces be free of drugs and alcohol) and for the clear health and safety benefits, employers want and need programs to prevent, treat, reduce, and eliminate substance use. The most obvious costs to employers are the financial ones: lessened productivity; increased workplace accidents with injuries and damaged equipment; poor-quality work; absenteeism and tardiness; increased costs of training and turnover; fights and violence; and increased workers' compensation claims (Bass et al., 1996). Studies by Ames et al. (1997) and Mangione et al. (1999) have supported the expected association of substance use with morale problems, problems with supervisors, arguments with coworkers, and similar personal and social losses.

Many companies already have DFW programs in place, but small and new companies will need programs, and both types of businesses can need ongoing and more sophisticated programs. Although you may have to provide some free educational efforts at the beginning, when you have established your credibility and skills, you can charge for consulting hours or DFW program development. Fees can be quite adequate on a flat-fee, hourly, or contract basis. You may also receive referrals for the treatment of individual clients in your private practice. Unless you already have experience with employee assistance programs (EAPs), you should consider working collaboratively with EAP professionals and with specialists, because of the legal complexities of DFW work. (See the "Cautions . . ." section, below.)

Experience in substance abuse work is not essential for providing DFW education or program development, but it is necessary for providing treatment.

- The federal government recognizes psychologists and others as Substance Abuse Professionals. Many employers recognize the Certified Alcoholism Counselor credential, and you might consider taking the coursework for this. Each state has a board that monitors this and the training is provided locally. The training is not extensive but quite a bit of supervision is required.
- If you wish to work with managed care organizations, you might consider earning the APA College of Professional Psychology's Certificate of Proficiency in the Treatment of Alcohol and Other Psychoactive Substance Use Disorders. This certificate requires independent licensure, a year of postlicensure experience in substance abuse treatment, payment of application and examination fees, and passing a multiple-choice item test. The knowledge required is described in the *Candidate's Guide*, available from the College at 202-336-6100 or http://www.apa.org/college/certificate.html.

Cross-References to Related Specializations

Niche 3.1. Treating Public Speaking Anxiety for Work Success
Niche 3.2. Consulting to Family-Owned Businesses
Niche 5.4. Sport Psychology, Exercise, and Fitness
Niche 5.5. Wellness and Positive Psychology

Subspecializations

Coaching Subniches

- Coaching women executives (see, e.g., http://www.womenofwisdom. com).
- Coaching minority executives.

- Coaching in a particular industry.
- See the summer 1999 issue of the *Independent Practitioner* ("Feature Issue on Coaching") for some other creative ideas on coaching subniches.

Diversity and Sensitivity Training

A particularly suitable area for working with businesses might be dealing with diversity, because a consultant psychologist can show the majority members the need for culture change; create a safe environment for learning; and model the skills necessary to lead a diverse, inclusive workforce through change processes (Katz & Miller, 1996). See Niche 5.3 for more details on diversity/sensitivity work in general.

Improving Training

Businesses make huge and continuing investments in training for staff members at all levels, and this training has to be designed, integrated, presented, evaluated, and improved. Psychologists have training in learning, cognition, motivation, measurement, and other relevant skills. There are many local opportunities everywhere and lots of resources, although there are competitors locally and nationally.

Practice Models

Consultation models are common, but it is quite possible to do executive coaching using a private practice model.

Financial Considerations

This is clearly a managed-care-free area. Although some of your clients may merit formal psychiatric diagnoses, you will not be working with them under their health insurance as a consultant.

If you decide to consult with business leaders, you can typically charge your usual fees, with additional charges for travel time or similar costs.

Cautions, Ethical Dilemmas, Culture Clashes, and/or Managed Care Issues

When we examine the roles coaches offer to play in the lives of their clients, it seems to us that boundary issues are likely to need continuous clarification.

[When done as intended,] coaching can be an effective means of improving business results while also contributing to executive development. [However, coaching] can grow beyond the control of top management as the demand grows for having a "personal trainer" coach, many managers are initiating their own ongoing (and expensive) relationships with external coaches as a survival strategy. Not only is this aspect of the practice adding considerably to the cost of doing business, there is also the risk of wrong advice by external coaches who do not really understand the business, sometimes resulting in disastrous consequences for both the manager and organization. (Hall et al., 1999, p. 49)

The workplace has acquired an extensive legal structure, including laws on disability, discrimination, and labor practices, so you should strongly consider partnering with EAP professionals or industrial/organizational psychologists before offering your services. Remember, you don't always know what you don't know.

PROSPECTS AND PROSPECTING

Where Is the Need?

The number of books, periodicals, and newspaper articles concerned with workplace effectiveness issues is testimony to the salience of these issues. Books applying psychological knowledge to such issues have received an enthusiastic reception (e.g., Weisinger & Williams, 1997; Goleman, 1998; Bennis, 1994; Covey, 1990). Tong (1998) observed that 35% of the books on the business best-seller list were about spirituality and psychological security. *Who Moved My Cheese?*, a book about transitions, has been a bestseller since 1998, with over 10 million copies in print.

Corporations are willing to pay for executive coaching because the limitations of executives can have a major impact on the bottom line, according to an *APA Monitor* article ("More Clinical Psychologists Move . . . ," 1998). For example, executive coaching can assure that knowledge acquired in training is converted into applied skills. Olivero et al. (1997) found that training sessions alone led to a 22.4% gain in productivity, whereas adding 8 weeks of coaching (including goal setting, collaborative problem solving, practice, feedback, supervisory involvement, evaluation of end results, and a public presentation) produced an 88% increase in productivity.

Competition

Competition from those without clinical training (persons with MBAs, human resources personnel, EAP professionals, etc.), will be intense. You will need to foster an awareness of the superiority of your knowledge, skills, and interventions (e.g., clinical and other psychological assessment, utilizing group dynamics in communication and conflict resolution, ways of doing outcome measurement and program evaluation, etc.).

There are currently thousands of professional coaches, only a minority of whom have backgrounds in the mental health fields. As a psychologist, you can bring a unique breadth of knowledge and resources to executive coaching.

Reaching Clients/Directions for Marketing

You can reach clients through company insiders and other professionals who advise businesses but are not your competitors, such as attorneys and accountants, and their acquaintances and family members. Your personal circle of friends, family members, and acquaintances probably includes many who could function as contacts for securing an initial interview. Networking through community and business organizations is another productive direction to explore. For marketing to businesses, the following all provide worthwhile perspectives: Heller (1997), Weiss (1992), Perrott (1999), Ackley (1997), Dean (1999), and Martin (1996). See also our introduction to this section for general marketing ideas. Some marketing approaches for specific opportunities are described below.

Coaching

Fox (1999, p. 121) emphasizes the importance of recommendations from people in the same business for executive coaching clients: "One of the things that weighs heavily in the minds of potential new clients is your familiarity with their particular type of business. Like most people in the role of customers, business leaders do not want to put themselves in the hands of an 'expert' who is unfamiliar with their realities."

Though convinced that the topic of executive coaching would be "old news" to the audience, Fox agreed to be interviewed for a story on National Public Radio. "As it turned out," Fox relates, "I could not have been more mistaken." Follow-up stories were featured in major business publications. "I received more calls, letters, faxes and e-mails about that interview than anything I had ever done" (p. 121).

Implementing the DFW

Employers who are interested in DFW programs have joined in local initiatives and coalitions that may provide sample policies, technical assistance, low-cost drug testing services, and ongoing training sessions for supervisors. For help with finding these coalitions look in the phone book for entries like

"Drug-Free Business Initiative" or "Coalition for Drug-Free Workplaces," or call on your local Chamber of Commerce. Other organizations that may know of DFW efforts include your state or county office of alcohol and drug abuse services, as well as your local mayor's office, police department's community relations office, office of economic development, or business relations office. This information will help you decide on the degree of unmet needs in your community, and thus will guide your marketing efforts. Local drug abuse organizations may or may not welcome you.

Go to the businesses in your community. When making these contacts, you can offer this kind of information: Implementing a DFW program is likely to produce reductions in health care and workers' compensation premiums of about 5%, as well as to reduce on-the-job injuries and lessen absences; for every dollar invested in an EAP/DFW program, companies can save between $5 and $16 (American Council for Drug Education, 1999). Even rural employers have a need for these program (Paz, 1998). The National Institute on Drug Abuse (1998) has a document, *The Economic Costs of Alcohol and Drug Abuse in the United States—1992* (see especially Section 1.4, "Impaired Productivity"), which will be helpful to you in developing marketing materials oriented toward business.

INCREASING YOUR FORMAL KNOWLEDGE BASE

Core Readings

Ackley, D. (1997). *Breaking free of managed care: A step-by-step guide to regaining control of your practice.* New York: Guilford Press.
    —This is the original book in this area, written by someone who has shed managed care and established a well-respected business consulting practice. It offers inspiration, experience, and expertise.
Gellerman, S. W. (1998). *How people work: Psychological approaches to management problems.* New York: Quorum Books.
Korman, A. K., & Associates. (1994). *Human dilemmas in work organizations: Strategies for resolution* New York: Guilford Press.
    —This volume offers nine case studies of the clinical problems seen in work settings.
Division of Workplace Programs, Substance Abuse and Mental Health Services Administration, U.S. Department of Health and Human Services. (2001). *Mandatory guidelines for federal workplace drug testing programs* [Online]. Available: http://workplace.samhsa.gov/drugtesting/MGuidelines.htm
Perrott, L. A. (1999). *Reinventing your practice as a business psychologist.* San Francisco: Jossey-Bass
    —The book is not industrial/organizational psychology. Instead, it guides you through the steps of preparation to become a business psychologist: market research, community networking, designing consultative services, creating mar-

keting plans, selling business consultations, and the retraining you will have to do.

Potter, B., & Orfali, S. (1998). *Drug testing at work: A guide for employers and employees.* Berkeley, CA: Ronin.

—It describes how the tests work, what the legal issues, are, and how employees can avoid a false-positive drug test. It shows employers how they can maintain a DFW without violating individual rights. It also describes the dangers employees face in testing; people using over-the-counter medicines, for example, can test falsely positive for narcotics. And tests can reveal personal information, such as health problems and pregnancy. Finally, the book reveals techniques employed by substance-using workers to "beat" the tests.

Sperry, L. (1996). *Corporate therapy and consulting.* New York: Brunner/Mazel.

—Sperry, a psychiatrist, brings highly clinical and dynamic perspectives to his work with corporations.

Journals

Consulting Psychology Journal: Practice and Research
Journal of Business and Psychology
Journal of Applied Psychology

Two special journal issues on coaching are worth mentioning here. *Consulting Psychology Journal* (1996) dedicated an issue to the topic of executive coaching, which provides an excellent opportunity to learn more about this topic. *Independent Practitioner's* summer 1999 "Feature Issue on Coaching" has several articles on coaching. As this is a rapidly developing area, new books are coming out all the time. Search under "executive coaching" at booksellers' Web sites for the latest.

Online Resources

American Council for Drug Education (ACDE)
1-800-883-DRUG
http://www.acde.org

—The ACDE offers training and specialized services, and provides discounted drug testing, along with a wide array of other services. Fees for services and materials are minimal, and in some cases they are free.

Internet Survival Guide of I/O Psychology
http://allserv.rug.ac.be/~flievens/guide.htm

—Links to some useful sites for human resources and industrial/organizational information.

Learnativity
http://www.learnativity.com

—This site provides access to over 40 journals, publications, Web sites, and organizations of interest to training/development and human resources professionals.

Training Magazine
http://www.trainingmag.com/training/index.jsp
—Here you can subscribe to journals, read news related to training, calculate salaries for training, or order books and other tools.

Training and Development Resource Center
http://www.tcm.com/trdev
—Though commercial, a site rich in resources for training and development.

U.S. Department of Labor's Working Partners for an Alcohol- and Drug-Free
  Workplace
http://www.dol.gov/dol/workingpartners.htm
—This is an amazingly large collection of materials and data on the benefits of DFW and costs of substance use. The database of materials (Substance Abuse Information Database) is enormous and rich (assessment, training, laws, surveys, tools, etc.). (Another U.S. Department of Labor site, http://www.dol.gov/dol/asp/public/programs/drugs/steps.htm, fully describes a DFW program's components.)

PROFESSIONAL ORGANIZATIONS

Society of Consulting Psychology. Division 13 of the American Psychological
  Association
750 First Street, NE, Washington, DC 20002-4242; 202-336-6013
e-mail: kcooke@apa.org   http://www.apa.org/divisions/div13
—Membership includes a nationwide information and referral network and the Division's journal. The division also offers training and conferences.

Society for Industrial and Organizational Psychology. Division 14 of the American
  Psychological Association
SIOP Administrative Office, P.O. Box 87, Bowling Green, OH 43402-0087; 419-353-0032
e-mail: LHAKEL@siop.bgsu.edu   http://www.siop.org/.
—The Division offers conferences and tutorials, and publishes *The Industrial/Organizational Psychologist* (back issues are available through the Web site).

International Coach Federation
888-423-3131
e-mail: icfoffice@coachfederation.org   http://www.coachfederation.org

Packaged Programs and/or Franchises

Many coaches offer training in becoming a coach through workshops, tapes, and, no surprise, coaching—usually online or by telephone.

Ben J. Dean, PhD, offers a 6-month seminar on "Saying good-bye to managed care: Complementing your professional practice with personal and professional coaching:

Different arena, same skills." Contact him through his Web site (http://www.mentorcoach.com) or via e-mail (ben@mentorcoach.com), or at Suite 1104, 4400 East–West Highway, Bethesda, MD 20814-4515; voicemail 301-986-5688.

Mel Silberman offers ready-to-use, out-of-the-box programs for use with clients that can be adapted for your needs. Some free materials, and descriptions of his several books, are available at his Web site (http://www.activetraining.com).

Coach University

P. O. Box 881595, Steamboat Springs, CO 80488-1595; 800-482-6224; fax 800-329-5655

e-mail: info@coachu.com   http://www.coachinc.com

—Coach University is a 2-year training program for those wishing to become coaches. It is not restricted to clinicians.

Institute for Life Coach Training (formerly Therapist University)

2801 Wakonda Drive, Fort Collins, CO 80521; 888-267-1206; fax 970-224-9832

e-mail: info@lifecoachtraining.com   http:lifecoachtraining.com

Consulting on Workplace Stressors

OVERVIEW AND OPPORTUNITIES

As noted at the beginning of this section, work is integral in sustaining life and identity. Yet, according to Cryer (1996), life at the workplace is 44% more difficult today than 30 years ago, as measured by the Holmes–Rahe scale (a gauge of the difficulties of adjusting to demands for change).

Recent history has witnessed massive corporate restructurings and lay-offs. According to a Brown University poll (reported in Jones, 1997), 70% of workers said that employee trust was at an all-time low; nearly 60% agreed that workers were not sharing in the success and profits of their companies; and 60% felt that their level of commitment to their jobs had decreased. Research on "survivor sickness" in downsizing organizations (Noer, 1993, 1997), and research on stress and coping with transition at AT&T (Bunker, 1997), demonstrate the pervasively negative effects of change and uncertainty in the workplace. Both the breakneck pace of technological change and the stressful effect of technologies on the structure and meaning of jobs are resulting in more miscommunications and mistakes. Conflicts and frustrations can enrage some, while others may suffer from their coworkers' misdirected and inappropriate anger. Those who experience work impediments because of harassment, abuse, or threats can be at a huge disadvantage—a disadvantage that can translate into missed opportunities, lost income, and low self-esteem.

The workplace has always been threatening, but the kinds of dangers have changed. The risks of accidental injury and death have lessened because of government interventions, legal decisions, and social pressures. However, the change from an industrial to a service-and-knowledge economy, the rise of terrorism, and the intrusion of personal conflicts into the workplace have created new pressures and threats. These changes are of concern to businesses because they create the potential for great financial loss. By working to lessen these risks, psychologists can improve function and satisfaction in the workplace. There are effective methods to help people cope with change: accept the new, find the resources to adapt, grieve for the losses, and help each other to learn and grow. Interventions can be at different levels: small-group efforts, organizational consultation, and work with individuals.

YOUR POTENTIAL SATISFACTIONS

This work involves transferring theoretical understandings and clinical skills from familiar clinical settings to the workplace. But it still deals with the problems of stress and adaptation, coping and burnout, depression and anxiety, fear and courage. These are topics you can get your clinical teeth into.

As in Niche 3.3, many of the improvements you can help make in this area are win–win–win situations (for the employers, the employees, and you), because your activities can reduce stress on workers, improve morale and productivity, and benefit the community at large.

YOUR SKILL SET

Recycling Your Current Competencies

Again as in Niche 3.3, the basic skills for many of these interventions are likely to be in your repertoire already. In this case, they include methods for managing conflict, anger, and grief; facilitating effective interpersonal communication; and learning and teaching problem solving. A wide range of techniques have been employed in dealing with workplace stressors, such as stress inoculation training, cognitive reframing, imaginal rehearsal, and assertiveness training.

Retreading for Additional Skills

In addition to the suggestions made in the introduction to this section, we make specific recommendations, when applicable, within each practice area below.

NATURE OF THE WORK

"Humanizing the workplace"—long the battle cry of such pioneers as Robert Allen (Allen & Pilnick, 1973) and Robert Levering (founder of The Great Places to Work Institute, and coauthor of *The 100 Best Companies to Work for in America*—(Levering & Moskowitz, 1994)—has become an achievable goal because studies have shown that while it is the "right" thing to do, it is also good for the "bottom line" (profits) (Levering & Moskowitz, 1994).

Areas of Practice

As in other niches in this section, you will need to remain mindful of the boundaries of your own knowledge and skills versus those of other professionals. For this niche we have identified three areas of practice that seem to draw uniquely upon clinical psychological skills in general and the skill set described in this section's introduction in particular:

- Coping with workplace changes and job stress.
- Coping with job loss and job finding.
- Creating a safe workplace.

Coping with Workplace Changes and Job Stress

Faced with the negative human consequences of corporate changes for employees, corporations have tried to develop strategies to reengage them and help them deal more effectively with these changes. One such intervention (Bunker, 1997) is a 5-day group format, The Leading Transitions Course, which targets senior executives who are experiencing the stresses of corporate restructuring. The program taps core clinical skills, such as grief work; helping clients tolerate vulnerability, develop authenticity, and process anger; and supporting reengagement. Noer (1993) provides another example of a four-level intervention treating highly stressed survivors of corporate downsizing; it includes helping clients recognize and work through their emotions, as well as reengagement. Maccoby (1995) demonstrates how psychology and psychoanalysis can be translated into a business vernacular. This can be useful in helping managers and workers understand how values affect work motivation, and how people differ with regard to the variety of intrinsic and extrinsic factors that motivate them to work.

Another aspect of this work is reducing resistance to workplace change. Corporations often invest tremendous amounts in technological improvements, only to hit the wall of human resistance to adopting the change. Many efforts at corporate change fail to address the "fundamentally psychosocial process" of human adjustment to change. As Diamond (1996) notes, "The successful adoption of innovations and technology transfer depends on the individual's openness to learning and change, and that openness requires minimal defensiveness and adequate self-competence" (p. 222). Clinicians can help corporate change agents understand these processes, and can then guide more sensitive efforts to design and implement changes.

High levels of stress are reported by American workers (Rigaud & Flynn, 1995). Stress management in the workplace is yet another vehicle for dealing with untoward workplace demands. Pelletier (1977) offers many useful suggestions that can help you fashion stress interventions for the workplace. HeartMath LLC (see "Online Resources," below) provides a brief stress management intervention that is particularly valuable because it can be applied "on the fly" in work settings, thereby preventing stress from accumulating and causing deteriorating work performance.

Coping with Job Loss and Job Finding

Recent economic downturns in the United States have led to unemployment for new groups, such as experienced white-collar professionals who have never had to look for a job (or at least not recently). They don't know how to do it or where to turn. You may want to offer your services to assist them.

For those whose positions have not survived downsizing, Nathan Azrin's "job club," has demonstrated striking effectiveness. It has been well researched and is highly effective in increasing employment, reducing depression, improving emotional and social role functioning, and creating an enhanced sense of mastery and inoculation against setbacks. It is a program of five 4-hour meetings of 15–20 unemployed people designed to teach job search skills. It is well described by Curran (1992), Price and Vinokur (1995), and Caplan et al. (1997). See also Joseph and Greenberg (2001), who demonstrated the efficacy (relative to a placebo) of a career transition program in increasing reemployment.

For 12 years, I (ELZ) presented a 2-hour workshop entitled "Overcoming Rejection in Job Searching" at a local job-finding club organized by a group of churches. Since the club already addressed job-finding skills, I focused on coping with the emotional aspects of job loss and job searching. I tried to inculcate rational beliefs, such as "You can only be refused by someone; rejection is self-created," and " 'No' means only 'Not presently interested in what I believe you are offering.' "

Retirement counseling is another area that has been created by corporate mergers, acquisitions, and general reengineering. Geriatric experience is valuable here.

Creating a Safe Workplace

Business owners have a legal obligation to provide a safe workplace for employees and others at the worksite. Many are turning to firms utilizing psychological principles to teach a package of skills related to safety; such skills can include identification of troubled employees, conflict resolution, anger management, criticism training, and critical-incident stress debriefing. Mossman (1995) suggests that "failure to use mental health professionals appropriately, to recognize the need for clinicians' input, to respond to behavioral changes that signal a potential for violence, or to implement antiviolence policies might form grounds for a suit against the employer of a violent worker."

We focus here on anger management. Multicomponent approaches to anger management may include relaxation training, self-talk, and stress inoculation training. Here are some examples:

- Ray Novaco (1977, 1980) demonstrated a psychologically sophisticated approach to anger in the workplace with his pioneering application of the stress inoculation approach with police offers, who have to maintain self-control in the face of high levels of provocation.
- The Institute for Management Studies (see "Online Resources," below) offers coursework in anger management solutions for business throughout the United States.
- Steven Stosny's Compassion Power programs (again, see "Online Resources," below) include anger workshops for business groups, individual treatment for court-referred clients, treatment for road rage, workshops for partner and child abuse, and groups for compassionate parenting and compassionate divorce.

Cross-References to Related Specializations

Niche 3.2. Consulting to Family-Owned Buinesses
Niche 3.3. Improving Work Performance
Niche 5.4. Sport Psychology, Exercise, and Fitness
Niche 5.5. Wellness and Positive Psychology

Practice Models

Although there are opportunities for solo consultation practice, combining your skills and knowledge with those of other professionals would enable you to offer a larger variety of services and benefit from the knowledge and expertise of others.

Financial Considerations

When you decide to consult with businesses on workplace stressors (or to work with businesses in other ways), you will have to reconsider how your expenses are to be integrated into your fees. You must take into consideration the substantial expenses of marketing, time devoted to networking and required travel, your needs for office staff, and time for writing reports and proposals. Other likely costs are upgrading office and communication equipment and services, costs for a business wardrobe, and the maintenance of a business vehicle. See the introduction to this section; for more in-depth treatments of this topic, see Ackley (1997) and Perrott (1999).

Cautions, Ethical Dilemmas, Culture Clashes, and/or Managed Care Issues

As companies come to know and trust in your skills, it is likely that they will ask you to do more and more for them. Learn to say, "I don't know," and to recognize when to refer clients to a content expert when asked for help with problems outside your areas of competence. As with all of the niches described in this book, obtain appropriate training and supervision before venturing into new areas. And consider partnering with someone who is experienced and trained in these new areas and combine your competencies.

PROSPECTS AND PROSPECTING

Where Is the Need?

- As mentioned in this section's introduction, studies have revealed the huge hidden cost of workplace conflicts and stress (International Labor Organization, 2000). Clearly, worker dissatisfaction and burnout have a negative impact on the bottom line.
- The best-selling management books acknowledge the importance of psychological factors as a component of corporate success or failure. Many of the popular speakers at management conferences espouse this, and some are even psychologists by training.
- On a visit to *Career* magazine's Web site (http://www.careermag.com), we found that more than half the articles were directly related to psychological impediments to work. Prominent among these were workpace frustrations, conflict, and other difficulties; workplace relationships and emotions; emotions associated with change; and general workplace well-being and/or satisfaction issues.

Competition

As noted in Niche 3.3., competition from those without clinical training or with less clinical training will be intense. Again, you will need to foster an awareness of the superiority of what you have to offer.

Reaching Clients/Directions for Marketing

Many of the approaches described in the introduction to this section are appropriate for reaching clients interested in these services. Offering entry-level services, such as an anger management workshop, for a reasonable fee provides a low-risk way for a company to sample your expertise. You should aim at developing several of the services mentioned above or in the other niches in this section, so that once you have an established relationship with a business, you will be able to build on that to meet their other needs.

INCREASING YOUR FORMAL KNOWLEDGE BASE

Core Readings

Davis, M., Eshelman, E. R., & McKay, M. (1995). *The relaxation and stress reduction workbook* (4th ed.). Oakland, CA: New Harbinger.
  —This book is extraordinarily popular, because it gives step-by-step directions for exercises and methods. It covers breathing, meditation, autogenics, visualization, cognitive methods, hypnosis, biofeedback, exercise, nutrition, and so on. A *Leader's Guide* is also available.
Keita, G. P., & Hurrel, J. L., Jr. (Eds.). (1994). *Job stress in a changing workplace: Investigating gender, diversity, and family issues.* Washington, DC: American Psychological Association.
Murphy, L. R., Hurrel, J. L., Jr., Sauter, S. L., & Keita, G. P. (Eds.). (1995). *Job stress interventions.* Washington, DC: American Psychological Association.
  —A very wide-ranging collection of articles.
Noer, D. M. (1993). *Healing the wounds.* San Francisco: Jossey-Bass.
Noer, D. M. (1997). *Breaking free.* San Francisco: Jossey-Bass.
Quick, J. C., Quick, J. D., Nelson, D. L., & Hurrell, J. J., Jr. (1997). *Preventative stress management in organizations.* Washington, DC: American Psychological Association.
  —A very comprehensive overview of stress in the workplace context.
Sauter, S. L., & Murphy, L. R. (1995). *Organizational risk factors for job stress.* Washington, DC: American Psychological Association.
Schwartz, M. K., & Gimbel, K. G. (2000). *Leadership resources: A guide to training and development tools* (8th ed.). Greensboro, NC: Center for Creative Leadership.

Journals

Journal of Occupational Health Psychology
Consulting Psychology Journal: Practice and Research
Journal of Business and Psychology

Online Resources

Society for Human Resource Management
http://www.shrm.org
—A resource-rich site for human resource professionals, with online publications and much other information available to nonmembers.

Center for the Study of Work Teams
http://www.workteams.unt.edu
—This site contains an annotated bibliography of books about work teams, 8 years of conference proceedings (including comprehensive abstracts of the presentations), research, and products.

Occupational Health Psychology
http://www.cdc.gov/niosh/ohp.html
—Over the last 30 years, the National Institute of Occupational Safety and Health and the APA have supported postgraduate training and conferences in the field of occupational health psychology.

HeartMath LLC
800-450-9111
http://www.heartmath.com
—Bruce Cryer, HeartMath's president and CEO, offers a Stress management program called "Inner Quality Management" that has been taught to many large companies.

Professional Organizations

See Niche 3.3 for information on Division 13 and 14 of APA.

Section 4

Forensics

Introduction, Overview, and Commonalities

Increasingly, psychologists have become involved in all aspects of the legal system—as assessors of both perpetrators and victims; as providers of treatments; and as consultants to attorneys, police, courts, and correctional facilities.

Trent (1998) notes that "clinical psychologists are turning to forensic psychology in search of a refuge from managed care," but he then emphasizes that clinicians "need *formal* training, which for many must include graduate study, an internship or other postdoctoral training while a few very well prepared clinicians can be successful with only [continuing education] experiences" (p. 8). We agree: Becoming expert in all aspects of the overlap between psychology and the law is Herculean. We believe that working in almost any part of the legal system requires specialized knowledge, sophisticated judgment, and significant educational efforts. Even in civil (noncriminal) cases, some practice areas are too complex (forensic neuropsychology, sexual harassment) or professionally hazardous (custody evaluations; see more below) for us to recommend them as practice specializations. Similarly, unless your expertise is especially well developed and you can perform in court, being an expert witness is hazardous, and we do not cover it here.

Of course, courts may refer clients for evaluation or treatment for all kinds of disorders. Examples include substance abuse treatment for clients convicted of driving under the influence; family therapy for adjudicated juvenile delinquents and for juveniles at risk; predivorce counseling or mediation in contested divorce cases; and many others. In particular child custody conflicts always lead to evaluations. However, in any custody decision, it is very likely that one party will be made very unhappy. As a result, psychologists doing this work frequently experience licensing board complaints and malpractice (professional liability) suits. If you can withstand the

211

hostility and abuse and still do a proper job, by all means explore this specialization, as it is needed by the courts and society.

In this section, we discuss two forensic niches in which we believe the modal practitioner (for whom this book is designed) can perform competently without significant additional training. These two areas of treatment are not commonly considered by psychologists, but each has its own satisfactions.

- Treating those convicted of shoplifting. Although this is considered a minor crime, it is often associated with antisocial patterns, dementia, kleptomania, or substance abuse.
- Providing assessment and treatment services in jails and prisons. Careful assessments can match inmates' psychological needs with the treatments available, and can support better probation and parole decisions. Psychologists can also develop and staff treatment programs.

Treating Shoplifting

OVERVIEW AND OPPORTUNITIES

We know what you may be thinking: "Shoplifting? Are you kidding? Shoplifting isn't a big deal. Just peer-pressured kids on a lark, or poverty-stricken folks. Situational behavior. Not worth psychotherapy."

Well, many kids do shoplift. But without the treatments we have available (and for which payment is available), many adolescent perpetrators will go on to more illegal activities and dysfunctional lives. The "THEFT TALK" Counseling Service Inc. Web site (see "Online Resources," below) reports that 50% will reoffend within 1 year. There are also substantial numbers of impoverished or cognitively impaired persons who shoplift food. Sorting them out of the criminal justice system would be good for everyone. And then there are those who qualify for a formal diagnosis of kleptomania; they often ruin their own and their families' lives with "unnecessary" stealing. Also, more than half of the merchandise that disappears from stores is systematically stolen by employees, and so businesses are very interested in reducing these losses. The costs to our communities are actually quite significant in both dollars and suffering, and the number of potential clients is quite large.

In a strict sense, stealing by customers is called "shoplifting"; stealing by employees is called "inventory shrinkage"; and both are crimes called "retail theft," a kind of larceny. (However, we continue to use "shoplifting" as a general term throughout, since it is the most familiar.) Common punishments are fines and, depending on previous convictions and the value of the items stolen, jail time. Law-abiding adults are likely to underestimate the commonality of shoplifting. People of all ages shoplift, including females in their 40s, teens, and a significant number of elderly individuals, whose stealing may be due to dementia or other psychiatric disorder than to economic hardship (Moak et al., 1988). Shoplifting is a behavior, whereas kleptomania is a psychiatric diagnosis whose full criteria only a few persons will meet. Although symptoms of thrill and impulsivity are often present, and dissociative-like experiences are sometimes present (Sarasalo et al., 1997), these are secondary and reactive for most. Identifying compulsion-disordered individuals with kleptomania, and treating this "addiction," are complex clinical tasks.

For many, shoplifting is an impulsive act committed during a period of great stress that involves identifiable losses and resulting depression (Cupchik & Atcheson, 1983). First-time offenders are the focus of diversion programs, while repeat offenders are treated with court punishments. Treatment programs that divert those convicted of shoplifting from the criminal justice system have been notably effective; Royse and Buck (1991) report reducing the rate of recidivism to one-sixth of that of their untreated peers. Although common, fines have had little effect in reducing recidivism (Sarasalo et al., 1997).

YOUR POTENTIAL SATISFACTIONS

- Treatment for shoplifting can change a client's life course to happier outcomes.
- Treatment is straightforward, is effective, and well justifies the costs.
- Significant numbers of clients exist in every locale.
- The skills needed are fairly common among clinicians or easy to master, and the literature to read is small.
- Treatment in groups is efficient, and you could provide supervision or consultation for such ongoing groups.
- Programs can be established that can run over periods of many years.
- Payment for services can be certain, easy to arrange, and repeated on a contractual basis.
- If you are intellectually curious, shoplifting is actually a complex set of behaviors, affects, cognitions, and social forces. It is isolatable and well defined, yet intricate and well worth exploring.
- This is a managed-care-free area.
- This can provide an excellent entry into consulting to local businesses, lawyers, and police departments.

YOUR SKILL SET

Recycling Your Current Competencies

- Skills at running psychoeducational groups, which constitute the most common approach, are valuable.
- Many treatment approaches have been used effectively (see Cup-

chik, 1997, for a review), so you may not need to acquire completely new skills.
- Consultation and program development skills would be useful in setting up a program.

Retreading for Added Skills

Familiarity with your local laws and court system procedures is essential, as is strict adherence to them. Your clients are likely to offer inaccurate, self-serving information about themselves or their crimes, which you must be able to check.

NATURE OF THE WORK

Assessment

If you operate a diversion program as an alternative to trial and punishments, you will need to do some psychological assessment. As noted above, people of all ages, diagnoses, and motivations are caught shoplifting. For example, shoplifting can be a way to feed a drug habit; part of a pattern of full-fledged kleptomania; a way to acquire items one wants but can't afford; a response to peer pressure to demonstrate one's courage; or a means of fulfilling many other needs.

In efforts to understand people who shoplift, psychological testing has had mixed results. Beck and McIntyre (1977) found much pathology and Moore (1983) found little, although both studies used the Minnesota Multiphasic Personality Inventory (MMPI) with college students. Bradford and Balmaceda (1983) found that people convicted of shoplifting closely resembled psychiatric outpatients. Taking a different approach, Schwartz and Wood (1991, p. 234) identified "five specific motivational factors: entitlement, addiction, peer pressure, stress, and impulsiveness" and offered ways to assess each.

Treatment

Group treatment is the method of choice, as it is efficient, addresses the social pressure issues, can best overcome denial and minimization, and can be run by people you supervise as well as by yourself. Once implemented, a treatment program can employ you and function for many years.

One effective and fairly typical group treatment approach (MacDevitt & Kedzierzawski, 1990) consists of six therapist-led meetings in which the context of the offense is examined. The stressors, rationalizations, and consequences are explored via group dynamics. In another program, rational–emotive interventions aimed at changing the irrational beliefs have been effective in an 8-hour group format (Solomon & Ray, 1984). Another example, Shoplifters Alternatives (Alabama Associated Resources Corporation, n.d.) is an educational program offered in three Alabama counties that includes versions for youth and adults. The program consists of a 6-hour home study course done through a packet given at the time of referral that consists of audiotapes, a workbook, and a test with instructions. Upon completion of the home study course, the student attends an 8-hour class/workshop. Cost is $75 per student.

In individual treatment, positive reinforcement for engaging in alternative behaviors (Kurlychek & Morganstern, 1978) and covert sensitization (Gauthier & Pellerin, 1982; Glover, 1985) have been found effective.

There are also some successful community interventions (rewarding employees and customers for reporting shoplifters, compelling public returning of stolen merchandise, etc.; Cupchik, 1997), and extensions of these interventions can be easily developed.

Cross-Reference to Related Specialization

Niche 3.3. Improving Work Performance

Financial Considerations

Local merchants and their organizations will sometimes pay for treatment of customers caught shoplifting. This is usually not the case for employees caught stealing, who are simply fired; however, those fired for stealing might be interested in private therapy.

PROSPECTS AND PROSPECTING

Where Is the Need?

Shoplifting is a very common problem, and many communities do not have effective ways of dealing with it. Police and courts see it as a minor crime and treat it lightly. Merchants simply raise their prices to cover its costs. Given this environment, few providers are offering treatment, yet available treatments are effective. Investigate your local situation to determine what is available, and consider setting up this kind of program with the court system. Educating police, courts, and merchants about the availability of effective treatments could greatly increase demand.

Competition

Your community may already have a diversion program, because there are few limits on who can perform this kind of treatment. If so, you may be able to receive referrals for those who have not benefited from a more generic treatment. These people would be self- or insurance-paid clients.

Reaching Clients

Self-referral is a possibility, because many people shoplift and do not get caught or prosecuted. Adults who qualify for a diagnosis of kleptomania may seek individual treatment if you are known to provide it.

Directions for Marketing

- Because so many shoplifting cases are processed by courts, they will usually be grateful for your interest in treating shoplifters and diverting them out of the courts. Make contact with court officials and discuss their present referral resources, if any.
- Contact your local business organizations to see whether a program sponsored by merchants might be organized in your community.
- Lawyers may be eager to refer clients arrested for shoplifting.
- Contact local schools and offer to do a prevention program for them. One such program (McNees et al., 1980) reduced losses by 54%.

INCREASING YOUR FORMAL KNOWLEDGE BASE

Core Readings

Cupchik, W. (1997). *Why honest people shoplift or commit other acts of theft: Assessment and treatment of 'atypical theft offenders.'* Toronto: Tagami Communications.
   —According to Cupchik, " 'atypical theft offenders' are generally honest and ethical persons who should—and do—know better, yet who risk their personal and professional reputations, and very possibly their working and/or family lives, for what is often (though not always) very little material gain, through stealing" (Cupchik, n.d.). This is the bible of shoplifting treatment. It speaks to clinicians, lawyers, the police, merchants making efforts at loss prevention, and human resources personnel. It offers clinicians many approaches for different orientations, and many assessment and treatment techniques.

Murphy, D. J. (1986). *Customers and thieves: An ethnography of shoplifting.* Aldershot, England: Ashgate.
   —This book provides a sociological insiders' view.

Online Resources

Why Do Shoplifters Steal . . . and Why Do So Many Continue to Steal Even After Getting Caught?
http://www.mindspring.com/~stancom/shop.html

—Written by Peter Berlin to sell protection services to businesses, this article is a complete, yet brief, overview of the psychological and social dynamics and treatment of shoplifting.

"THEFT TALK" Counseling Service Inc.
3530 S. E. 52nd, Portland, OR 97206; 503-771-2542, 800-888-4338
e-mail: mail@thefttalk.com   http://www.thefttalk.com
—Certified "THEFT TALK" counselor training is available. The Web site offers several useful articles, and the links are very educational.

Patient Education Materials: Online Resources, Printed Resources, and Organizations

CASA (Cleptomaniacs And Shoplifters Anonymous)
http://www.shopliftersanonymous.com
—A self-help group with fact sheets, links, and book reviews.

For Businesspersons

Caime, G., & Ghone, G. (1996). S(h)elf help guide: The smart lifter's handbook. Toronto: Trix.
—This book presents shoplifting techniques from a perpetrator's point of view. If you want to learn how people shoplift, here it is. It is obviously also useful to security and loss-control staff.

Farrell, K. L., & Ferrara, J. A. (1985). Shoplifting: The antishoplifting guidebook. New York: Praeger.
—Written by a clinical psychologist and a retired police captain, this book offers retailers antitheft techniques based on psychological research and expertise.

Working in Correctional Facilities

OVERVIEW AND OPPORTUNITIES

First, some clarification of terminology is in order. By "correctional facilities," we mean local jails, state prisons, and federal prisons, at all levels of security. (In general, jails hold those not yet tried or convicted, as well as those serving sentences of less than a year.) We do not mean law enforcement (police forces of all kinds, U.S. marshals' staffs, or sheriffs' departments) or the justice system (courts or prosecutors' offices).

Correctional facilities have been called the "new mental hospitals" because of the high rates of psychopathology among incarcerated populations. Clearly, the jails and prisons have high levels of needs and are expanding in number and staffing (Maurer, 1997). The work involves conducting individual assessments, providing group (Morgan et al., 1999) and individual therapy, evaluating programs, and consulting with and training coworkers.

Imprisonment does not reduce recidivism, and it does not deter criminals who are at high risk of reoffending. Indeed, longer sentences slightly increase reoffending (Gendreau et al., 1999). However, psychologists can improve correctional systems in several ways:

- Improving the match of criminals' characteristics with the treatment options (i.e., making the treatment fit the criminal rather than the crime) in each case.
- Developing and implementing psychological treatments for the large number of mentally ill people in prisons and jails.
- Developing programs outside prisons and jails that can be truly rehabilitative.

- Supporting better treatment, probation, and parole decisions (Gendreau et al., 1996).
- Training staff members in interpersonal skills, and so reducing violence and damage.

This is not happy work, but it is complex and challenging, and it can be beneficial. If you find yourself unable or unwilling to deal with psychic pain, evil, stupidity, injustice, and almost unalterable organizational rules, this niche is not for you. If you can maintain professional distance and offer professional caring; if you enjoy struggling with difficult problems, and addressing goals limited by history and the context; and if you want a comfortable, predictable, often rural work setting, you may be right for this work.

YOUR POTENTIAL SATISFACTIONS

- For those who are interested in the challenges and dynamics of individuals with schizophrenia or other serious and persistent mental illness, there are many opportunities to work with those in correctional facilities. Long-term treatment is not only available but likely.
- Jobs are available across the United States, many in pleasant rural areas.
- Jobs are in the civil service or with private contractors; are secure and clearly defined; offer excellent benefits; and pay rather well.
- The work is managed-care-free, with no marketing needed.
- Contrary to myths, working in correctional facilities is as safe as or safer than working in most other settings.
- It is possible to enter this work after one's internship and receive supervision for licensure while making a decent living.

YOUR SKILL SET

Recycling Your Current Competencies

- State licensure is usually not required for entering civil service positions, but it is required for working for the private agencies contracting with prisons to provide psychological services.
- No additional specialized training or credentials are required for being hired.
- Skills in assessment are essential.
- Gender is not an issue for hiring.
- Your age may be an obstacle for being hired in all federal and some state positions, but not for jobs with the private organizations that provide psychological services or in administration and training

functions outside the prison. The federal system allows hiring only before age 40, but the rules are complex so, if this applies to you, inquire when you apply.

NATURE OF THE WORK

Areas of Practice

From the U.S. Bureau of Prisons (2003) comes this description of the work:

> Clinical Psychologists work closely with inmates in federal prisons. They participate as members of an interdisciplinary healthcare team, administer a wide variety of psychological assessment techniques, interpret results, and prepare comprehensive reports.

They are also involved in the development and organization of individual and group therapy and other rehabilitative programs for the treatment of prisoners with many kinds of problems. The literature on all these topics is fairly extensive, and the issues are complex. Megargee (1995), perhaps the best-informed psychologist writing on assessment issues in this area, has noted that individual assessments are essential to allocate scarce service resources most wisely, to be most helpful to inmates, and to protect inmates and staff. His overview article describes the need for research in this area and indicates some of the challenges. The *Diagnostic and Statistical Manual of Mental Disorders* is of little assistance, because it offers just a few personality diagnoses. Evaluators are asked to predict violence and recidivism (using risk factor and statistical approaches); to deal with forensic issues, such as working with those adjudicated "not guilty by reason of insanity"; and to treat those with all kinds of mental illnesses.

Psychologists can also assist with personnel selection and training; instruments have been developed for these tasks. The Correctional Officer Screening Inventory is available from the International Mental Health Network (contact Robert Christopher, PhD, at 619-486-9745). Dr. Robin Ford of the Maricopa County Sheriff's Office in Arizona has developed a corrections screening tool using the Sixteen Personality Factor Questionnaire, and the Behavioral Personal Assessment Device (B-PAD), a video-based test of interpersonal competency and judgment (800-424-2723 or http://www.bpad.com). The Inwald Personality Inventory, the MMPI, and the MMPI-2 are all in wide use. Counseling of staff and their families during and after prison/jail disturbances may be yet another area of professional work (Hawk, 1997).

Hawk (1997) describes her experience as a psychologist working at the U.S. Bureau of Prisons, which ultimately led to her becoming its director:

> Nothing could have prepared me for [the director's] position more effectively than my training as a psychologist. Unfortunately, even though not many fields could be as demanding and as rewarding for psychologists as corrections, few psychologists ever consider a career in prison work. (p. 335)

Subspecializations

There are also opportunities for developing mental health courts, which aim to get nonviolent mentally ill defendants into treatment instead of jail. Most communities do not yet have such services, but funding has become available under the America's Law Enforcement and Mental Health Project Act of 2000. Grant funding is also available to train and support law enforcement professionals.

Practice Models

Although there may be some consulting work, almost all of these jobs are either in the civil service or with contractor organizations providing services to prison populations, as noted above.

Most jobs are "inpatient," but more are opening in such settings as detention centers, probation/parole agencies, and community corrections/halfway houses.

Many psychologists find that they can develop an outside part-time practice with a corrections job as a basis.

Financial Considerations

Many openings exist in federal and state prisons, and starting salaries are in the $42–$60,000-per-year range with excellent benefits packages. Salaries differ by grade (psychologists are GS-11/12/13) and location as well, and generally top out around $87,000. As of August 2000, a national private organization that provides psychological services was seeking lead psychologists at $70–$75,000 per year and staff psychologists at $63–$67,000 per year with a benefits package. (These figures are from a mailing from the Center for Family Guidance in Northfield, NJ.)

Cautions, Ethical Dilemmas, Culture Clashes, and/or Managed Care Issues

Working in correctional facilities presents unique ethical challenges and conflicts for psychologists. In an overview article, Weinberger and Sreenivasan (1994) discuss the issues, offer case vignettes, and examine existing guidelines.

PROSPECTS AND PROSPECTING

Where Is the Need?

Crime and imprisonment are growth industries in America. We imprison a larger percentage of our citizens than any industrialized country except Russia (Maurer, 1997). Hawk (1997) states that "Psychologists . . . are in high demand in the country's prison system, and there is enormous potential for them to exercise considerable influence over the development of corrections policies" (p. 335).

There are hundreds of job openings across the country. This situation is due to (1) the fact that many jails and prisons are in either inner cities or very rural areas; (2) widespread public pessimism about our ability to change the life trajectories of criminals; (3) perceptions that such work is dangerous and frustrating; and (4) the low status of the work setting. In fact, salaries, opportunities for training and advancement, and job security and benefits are all quite good.

Jobs with federal prisons usually pay better and are in more pleasant situations than work in state prisons or local jails. Federal openings are posted on the Internet (see "Online Resources," below, for the two major federal Web sites), and state and local positions are obtainable from the respective personnel offices.

Competition

There is little or no competition from nonpsychologists.

Reaching Clients

Since correctional psychologists work in organizations, you need only find potential employers, and job openings can be located as described above.

Directions for Marketing

One of the main advantages of this specialization is that, beyond the job interview and resumé, there is no marketing to be done.

INCREASING YOUR FORMAL KNOWLEDGE BASE

Core Readings

Ashford, J. B., Sales, B. D., & Reid, W. H. (Eds.). (2001). *Treating adult and juvenile offenders with special needs*. Washington, DC: American Psychological Association.

—Chapters address all kinds of offenders with all kinds of crimes, diagnoses, and needs.

Landsberg, G., Rock, M., & Berg, L. K. (Eds.). (2002). *Serving mentally ill offenders: Challenges and opportunities for mental health professionals*. New York: Springer.

—This book describes many programs and thus provides good background knowledge.

Quinsey, V. L., Harris, G. T., Rice, M. E., & Cormier, C. A. (1998). *Violent offenders: Appraising and managing risk*. Washington, DC: American Psychological Association.

—This is the ideal book if you will work with violent offenders and you accept the actuarial judgment model. Based on 25 years of data from a maximum-security psychiatric hospital, the authors developed ways to collect and integrate objective data for the prediction of recidivism—ways that can balance the individual's rights with society's needs for protection. This is an example of the best of science in the best interests of all concerned.

Toch, H., & Adams, K. (1994). *The disturbed violent offender* (rev. ed.). Washington, DC: American Psychological Association.

—These authors used a sample of 1 year's new prisoners in New York State who were violent and mentally ill, and did a cluster analysis of their psychological problems and patterns of behavior and criminal offense. The resulting typologies are employed to examine and recommend polices, practices, and prediction. Toch's previous books are also of value.

Wettstein, R. M. (Ed.). (1998). *Treatment of offenders with mental disorders*. New York: Guilford Press.

—This volume provides an excellent overview of settings, problems, and interventions. It reviews administrative and legal issues and addresses therapeutic work with inpatients, outpatients, and incarcerated persons. Chapters cover issues in treatment of sexual offenders, offenders with mental retardation, and juvenile offenders. The methods are interdisciplinary and eclectic, incorporating biological and psychological perspectives.

Journals

Journal of Research in Crime and Delinquency
Journal of Criminal Justice
Psychology, Public Policy, and Law
Law and Human Behavior (for contents, see http://www.unl.edu/ap-ls/ LHBXYear.htm)
Psychology, Crime and Law

Online Resources

U.S. Department of Justice
http://www.jobsearch.usajobs.opm.gov/a9dj.asp

—A list of job openings with the Department of Justice (completely searchable by pay range, location, etc.).

U.S. Bureau of Prisons
http://www.bop.gov
—Go to "Employment" for everything you need to know and do to find a job in a federal prison as a clinical or counseling psychologist, drug treatment specialist, or teacher.

Criminal Justice MegaLinks
http://faculty.ncwc.edu/toconnor
—Links to "Corrections" are down the page.

Professional Organizations

American Correctional Association
4380 Forbes Boulevard, Lanham, MD 20706-4322; 800-222-5646
http://www.corrections.com/aca
—Members number about 20,000 professionals in all kinds of correctional facilities, including federal, state, and military prisons. Members also include representatives of the criminal justice system.

Section 5

Underserved Populations and Developing Needs

Introduction, Overview, and Commonalities

HOW TO IDENTIFY AND MINE NICHES ON YOUR OWN

We were able to define the niches in this section (and some of the preceding ones) by using three classic ways of "building out" one's psychological practice. In this introduction, we describe and flesh out these approaches. Then, in the rest of the section, we show what we found when we applied them. You can identify promising practice specializations on your own by using these three approaches:

1. *Find barriers to treatment and remove them.* Seek out barriers to treatment created by logistics (e.g., distances in rural areas), by physical factors (e.g., disabilities), or by cultural factors (e.g., the unique problems of ethnic minorities and homosexuals in mainstream U.S. culture). Then design your services to remove those barriers and meet clients' needs.
2. *Extend what you know to enhance other human activities.* Apply your psychological skills to optimize some aspect of human functioning—for instance, to improve sports performance, to increase health and wellness, or to enhance interdependent relationships (even the human–animal bond, which can be worked with in its own right or used to improve functioning in other ways).
3. *See trends as your friends.* Changes in society are also opportunities. Look for trends such as rapidly increasing knowledge, continually adapting economics, and continually changing power distributions. Then consider how the changes create additional applications for your knowledge, skills, and abilities.

Now we take a more detailed look at each of these approaches.

FINDING BARRIERS TO TREATMENT AND REMOVING THEM

Sizeable numbers of potential clients have been kept from treatment by various barriers. Removing those barriers creates opportunities to expand your work to those who are not seen in traditional clinical practice. The groups that presently underutilize clinical services, or those that have been dissatisfied with traditional services, represent pockets of actual demand (not just need) and potential professional gratification.

And there is more good news: You may already possess many (if not all) of the skills for working with a specific group, and you may simply need to develop strategies for reaching out to the population that you would like to serve. For example, we have found rich and rewarding areas for practice expansion in geriatrics (see Niche 5.1), in serving rural areas (see Niche 5.2), and in addressing clients' cultural differences sensitively (see Niche 5.3).

Barriers to treatment can be logistical, such as distance, schedule, and time constraints; physical, such as disabilities or age-related factors that interfere with individuals' getting to the usual treatment settings; or cultural, such as differences in ethnicity, language, or other characteristics that inhibit people from seeking treatment.

Try to find solutions to the various types of barriers that some clients present. Here are some examples:

- Some logistical and physical barriers to access yield to straightforward solutions, such as locating your office close to the homes of the population you wish to serve, or making your office accessible to clients who use wheelchairs or walkers.
- New forms of technology (such as telehealth, the Internet, and various recordings) may enable you to overcome some barriers of time and distance.
- Offering your services in some clients' homes may be productive. This can improve access for those whose behavioral impairment is itself an impediment to treatment. Some patients simply might not come to an office—for example, those with agoraphobia or anergic depression. Some might come, but only with great difficulty (e.g., persons with disabilities, frail elderly individuals, or caregivers who lack access to respite care).
- Cultural barriers can be reduced by placing information about your practice in the appropriate community newspapers, by putting culture-affirmative materials in your office's waiting room, and by providing voice mail greetings and office forms in the appropriate languages for clients whose English is limited. This helps communicate your familiarity with and sensitivity to each group and its needs.

EXTENDING WHAT YOU KNOW TO ENHANCE OTHER HUMAN ACTIVITIES

Forget those old images of encounter groups and gurus: "Personal growth psychology" today is about helping people to live well, achieve optimal functioning in all areas, and prevent decline and disorders. We can extend our services to support and enhance wellness, prevention, spirituality, and growth.

Americans have begun embracing these positive concepts. Surveying users of alternative medicine, for example, Astin (1998) found that prevention was a frequently cited benefit. Prevention researchers have found that psychological traits such as courage, optimism, interpersonal skill, hope, honesty, future-mindedness, and perseverance are the most likely buffers against mental illness (Seligman, 1998a), and many interventions have been shown to be effective in building competencies that can reduce the risk of adverse mental health outcomes (see, e.g., Cowen, 1994; Pedro-Carroll, 1998; Gillham et al., 1995; Saunders et al., 1996).

Possible Types of Interventions

You might design interventions to help clients do the following:

- Improve physical or mental performances through peak performance training, sport psychology, or coaching for talented artists or performers.
- Further creativity by resolving writer's block, perfectionism, performance anxiety, or other work inhibitions.
- Optimize life's transitions, such as navigating adolescence, making midlife "course corrections," making a career change, or assuring "generativity" in aging.
- Improve interpersonal effectiveness by overcoming shyness, becoming more assertive, or improving couple or family relationships.
- Enhance various competencies through skill training and adopting cognitive strategies that buffer stress, such as learned optimism, hopefulness, and delay of gratification.
- Pursue approaches to integrating mind, body, and spirituality. People are seeking more spiritually fulfilled lives.
- Seek personal fulfillment and relief from inner emptiness. Personal growth approaches emphasizing authenticity, self-actualization, and connectedness may be useful in this regard.
- Use the intense bond between humans and animals to improve functioning or gain emotional support—or deal with the trauma of an animal's illness or death.
- Integrate physical health and economic security with subjective, ex-

periential, and philosophical aspects to produce happiness, meaning-fulness, and "flow." People want a higher quality of life, and psychologists are equipped to help them achieve this.

Reaching Clients

Based on focus groups and survey responses from a large representative sample of Americans, sociologist Paul Ray (1997; see also Ray & Anderson, 2000) has identified a growing segment (25%, up 5% from a generation ago) of the U.S. population whom he calls "Cultural Creatives," and whom he views as being at the forefront of cultural change. This group values self-actualization, holistic health, alternative health practices, altruism, feminism, and environmentalism. Valuing inner life and self-exploration, Cultural Creatives emphasize new and unique experiences, and thus they are drawn to personal growth psychology. In fact, according to Ray (1997), they constitute the "core market" for psychotherapy services in general, and are discriminating utilizers of these services.

SEEING THE TRENDS AS YOUR FRIEND

Trends are opportunities. In this book we offer information on viable, currently unfilled, or underfilled niches, but society is dynamic; it continually generates opportunities for those who are looking. Below we first present some ideas about the forces that are creating opportunities for clinicians, and then suggest where you might look for emerging societal trends leading to opportunities in the future.

A Selection of Current Trends

- Immigration and population trends are always significant. According to the U.S. Bureau of the Census (2001), minorities (including Native Americans, African Americans, Asian Americans, and Hispanics) constituted almost 25% of the U.S. population in the year 2000. Although these groups have not traditionally accessed mental health services at the same rate as European Americans, incidence and prevalence data suggest that there is a substantial need for mental health services among these populations.
- Intermarriage among racial and ethnic groups is increasing. The Statistical Assessment Service (1997) reported that the trend toward interracial marriages between African Americans and European Americans was greatest among the youngest generation marrying; this suggests that the future may hold even greater increases. Interracial

and interethnic marriages (and their biracial and interethnic off-
spring and families) have unique needs, and clinicians who can address those needs will be increasingly valued as this trend continues.

- Sexual minorities seek treatment that is free of biases. Gays and lesbians have higher therapy utilization rates than the average, but
many have been dissatisfied with their therapy experiences, (Ritter
& Terndrup, 2002).

- A large percentage of Americans have a disability that can interfere
with their mobility. Nineteen percent of noninstitutionalized Americans over the age of 21 are classified as having a disability (U.S. Bureau of the Census, 1997) that may restrict their ability to function.

- Rural populations have little or no access to high-quality mental
health services. A surprising total of 55 million Americans, one in
five, live in rural areas. Sixty percent of rural areas are underserved
by mental health professionals (Benson, 2003).

Sources of Information on Trends and Patterns of Change

Just as Peter Lynch, the famous mutual fund manager, productively used
what he saw happening around him, you can pay attention to changes in
your own life. What are you reading now? What do you see advertised?
What relationships and populations do you see more of in the movies and on
television? What are you and your friends and family talking about? Make
some notes, collect some data, and let your curiosity run.

Besides doing these things, you might look at sources that have already
collected and processed information. We have found bookstores (both "free-
standing" and online) and the Web to be rich sources of information about
trends.

Your Local Bookstore as a Source of Trend Information

Spend some time in the "Self-Help" or "Psychology" section of your local
bookstore, or research the recent best-sellers in nonfiction, and you will discover a great deal about unmet needs. These books were written, produced,
and marketed at significant expense. For this to happen, many people had to
agree that a demand exists in a sizeable part of the population.

- Look at each book and try to understand its focus. What is the book
trying to do for its readers? What is the need that buying it would
meet? Disregard the author's credentials, the publisher's reputation,
and the production values of the actual book. Focus only on the need
the author saw. Then evaluate how he or she tried to meet that need.
Do not yet work on how you might meet that need, or how well or

poorly the author has met it. Look at all the books and simply formulate a sentence or two about each one's goals.

- Step back and see how many books are aimed at each need. This may
give you a sense of the importance of the need, but remember that
more books appear over time although the need does not change.
- Compare the books and try to distinguish trends within topics.
- Compare the newer titles, which may indicate a direction to investigate.

Select a few books for careful study that appeal to your YEARNings, from
which you could LEARN some things of value, and whose activities could be
a source of EARNings for you.

Web Bookstores as Sources of Trend Information

Both Barnes and Noble (http://BN.com) and Amazon (http://amazon.com) allow unlimited free searches by topic; just type the topic as a keyword in the
"search" box.

- Note how many books were found for the topic you entered.
- How many are professional or technical books (to give you a sense of
the scientific base for interventions), and how many were mass market or trade books (to see aspects of the audience)?
- Quickly review each book. Click on the title to read about it. There is
a lot of information about trends on each page. Is this a second or
third edition (suggesting continued interest)? What is its "sales rank"
(a rough index of popularity)? Be sure to read any readers' comments
for indications of their needs, parts they liked, things they found
missing, and so on. Look at what buyers of this book also bought. You
can often see a book's introduction and/or table of contents, a review
(or even several) by readers, and links to similar books.

The Web as a Source of Trend Information

Surf the Web to see the proliferation of support and discussion groups on
topics that may give you clues to possible niches. For example, Topica (http://
www.topica.com) is a directory of Internet discussion groups with a search
function that will allow you to locate discussion lists by keyword. For example, a recent search of Liszt under the keywords "family," "parent," "aging,"
"midlife," and "divorce" located hundreds of lists on such topics as blended
families and stepfamilies, gifted/talented children, families of special-needs
children, aging parents, adoption, the "sandwich generation," single parents, divorce, custody, and so on (and on).

When you find groups that seem most relevant, join them; read recent postings, and perhaps the archives to see what concerns are being addressed. Pay particular attention to any discussions that relate to dissatisfactions or obstacles faced by the potential client population. Eliminating these could constitute a practice niche in itself. For example, stepfamilies are highly stressed family systems. Learning about their issues could lead you to create a niche that eases access to services for this potential client base. You can also participate in a list and get feedback about your ideas.

Another indication of need can be found via Web sites. The number of people who have visited a site is often captured by a "counter" (usually at the bottom of the home page) that tallies the number of visitors (hits) over a designated time period, and can give you an estimate of interest in the topic.

If you enter a keyword (or topic of interest) in Google (http://www. google.com), it will return links to all the pages containing this word. (If the number is too large to review, enter more keywords; if too few, add variations on the keyword.) These links are ranked by the number of other pages that are linked to it (not by money paid to the search engine, as with some other engines). The ranking will give you a sense of the importance of the topic. For example, if the first few links found by Google are not relevant to your interest (even after variations of the keyword) then there is probably no sizable body of information out there or little interest in this topic.

Google now incorporates the postings made over the years to public mailing lists, which were previously available at DejaNews. If you find relevant information as postings, go to the mailing list and join for more current information.

Finally, see our own Web site (http://www.nichesforclinicians.com) for more information on trend spotting in general and technology and practice in particular.

Gerontology
and Services
to Aging Individuals

OVERVIEW AND OPPORTUNITIES

Thirty years ago, in what has become a classic article, Robert Butler (1974) described the value and nature of psychological work with elderly individuals. He was one of the first professionals to rebut the negative social stereotypes about aging and assert the positive aspects. He contended that the common view of aged persons as unproductive, inflexible, and demented is false and must change if one is to age well. Old age can be a time in which one can find uses for a lifetime's learning.

Many people, including professionals, are still shackled by the stigma of aging—those stereotypes that limit the exercise of options and reduce perceived choices. "Gerontology" is not the study of "dementia, depression, and disease." If you have shed your own limiting attitudes, assumptions, and prejudices about aging, you can help others to do so as well. Nothing is more powerful than knowing people who have adjusted positively and successfully to aging; as partial substitutes, we heartily recommend reading Friedan's (1993) *The Fountain of Age*, Rowe and Kahn's (1998) *Successful Aging*, and Jacobs's (1997) *Be an Outrageous Older Woman*.

A clinical adage with much truth to it is this: "When you have seen one older adult, you have seen one older adult." Although elderly people are indeed an astoundingly diverse group, we can distinguish three general groups because their needs, abilities, and lifestyles are so different. Those aged 65–75 are called "younger old" people; those 75–85, "older old" individuals; and those over 85, the "oldest old" persons. In terms of their needs, consider this (usually surprising) statistic: Although 24% of those aged over 85 reside in nursing homes, only 6% of older old people and only 1.4% of younger old persons do (1990 data, cited by Ables & American Psychological Association [APA] Working Group on the Older Adult, 1997).

Psychology has much to contribute to smoothing the passages of aging, enhancing the outcomes, and reducing the impact of unavoidable losses. The truths are not so bleak, unchangeable, or depressing as you may believe. For example, based on a monumental study of more than 5,000 adults for up to 35 years, Schaie (1994) concluded:

> . . . average decrements in psychometric abilities cannot be reliably confirmed prior to age 60, except for word fluency which shows significant decline by age 53 [citation omitted]. . . . Average decrement before age 60 amounts to less than .2 SD, but by age 81, average decrement increases to approximately one standard deviation for most abilities. . . . As compared with age 25, at age 88, there is virtually no decline in verbal ability; however inductive reasoning and verbal memory have declined by better than 0.5 SD, spatial orientation by almost 1 SD, and numeric ability and perceptual speed have declined by more than 1.5 SD. (p. 308)

Pessimism about loss of mental abilities is hardly warranted by this evidence.

In regard to preventing or slowing the cognitive changes of aging, we know that level of education, physical activity, "engagement with the environment," and self-efficacy all contribute significantly (Albert et al., 1995) to course and outcome, and that as psychologists we can affect all but the first of these. More commonly known as the "use it or lose it" theory of cognitive decline, this principle has enough empirical support (Snowdon et al., 1996; Schaie, 1996; Hultsch et al., 1999) for us to act on it. Most recently, preliminary research has suggested that age-related cognitive declines can be substantially remediated by cognitive therapy retraining techniques (Logan et al., 2002).

YOUR POTENTIAL SATISFACTIONS

- A long life should be a gift, not a burden. Aging is a multifaceted process—a dynamic between an individual's particular strengths, resilience, and support system on the one hand, and the toll taken by social losses, trauma, and physical and cognitive changes on the other. With our particular skills, we can help elderly people achieve a positive balance between these two sets of factors, and enjoy the gift of long life.

- It has been wisely said that aging is only a problem if we fail to make the appropriate adaptations. We can help with optimal adaptation for productivity, generativity, and social inclusion.
- Did you ever have an English teacher who asked you to rewrite the ending of a story or book that you didn't like? I (RLL) loved doing that! That's essentially what we can do in working with older adults—rewriting their stories with and for them.
- Working with elderly people can help us prepare ourselves and our loved ones for the difficulties as well as the joys of a long life.
- Training in gerontology will raise your understanding of complex interactions among the effects of cohort, "organic" cognitive deficits, education, work history, toxin exposure, language history, gender, race/ethnicity, and many of the results of living a long and full life.

YOUR SKILL SET

Recycling Your Current Competencies

Competencies in conducting clinical interviews and in administering, scoring, and interpreting psychological and neuropsychological tests are necessary but not sufficient for this specialization. A Task Force of the APA (cited in Qualls, 1998) identified the following areas of needed knowledge:

1. Research and theory in aging;
2. Cognitive psychology and change.
3. Social-psychological aspects of aging.
4. Biological aspects of aging.
5. Psychopathology.
6. Problems in daily living;
7. Sociocultural and socioeconomic factors.
8. Assessment, including the methodology of assessment in older adults, specific issues in assessment of older adults, and the assessment of therapeutic and programmatic efficacy.
9. Treatment, including individual, group, couple, family, and environmental psychotherapeutic interventions; specific applications of psychotherapeutic interventions for the aging; and issues in providing services in specific settings.
10. Prevention and crisis intervention services.
11. Providing consultation.
12. Interfacing with other disciplines, including appropriate referral to other disciplines, and working within multidisciplinary teams and across a range of sites.
13. Special ethical issues in providing services to aging individuals.

In our view, possessing the skills listed above would qualify you as a "geropsychologist generalist." We follow Taylor's (1992) model of such a generalist, who "would be able to handle 80% of the problems that come to her/him, to discern the 20% that are beyond her/his kin [*sic*], and to have the support system to refer those 20% on to a specialist in geropsychology." Specialty areas might include skills and knowledge in geroneuropsychology, human sexuality, or medication consulting.

Retreading for Added Skills

> Failure to recognize the unique aspects of geropsychology practice creates a barrier to competent practice. . . . [And] the first barrier to obtaining training may be a professional's belief that older adults are not so very different from younger adults—a belief that leaves the clinician with the privilege of using familiar clinical tools and theories without considering appropriate standards of care. (Qualls, 1998)

As Qualls points out, additional training is needed to practice in this area. Of what should this training consist? Moye and Brown (1995) surveyed post-doctoral programs and reported the following content areas (all quotations below are from their article, p. 593):

- Lifespan development, to "address myths and cultural stereotypes about aging" and "the opportunities and pathways for development and growth within individuals and families in the many years encompassing old age."
- "Emotional problems" and "the epidemiology and symptomatology of psychopathology in old age, typical and atypical presentations of emotional problems, and issues in adjustment and bereavement," as well as the "assessment and prevention of suicide among elderly adults."
- An "introduction to the most common neurological syndromes seen in old age. . . . [with a] focus on discrimination of dementia from other conditions, including depression; sleep disturbance; and the side effects, interaction, or mismanagement of medication." Moye and Brown add conditions like strokes and progressive disorders (e.g., Parkinson's disease, Huntington's disease, and multiple sclerosis).
- "Ethical and legal problems specific to old age," such as "reduced competency and vulnerability to elder abuse," This area also includes advanced directives and knowledge of local state statutes and landmark cases.

To this list, we would add these specific topics for additional education, training, experience and/or supervision: bereavement (see Niche 1.3); caregiver burdens (see Niche 1.2); pain management (see Niche 1.4); cultural attitudes and differences (see Niche 5.3); and compliance with medical evaluations, procedures, and treatments (see Niche 1.6). In addition, some elderly persons need treatment for loneliness and coaching in the skills needed to enter self-help groups.

NATURE OF THE WORK

Perhaps more than at any other time in life, adaptive skills are crucial in successful aging. Much psychological work with elderly persons is aimed at ameliorating the stressors of aging, encouraging the potential for growth, training compensating strategies for inevitable and irredeemable losses, supporting caregivers, and helping to smooth the trajectory of dying and the impact of death on the survivors. In addition, as we discuss later, research suggests (contrary to popular beliefs) that elderly people benefit from treatments for depression, family conflicts, sexual dysfunctions, and anxieties.

Areas of Practice

Assessment

The most common reasons for referral of elderly persons are these: (1) separating the contributions of depression and dementia; (2) evaluating degree and types of dementia; (3) evaluating competence to manage finances and make health care decisions; and (4) integrating all of these, in a biopsychosocial model, to assist the making of life-planning decisions. Because of our wide training and our specialization in evaluation, we psychologists can properly weigh the strengths resulting from previous successful adaptations on the one hand, and the effects of medications, drug and alcohol abuse, social stressors, family dynamics, and medical conditions on the other.

For each individual, we can help to separate the remediable from the unalterable. For instance, does an elderly patient have a resolvable delirium or a dementia? If it is a dementia, is the cause reversible or irreversible? Is it a dementia or a pseudodementia due to generally improvable depression? And even when the most pessimistic findings are obtained, we can do a lot to ameliorate the personal, familial, and social consequences.

For assessing depression in elderly people (an important diagnosis— see below), the Geriatric Depression Scale is in the public domain and is available in the *Merck Geriatric Manual* (Abrams et al., 1995), in Farrell (1996), and at two Web sites (http://www.stanford.edu/~yesavage/GDS.html, with much additional material, and http://www.acsu.buffalo.edu/~drstall/ gds.txt). The second Web version is reviewed by Stiles and McGarrahan (1998).

In quite a different realm, the following is a creative use of experimental psychology that can serve as a model for other psychological contributions to gerontology and may offer a subspecialization of geropsychology. We know that at some point aging drivers become incapable and dangerous, but using a general rule such as "Give up driving at age 70" will punish some who can in fact operate safely, and will fail to identify some who are incompetent to drive although younger. Instead, Ball and Owsley (see Ball, 1996) have developed a simple test of "useful field of view" (UFOV) to assess visual attention and cognitive processing speed. Drivers with reduced UFOV "were 16 times more likely to have been involved in a crash during the previous five years than those without reductions" (Ball, 1996). Even for those who fail this test, training on a computer may raise their UFOV to normal in a few sessions. Although the UFOV test currently has no legal standing, many elderly drivers and their children might welcome such an objective assessment of driving ability and accident risk, and might be willing to pay for it on an independent basis.

Psychotherapy

Although there is widespread pessimism about doing therapy with elderly people, this permission is simply not supported by the evidence. In a meta-analysis of psychosocial treatments for depression, Scogin and McElreath (1994) found effect sizes comparable to those found for treatments of depression in younger individuals. Psychotherapy is an important treatment option, because elderly persons generally have increased sensitivity to all medications and their side effects, including antidepressants.

The first step in treating depression in elderly individuals is to recognize it as a treatable disorder and not a normal response to old age. Zeiss et al. (1996) make this point forcefully:

> . . . major depression is neither statistically nor clinically normal in the medically ill [older population]. Even in the group with the most functional impairment and the highest incidence of onset of depression, only 25% of participants in the present study developed an episode. Depression in an older adult should never be viewed as natural, regardless of the person's health status. However, health professionals who treat older adults should be sensitive to the fact that those who have functional impairment, with or without a clearly diagnosed disease, are at increased risk for depression.

In particular, every older adult presenting with apparent dementia deserves a full psychological evaluation. Not only are many such adults suffering from masked depression, but we can do much even for those elders with actual dementia who have little likelihood of returning to their previous level of function, by offering cognitive and behavioral therapies of proven effectiveness for their depression (e.g., Scogin et al., 1989; Scogin & McElreath, 1994; Thompson et al., 1987). Amelioration of their anxiety is also possible (Koder, 1998). Finally, the area of sexuality and aging is full of myths and in need of better views (see Hillman, 2000), and work in this area can also be very rewarding. Brief and essential orientations to therapy with older adults are provided by Knight and McCallum (1998) and by Zarit and Knight (1996). A more comprehensive presentation is the book by Zarit and Zarit (1998).

In addition to our psychological therapies, we should attend to and arrange the treatment of functional impairments by appropriate professionals (e.g., occupational and physical therapists), and should support the compensatory functions of such community services as Meals on Wheels.

Common Health Problems

Two of the most common health complaints of elderly people, insomnia and incontinence, can be effectively treated by psychological interventions (see Morin et al., 1993, and Burgio, 1990, respectively). Incontinence is a common cause of admission to a nursing home, and yet Burgio (1990) states: "The data indicate that behavioral treatment of stress or urge incontinence results in improvement rates which range from 78 to 94%." Interventions are also available for other common medical problems that affect elderly persons, such as tinnitus. Collaboration with primary care physicians (PCPs) is of course important in all such cases (see Niche 1.6).

Consulting about Retirement

Although most people would first consult a financial planner for retirement considerations, some people will also benefit from psychotherapeutic interventions. Counseling and assisting workers nearing retirement age is one potential practice niche; some may need assessment and feedback about the best time to retire, ways to capitalize on their strengths, self-efficacy versus learned helplessness, and so on. Those who own a business and have difficulty with letting go of it or planning for their succession (see Niche 3.2), or those who have retirement thrust upon them suddenly (see Niche 3.4), can benefit from therapy for their loss, grief, or depression. A fine overview of the difficulties and of possible interventions is provided by Richardson (1993).

The research findings in regard to work and the aging process are complex (Hansson et al., 1997). It's safe to assume that some decline in work function, through variable, does occur for many older employees (see Kubeck et al., 1996, for a meta-analysis), probably paralleling declines in cognitive and physical abilities. However, the advantages of such things as greater experience and better work ethics may mitigate these losses.

Consulting to Nursing Facilities

Consultation to nursing homes can represent an opportunity to augment and diversify your private practice. This can be combined with direct care. However, be aware that personal care homes and similar programs have needs for your services well beyond their ability to pay you; that staff members are undertrained, undermotivated, and overburdened; and that physicians and others may not welcome you. Meeks (1996) gives an account of doing such consulting as a specialization for psychologists.

Direct services needed by nursing homes include the following:

- Consultations with family members on a variety of subjects.
- Evaluating dementia, depression, delirium, and other psychological states; seeking their causes; and offering treatments.
- Designing cognitive-behavioral interventions (Marita & Mermelstein-Lopez, 1995) for confused, disoriented, depressed, and/or anxious patients.

Consultations can focus on such topics as these:

- Environmental redesign for improving orientation, slowing the loss of cognitive skills through disuse, and lessening the learned helplessness felt by residents (Foy & Mitchell, 1990).
- There are opportunities in job redesign and staff training as well (see, e.g., Burgio, 1990).
- Even though federal law (the Omnibus Budget Reconciliation Act of 1987) requires facilities to achieve zero physical restraint usage and a reduction in medications at least twice yearly, few facilities have implemented this difficult transition. Psychologically informed prevention and intervention programs are possible means of moving toward compliance with this law. A creative and comprehensive solution on which you could base the design of your interventions is presented in Mlynarek and Mondoux (1996).

Cross-References to Related Specializations

Niche 1.1. Treating Sleep Dysfunctions
Niche 1.2. Supporting Caregivers and Working with Chronic Illnesses

Niche 1.3. Working with Dying and Grieving People
Niche 1.4. The Psychological Management of Chronic Pain
Niche 5.5. Wellness and Positive Psychology

Practice Models

Working in a multidisciplinary setting with physiatrists and geritricians is recommended, as it would favor continuity of care.

Particularly for elderly patients, even small barriers to access can prevent their following through on referrals from PCPs, so make certain that your office and routines are "elderly-friendly."

Perhaps you could gradually integrate your services with those of one or more gerontological practices by providing your services for several hours and increasing your time commitment as referrals increase.

Financial Considerations

Working with older people can take place in the usual settings; referrals can come through the common channels; and payment for your services can be in the usual amounts and from typical sources, depending on the services offered. Do not automatically assume that elderly individuals are poor or destitute. In addition, psychotherapy with elderly patients is often partly reimbursable under Medicare. Becoming a Medicare provider is somewhat complex but can be financially rewarding; contact your local Social Security office for details. It is almost completely managed-care-free, and payments are reliable. In late 2001, the Bush administration agreed to stop automatically denying Medicare reimbursement for psychotherapy with individuals with Alzheimer's disorder (Pear, 2002). Research has demonstrated that numerous treatments (including psychotherapy) are helpful and effective with such patients.

Cautions, Ethical Dilemmas, Culture Clashes, and/or Managed Care Issues

The most common problem in assessment is that age-appropriate norms for the familiar instruments are minimal or even absent. There is no substitute for these, but your own locally collected data will be a start.

Since most services to this group are provided by networks and teams you face the double issue of differentiating your skills from what other professionals can offer and yet participating in a team of professionals with differing approaches, skills, and attitudes.

PROSPECTS AND PROSPECTING

Where Is the Need?

The numbers alone are impressive. The over-65 population of the United States in 1990 was about 31 million and increased by 12% in only 10 years to almost 35 million (U.S. Bureau of the Census, 2000) It is expected to be 59 million, or more than 20% of the total population, by 2025 as the "baby boomers" age (Meyers, 1990, cited in Moye & Brown, 1995). Furthermore, the "baby boomers" have shown a higher rate of depression than their predecessors and should carry this into their older years (Klerman & Weissman, 1989). In 1990, the "oldest old" segment of the U.S. population (those aged over 85) numbered almost exactly 3 million, but in just the 10 years since then it increased by more than one-third, as there were over 4 million in 2000 (U.S. Bureau of the Census, 2000). This group will continue to be the fastest-growing part of the population, and its members are projected to number 8.5 million in 2030 (U.S. Bureau of the Census, 1996, cited in Ables & APA Working Group on the Older Adult, 1997). These are among the frailest and neediest persons.

Competition

Other mental health professionals can specialize in this area, but the needs greatly exceed the supply and will continue to do so. Halpain et al. (1999) offer the following data: There are about 2,700 psychiatrists board-certified in geriatrics; about 13,000 nurses and about 6,000 social workers have training in this specialty. Only about 1,000 psychologists have any recognized certification in geriatrics. Therefore, the opportunities are wide open.

As noted above, most services you would offer would be as part of a team, and so you must find activities in which you can specialize and not overlap with the functions of other professionals.

Reaching Clients/Directions for Marketing

You will need to put effort into making physicians aware of the special or even unique services you have to offer. Most PCPs are swamped dealing with the medical needs of their patients and are not trained to evaluate or deal in depth with psychosocial needs, even though they know that many of their patients need this care. Even geriatricians and other gerontologists, while sensitive to the psychosocial issues, may not know of all the efficacious interventions we can offer. This is no time to be shy!

- Network with health care providers who serve this population, and let them know that you can augment traditional medico-pharmacological services for their patients. Being available for consultations on an "on-call" basis will create mutually beneficial connections with physicians.
- Marketing efforts should include letters of introduction, newsletters, brochures, and whatever it takes to keep your services in the minds of PCPs and other health care workers dealing with this population.

Here is a unique idea for marketing and networking as well as providing needed services: Put together a group of small business providers who focus on services for disabled and elderly individuals. One such network, the Special Needs Network, in Albuquerque, NM, included a psychologist, Joan R. Saks Berman, PhD, who provided counseling services for families of the elderly or persons with disabilities. Other needed services, such as evaluating seniors or persons with disabilities; making appropriate referrals for alternate placements and services; arranging "meals on wheels"; scheduling personal help such as in-home assistance and help with errands; obtaining medical supplies and mobility devices such as wheelchairs, scooters, or conversion vans; and doing home renovations for greater functional accessibility were available from other businesses in the network. This group approach supports truly integrated treatment in its community.

INCREASING YOUR FORMAL KNOWLEDGE BASE

Core Readings

General Background

Ables, N., & American Psychological Association (APA) Working Group on the Older Adult. (1997). *What practitioners should know about working with older adults.* Washington, DC: American Psychological Association.
   —In just 28 pages, this brochure will replace myths and stereotypes so that you can see ways to provide, and the value of providing, services to elderly individuals. This may be one of the best APA publications.

Birren, J. E., Marshall, V. W., Cole, T. R., Svanborg, A., & Masoro, E. J. (Eds.). (1996). *Encyclopedia of gerontology: Age, aging, and the aged.* San Diego, CA: Academic Press.
   —This is the most comprehensive professional reference (two volumes, 1,500 pages) to all aspects of gerontology: biology, psychology, social sciences, health science, and humanities.

Birren, J. E., Schaie, K. W., Abeles, R. P., Gatz, M., & Salthouse, T. J. (Eds.). (2001). *Handbook of the psychology of aging* (5th ed.). San Diego, CA: Academic Press.
   —A shorter volume by Birren and colleagues, confined to psychology.

Busse, E. W., & Blazer, D. G. (Eds.). (1996). *The American Psychiatric Press textbook of geriatric psychiatry* (2nd ed.). Washington, DC: American Psychiatric Press.

Kane, R. L., Ouslander, J. G., & Abrass, I. B. (1994). *Essentials of clinical geriatrics.* New York: McGraw-Hill.

—Written from a medical point of view, and organized by problem rather than diagnosis, this book is a comprehensive resource for managing medical treatments.

McIntosh, J. L., Santos, J. F., Hubbard, R. W., & Overholser, J. C. (1994). *Elder suicide: Research, theory, and treatment.* Washington, DC: American Psychological Association.

Spar, J. E., & La Rue, A. (1997). *Concise guide to geriatric psychiatry* (2nd ed.). Washington, DC: American Psychiatric Press.

Assessment

American Psychological Association (APA) Presidential Task Force on the Assessment of Age-Consistent Memory Decline and Dementia. (1998). *Guidelines for the evaluation of dementia and age-related cognitive decline.* Washington, DC: American Psychological Association.

—This publication reviews competencies, ethical considerations, and what you should know before doing assessments.

La Rue, A., & Watson, J. (1998). Psychological assessment of older adults. *Professional Psychology: Research and Practice, 29*(1), 5–14.

—This article is the best brief introduction to assessment of older adults, because it covers all interviewing as well as testing and guides the process of diagnosing and planning interventions.

Storandt, M., & VandenBos, G. (Eds.). (1994). *Neuropsychological assessment of dementia and depression in older adults: A clinician's guide.* Washington, DC: American Psychological Association.

—Dementia versus depression is always a tough differential diagnosis; this book provides guidance.

Zarit, S. H., & Zarit, J. M. (1998). *Mental disorders in older adults: Fundamentals of assessment and treatment.* New York: Guilford Press.

—This is the book to start with and to stay with; it is detailed, authoritative, and complete (topics include normal processes, effects of medications, evaluation of competence, collaborating with physicians, common disorders, etc.).

Do you need a guide to almost all the geriatric assessment tools? The Department of Veterans Affairs has compiled a guide to them that offers detailed information on each instrument, as well as a template for comparisons of instruments. *Geropsychology Assessment Resource Guide, 1996 Revision* is available from the National Technical Information Service (NTIS). To order, call the NTIS sales desk at 1-800-553-6847/NTIS. If you will be doing competency evaluations, the same organization has developed the *Assessment of Competency and Capacity of the Older Adult—A Practice Guideline for Psychologists.* Published in March 1997, in 72 pages it offers a conceptual framework and procedures, ethical and legal aspects, and reliability and validity. It is available from the National Center for Cost Containment, 5000 W. National Avenue, Milwaukee, WI 53295-3517 (catalog no. PB97-147904INZ).

Therapy

Knight, B. G., & McCallum, T. J. (1998). Adapting psychotherapeutic practice for older clients: Implications of the contextual, cohort-based, maturity, specific challenge model. *Professional Psychology: Research and Practice, 29*(1), 15–22.

Link, A. L. (1997). *Group work with elders: 50 therapeutic exercises for reminiscence, validation, and remotivation.* Sarasota, FL: Professional Resource Press.
—The title says it all. This book is useful for program design and group treatment in almost any setting.

Zarit, S. H., & Knight, B. G. (1996). *A guide to psychotherapy and aging.* Washington, DC: American Psychological Association.

Journals

Aging and Mental Health
Archives of Gerontology and Geriatrics
Clinical Gerontologist
The Gerontologist
Journal of Applied Gerontology
Journal of Clinical Geropsychology
Journal of Gerontology: Psychological Sciences
Journal of Gerontology: Social Sciences
Psychology and Aging

Online Resources

U.S. Administration on Aging
http://www.aoa.gov
—This is an enormously rich site and an excellent starting place.

Alzheimer's Disease Education Referral Center (ADEAR), a service of the National Institute on Aging
http://www.alzheimers.org/index.html
—At the ADEAR site, you will find about 10 brochures that may be useful to clients. The Combined Health Information Database contains more than 4,400 health education and information materials related to Alzheimer's disease, along with subfiles on 17 other health topics

New York Online Access to Health (NOAH), Aging and Alzheimer's Disease
http://www.noah-health.org
—If you need any kind of health information on aging or dementia, the NOAH site is the place to start. It includes a very rich set of papers, links, and informational handouts with full search, as well as a clearly organized table of contents.

Alzheimer's Association
http://www.alz.org
—A well-organized site with lots of accurate factual information, guidance and support, information on research, caretaking, guidance for professionals, and medical issues. The materials are suitable for patient, family, and professional education.

Professional Organizations

American Society on Aging, Mental Health and Aging Network, 833 Market
    Street, Suite 511, San Francisco, CA 94103-1824; 415-974-9600
http://www.asaging.org
—This group is more issue-oriented than disease-oriented. The Web site covers such topics as productivity and aging, end-of-life issues, pain management, alcohol abuse, and cultural diversity.

Gerontological Society of America, Mental Health Practice and Aging Interest
    Group
1275 K Street N.W., Suite 350, Washington, DC 20005; 202-842-1275
http://www.geron.org

Division 12, Section 2 (Clinical Geropsychology) of the American Psychological
    Association
http://bama.ua.edu/~appgero/apa12_2/

Division 20 (Adult Development and Aging) of the American Psychological
    Association
http://www.aging.ufl.edu/apadiv20/apadiv20.htm
—Many postgraduate training opportunities are listed on this Web site. Click on "Newsletter" for a direct link to the Division 20 newsletter, *Adult Development and Aging*, and back issues.

Patient Education Materials: Online Resources, Printed Resources, and Organizations

The American Association of Retired Persons (AARP)
http://www.aarp.org
—They offer many self-help materials (which can be searched for under their Topic Guides).

ElderWeb
http://www.elderweb.com
—A research site for professionals and family members, with over 4,500 links to information on eldercare and long-term care; legal, financial, medical, and housing issues; as well as policy, research, and statistics.

Geropsychology Central
http://www.premier.net/~gero/geropsyc.html

—Slow loading because of graphics, the Senior's Corner offers the best short lists of links about health, retirement, news, and bulletin boards. The next section offers many valuable links to professional resources.

Administration on Aging
http://www.aoa.gov

—This is a federal site with lots of information. National Institute on Aging Age Pages offer many brochures of accurate information on health, alcohol, exercise, sexuality, and so forth. Some 20 AOA Fact Sheets are two- to three-pagers with facts and references designed for the educated reader.

Clinical Practice in Rural Areas

OVERVIEW AND OPPORTUNITIES

Whether you would like to return to the bucolic life of your childhood, or you have always dreamed of escaping the city, rural practice may provide an ideal opportunity. You can apply your skills to important unmet needs while also making significant lifestyle changes.

Fifty-five million Americans live in rural areas; and 60% of rural areas are underserved by mental health care providers. Areas considered to be "rural" range from those within a half-hour's drive of urban centers, to "isolated rural areas," to those more aptly described as "frontier areas" with under six or seven persons per square mile. The Frontier Mental Health Services Resource Network's Web site (see, "Professional Organizations," below) provides an informative discussion of the many differences among these types of areas.

Behavioral health care and treatment of drug and alcohol abuse are sorely needed by rural residents. According to a National Mental Health Association (1988) study, the mental health needs of rural Americans, particularly with respect to depression and anxiety, are significantly undertreated. Because rural physicians are stretched and have difficulty meeting the needs of this population, "rural practice presents the ideal venue for expansion of psychology's role in primary health care" (Newman, 1995). An estimated 40–60% of primary care medical diagnoses have a major behavioral component, and so mental health clinicians can make an important contribution by applying their expertise to the behavioral side of many illnesses (Newman, 1995) and extending the effectiveness of PCPs.

YOUR POTENTIAL SATISFACTIONS

- If you enjoy operating on your own and being a mental health "generalist," rural practice can afford you this opportunity. You may gain a sense of mission and importance from being the only provider in a given geographic area. Indeed, you are very likely to have to function without direct consultation or immediate backup.
- You can provide valuable services to a population that, without you, would have no services at all.
- Moving to a rural area can simplify your lifestyle in some (but not all) ways, and may lower your costs of living—or at least change them. For example, instead of paying for water a month at a time, you may need to invest 7 years of payments all at once in a new well.
- Rural practice has much less managed care. See "Financial Considerations," below.

YOUR SKILL SET

Recycling Your Current Competencies

Rural practice is varied, and the absence of other practitioners will require you to utilize all of your clinical skills. Generally, competencies in child, adolescent, and adult treatment are needed, as well as in dealing with substance abuse and domestic violence. Short-term, behaviorally oriented interventions will probably be the mainstay of your practice. In addition, familiarity with regional and ethnic issues will be most valuable.

Perhaps more than with other practice specializations, there is no substitute for experience, because there is so little formal information available. If you haven't lived in the area to which you want to relocate, try to spend time there to become familiar with the culture, values, mores, and informal support networks prior to beginning your practice. Although rural areas differ in culture and mores from urban areas, they also differ from one another (see "Cautions . . . ," below). Keeping an open mind and being flexible about practice parameters are essential attitudes for rural practice.

Retreading for Added Skills

Supervision, mentoring, and/or informal relationships with other caregivers can be extremely helpful in accelerating your learning curve for work with rural populations. Try to arrange for a mentoring or consultant relationship with another health care provider in the area, preferably someone with a sensitivity to mental health issues. Such a relationship with an experienced practitioner can provide valuable insights into the culture and help-seeking behaviors of residents, as well as help in networking, locating your practice, and marketing. Locate such individuals through networking at state rural health associations or through state association newsletters or directories.

Telecommunication may be essential. When you are working in a remote area, Internet access, fax capabilities, and e-mail can reduce professional isolation and add needed resources. Being connected to the Internet can stimulate you and improve your practice by facilitating collegial support and informal peer supervision around cases and practices, easing the exchange of information with agencies in your area, allowing access to professional information and information for clients, and obtaining access to continuing education classes online. High-speed Internet access may be obtainable at low cost through a Federal Communications Commission (FCC) program that provides discounts for rural health care clinics and similar providers (but not individuals) (see FCC, 2002).

INCREASING YOUR FORMAL KNOWLEDGE BASE

If you do not already have a solid foundation in substance abuse assessment and intervention, you should seek to upgrade your training in this area (Cellucci & Vik, 2001). Training in relevant diversity issues may also be needed. There are many guidelines available, depending upon the group(s) to which you would be offering services (see Niche 5.3 for more details).

NATURE OF THE WORK

You may be the only mental health care provider within driving distance, and so you will have to be or become a generalist. Coyle (1999) describes several necessary and useful modifications for clinical practice. For example, shorter-term, solution-oriented interventions or crisis intervention will be more in keeping with rural cultural norms (Murray & Keller, 1991). Mitigating against the traditional weekly and longer-term interventions are the distances between rural communities, weather conditions, challenging terrain, and the absence of public transportation. Also, clinicians must more fully utilize all the existing support systems. For example, Leukefeld et al. (1999) describe an approach to modifying a substance abuse program to better fit the needs of rural residents. Heckman et al. (1999) describe the use of telephone-delivered cognitive-behavioral therapy interventions for rural residents living with HIV/AIDS. Lewis (2001) describes providing specialty services in a community hospital.

Cross-References to Related Specializations

Niche 1.6. Collaborative Practice with Primary Care Physicians
Niche 5.3. Culturally Informed Diversity-Sensitive Practice

Subspecializations

If you enjoy doing evaluations with and without testing consider doing consultative examinations for the Social Security Disability Division. Call a nearby Social Security district office to find out how to reach the director of medical services, to see where the office is in need of evaluations and how to get onto its panel of consultants. Current fees are not high (at $100–$125 for testing, interview, records review, and dictating a report), but the clientele is diagnostically fascinating. Some areas that are not near a large city can need several hundred a year. You can, after you get into the routine, do two to four a day. The SSA site, at http://www.ssa.gov/disability/professionals, will explain more and offers information, guidelines, and links to all of the above.

Practice Models

Several models of practice are being used in rural areas.

1. Staff and administrative positions at area facilities may make for the simplest entry into professional life in a rural area. Many facilities have been deliberately located in rural areas for cost efficiencies. Psychiatric inpatient facilities (e.g., state mental hospitals), juvenile facilities, prisons, and rural community mental health and mental retardation centers are all generally understaffed. Openings can be part-time, full-time, consulting, or per diem arrangements, with the probability that a significant portion of your time will be spent in administrative and supervisory functions. Such a job could serve as a base from which to build a private practice and continue as a reliable supplement to your private practice.
2. If you have clinical experience and interest in working with children, explore the possibility of a part-time or consultant role with a rural school system. The entire spectrum of child and adolescent disorders is seen in schools. It is likely that you will assess and treat cases of suspected child abuse, neglect and endangerment; suspected domestic violence cases; parenting inadequacies; attention-deficit/hyperactivity disorder (ADHD); all kinds of learning disabilities; suicidality; substance abuse; and so on (and on).
3. Several types of part-time practice opportunities may exist. A rural area adjacent to your present location may have some needs on

which you can build with an office in the rural area. Rural areas that are a reasonable distance from a small city could also constitute a practice combination if you moved to that city. You might be able to provide services to several adjacent areas on an itinerant basis, and so combine part-time practices or a specialization into a full-time practice.

4. Collaboration with a PCP is a very viable format for rural practice, as it may be advantageous to you both. Collaborators can include pediatricians, obstetricians/gynecologists, and geriatric specialists addressing such areas as disease prevention, health promotion, smoking cessation, eating disorders, somatization, anxiety, depression, substance abuse, ADHD, caregiver burden, critical and traumatic incidents, domestic violence, and child abuse. For more on several of these topics, see the corresponding niches in this book.

5. Opportunities also exist to become part of the health care team at hospitals located in rural areas. See Lewis (2001) for a description of two such programs, and Morris (1997) for comprehensive guidance in entering rural hospital practice.

6. Rural practice will involve travel on your part. Mobile units and house calls are some of the ways rural practitioners have tried to overcome the obstacles to reaching some rural residents. For example, in an online article discussing ways of dealing with rural domestic violence, Mulder and Chang (1997) note:

> Mobile medical units, schools, and churches are all potential "office" sites. These same sites are often appropriate, non-threatening meeting places for offender and substance abuse self-help meetings, can be excellent resources during volunteer and paraprofessional recruitment activities, and are invaluable in attempts to broadly disseminate information. Self help literature should be available at locations which are readily accessible.

7. In extremely remote areas, telehealth applications may be useful, particularly when weather conditions or domestic or work responsibilities make traveling to a clinician's office impractical for patients. Ermer (1999) reports on a successful "telepsychiatry" project for rural children and adolescents.

Financial Considerations

- Pay scales may be lower than in cities, but the cost of living in rural areas can be lower as well. Based on my (ELZ) experience, the following are likely. Generally, taxes will be much lower; food and clothing cost about the same (but you will eat out less); utilities cost less, but automobile expenses cost more. You will probably need to do more house maintenance yourself and will probably have to buy larger or different lawnmowers, automobiles, and tools of all kinds. The overall cost of living may be a quarter less than in a medium-sized city.

• The expenses involved in relocating may be worthwhile if this change fits other needs in your life, such as the desire to live in a particular area; the wish to make a family, age-related, or lifestyle change; the wish to work in primary care; or the desire to work with small agencies or organizations.

• Do you want to get on panels, but can't? Managed care organizations are often looking for rural clinicians, and this has been suggested as a way to get on closed panels. However, managed care has less "penetration" in rural areas, and a Robert Wood Johnson Foundation study found that rural primary care practices reported deriving only a small fraction of their income from managed care (Parente et al., 1998). Rural areas are, however, affected by managed care for Medicare or Medicaid, so investigate the current status of managed care in the areas you are considering for relocation. Check the Web sites of the National Association for Rural Mental Health and the National Rural Health Association ("see "Professional Organization," below). Rural community health plans are nonprofit organizations that sell health insurance products. A directory of such plans is available from the Office of Rural Health Policy, 5600 Fishers Lane, Room 9A-55, Rockville, MD 20857; 301-443-0835. Many states have offices of rural health, and you can contact them for localized advice.

• The National Health Service Corps provides school loan repayment options to healthcare professionals who work with underserved populations, which include many rural areas. (For more information, go to http://www.bphc.hrsa.gov/nhsc, or phone 800-221-9393.)

Cautions, Ethical Dilemmas, Culture Clashes, and/or Managed Care Issues

Rural Americans are a very heterogeneous group with differing needs, cultures, and histories. Rural Florida is not like rural Pennsylvania or the Dakotas. The culture of Native Americans on reservations differs from that of Hispanic Americans or European Americans living nearby. Interventions should be culturally sensitive and community-based, so a thorough appreciation of the importance of the religious beliefs and cultural identities of the individuals receiving services is a necessity, as is your being able to accept working within this normative structure (which is usually a conservative one). Distrust of outsiders, valuing of self-sufficiency, and lack of familiarity with the benefits of mental health services are often barriers to be overcome by therapists.

Confidentiality is a concern for residents in rural areas, where anonymity is virtually impossible, and where the label of "mental illness" can carry inescapable stigma as well as creating issues of shame for family members. Ethical management of dual relationships is an essential skill. In a small town or rural area, social contacts between a therapist and client are much more likely, and often even unavoidable (Schank & Skovholt, 1997; Schank, 1998).

PROSPECTS AND PROSPECTING

Where Is the Need?

The needs are enormous. According to an online article in *Rural Health News*, 76% of all mental health provider shortage areas are nonmetropolitan areas; over one-fifth of rural counties have no mental health services whatsoever; and only 13% of rural hospitals offer outpatient psychiatric care ("Rural Mental Health: Familiar Problems . . . ," 1998). You can learn more about the location of health professional shortage areas at two Web sites (http://belize.hrsa.gov/newhpsa/newhpsa.cfm and http://www.shusterman.com/hpsa.html), so you can evaluate a move. A great deal of information is also available through *FedStats* (http://www.fedstats.gov), where links are available to such information as the number of psychologists per 100,000 population, and each state's rank in terms of health insurance coverage.

Another indication of need is that suicide rates in rural areas are double those of more populous regions and "soaring" (Wagner, 2000)—a disparity that is partly attributable to isolation and lack of services in rural areas, and is probably also related to high levels of substance abuse. Rokke and Klenow (1999) offer further information on needs for mental health services, particularly depression, among elderly rural residents. Reliable and current sources of information about need are job ads in professional organizations' newsletters.

The U.S. federal government has recognized the importance of meeting rural needs for mental health services. The Omnibus Budget Reconciliation Act of 1989 mandated that the Office of Rural Health Policy facilitate the development of services related to rural mental health.

Chamberlin (2003) quotes Rick McGraw, PhD, a rural psychologist in Fort Concho, Texas:

> at a time when many psychologists are looking for ways to attract more clients and market their practices, they might find this fact most alluring: "I could eas-

ily put five psychologists to work full time if I could get them to move here."
(p. 69)

In summary, rural mental health is an underserved area and is likely to
continue as such in the foreseeable future.

Competition

- To assess competition from other mental health care providers in
  your chosen area, the start with local Yellow Page listings. Check
  under all subject headings ("psychologists," "counseling," "marital
  counseling," "social workers," etc.).
- Look into your professional association's membership directory with
  entries by location or county.
- If you are in the rural community, look at the "professional services"
  ads in local newspapers, on bulletin boards in stores and churches,
  and in other public gathering places.
- School principals and religious leaders may be willing to share their
  perspective on the community's needs and resources, as may local
  politicians.

Reaching Clients/Directions for Marketing

If the local telephone directory has Blue Pages, review entries under "Human Services," "Drug and Alcohol Services," and similar headings to see
what already exists. A phone call to the directors of some of the listed agencies asking about their needs may be all the entrée you need in the less formal rural environment.

You can learn a great deal about a community by subscribing to the local newspapers for several months prior to making any decision about relocating. If you have the opportunity, speak with people who live in the community to try to get a sense of what services are available, how they are
accessed, and how they are understood and valued. If you can get a sense of
residents' satisfaction with available psychosocial services, this will be very
helpful. For an eye-opening critique of mental health service availability in
one rural area, see Cooper and Wagenfeld (n.d.).

Physicians, hospitals, school counselors and other school personnel,
clergy, law enforcement personnel, and volunteer firefighters and emergency medical technicians services are all gatekeepers who should be approached, as they all come in contact with many individuals needing mental
health services. You can meet them when you seek a local personal physician, register your child for school, pay your taxes, attend church, obtain licenses or building permits, or the like.

In addition, you could cultivate relationships with inpatient units in the area, as well as seeking admitting privileges or working in conjunction with a physician or psychologist on staff. According to Mulder and Chang (1997),

> Acceptance of mental health interventions in rural communities is enhanced by interdisciplinary associations with other primary care providers. It is also a basic necessity to establish collaborative and cooperative relationships with local religious authorities, shamans, healers, teachers, school administrators, law enforcement personnel and other individuals identified by the indigenous population who may have equally important, if less formalized, leadership positions in the community.

Suggestions for Relocating

- You may be able to find desirable locations for rural practice within your own state, so that credentialing will not be a problem. Your state office of rural health care, or state association of rural health may also be able to assist you in finding information with regard to need, managed care penetration, and available services.
- For information across the country, the Rural Information Center Health Service (National Agricultural Library, Room 304, 10301 Baltimore Blvd., Beltsville, MD 20705-2351; 800-633-7701; e-mail: ric@nalusda.gov) is the specialty arm of the Rural Information Center that provides a database and search service for persons interested in rural health and mental health. Its Web site (http://www.nal.usda.gov/ric/richs) has many publications online.
- The 3R (Rural Recruitment and Retention) Net provides information to health professionals who are interested in relocating to rural areas (http://www.3rnet.org).
- An excellent description of how one clinician planned and executed a move to a rural area in Florida is provided in a *Psychotherapy Finances* article ("How One Provider Revitalized . . . ," 1995).
- There are national real estate chains (e.g., United Country and West Realty) coordinating local agencies. Their catalogs can tell you a lot about a region, and rural real estate agents are very approachable and well informed.

INCREASING YOUR FORMAL KNOWLEDGE BASE

Core Readings

American Psychological Association (APA) Office of Rural Health. (1995). *Caring for the rural community: An interdisciplinary curriculum.* Washington, DC: American Psychological Association.

Holaday, M., & Greene, M. (1997) Resources for rural practitioners. *Psychotherapy in Private Practice, 16*(1), 15–20.
—This article provides a list of 22 resources for rural psychologists.
Lambert, D., Bird, D. C., Hartley, D., & Genova, N. (1996). *Integrating primary care and mental health services in rural America: Current practices in rural areas.* Kansas City, MO: National Rural Health Association.
Monsey, B., Owen, G., Zierman, C., Lambert, L., & Hyman, V. (1995). *What works in preventing rural violence: Strategies, risk factors, and assessment tools.* St. Paul, MN: Amherst H. Wilder Foundation. (Available from the Wilder Foundation, Publishing Center, 919 Lafond Avenue, St. Paul, MN 55104, 800-274-6024)
Morris, J. A. (Ed.). (1997). *Practicing psychology in rural settings: Hospital privileges and collaborative care.* Washington, DC: American Psychological Association.
—A very complete guide to educating and joining rural hospital practice, and to collaborating with PCPs, emergency rooms, and other care providers.
Sloboda, Z., Boyd, G., Beatty, L., & Kozel, N. (1997). *Rural substance abuse: State of knowledge and issues* (NIDA Research Monograph No. 168, NIH Publication No. 97-4177). Rockville, MD: U.S. Department of Health and Human Services. (Also available online at http://165.112.78.61/PDF/Monographs/Monograph168/Download168.html)
Stamm, B. H. (Ed.). (2003). *Rural behavioral health care: An interdisciplinary guide.* Washington, DC: American Psychological Association.

Journals

Journal of Rural Community Psychology (a tremendous resource; the current issue and many archived articles are available online at http://www.marshall.edu/jrcp).

Rural Health Bulletin (a publication of the APA Practice Directorate; several back issues are available online through the Resource Center for Rural Behavioral Health—see "Professional Organizations," below)

Online Resources

Contact information for the various state offices of rural health and state rural health associations can be accessed at the Office of Rural Health Policy's Web site (http://ruralhealth.hrsa.gov/funding/50sorh.htm).

Rural Net (http://ruralnet.marshall.edu) contains resources for rural health practitioners, including MEDLINE access and their online rural health magazine, *Country Doc.* This publication can give you insight into the issues facing health practitioners in rural areas and how to interface with them.

Rural Care, a low-volume interdisciplinary list for those interested in rural health care, is a place to ask questions and learn from professionals actually working in rural areas (to subscribe, send an e-mail to rural-care-request@lists.apa.org).

Professional Organizations

The American Psychological Association, through its Resource Center for Rural Behavioral Health (http://www.apa.org/rural) is a resource center offering papers, links, and many training opportunities. There are 38 APA-approved predoctoral training programs indicating that they have a "rural emphasis."

Frontier Mental Health Services Resource Network, Western Interstate
  Commission for Higher Education
P.O. Box 9752, Boulder, CO 80301-9752; 303-541-0256; fax 303-541-0291
http://www.wiche.edu/MentalHealth/Frontier

National Association for Rural Mental Health
3700 W. Division Street, Suite 105, St. Cloud, MN 56301; 320-202-1820; fax 320-
  202-1833
e-mail: narmh@facts.ksu.edu   http://narmh.org

National Rural Health Association
One West Armour Blvd., Suite 203, Kansas City, MO 64111-2087; 816-756-3140
e-mail: mail@NRHArural.org   http://www.nrharural.org

Culturally Informed, Diversity-Sensitive Practice

OVERVIEW AND OPPORTUNITIES

Much of psychology and psychotherapy has been formulated and evaluated for clients who are European American, heterosexual, middle-class, and English-speaking. Yet the U.S. population is far more diverse than this description suggests. Therapy must acknowledge these differences and their effects on expectations and understandings of self, relationships, emotions, and actions.

No matter what kind of therapy we do, for whom, or for what kinds of problems, our interactions with clients are enhanced by familiarity with the clients' cultures and world views. Conversely, lack of awareness of and/or sensitivity to different cultural norms, lack of experience with minorities, ethnocentrism, heterosexism, and prejudice can all present obstacles to effective treatment. Many have argued (see, e.g., Sue & Zane, 1987) that therapist–client differences in cultural background and/or beliefs can negatively affect the outcome of therapy. Years ago, Sue (1977) reported that therapy dropout rates for ethnic minorities were 50% higher than for members of the majority group, causing concern in the mental health community about whether minority group members' needs were being met within traditional treatment facilities. Supporting Sue's point, Takeuchi et al. (1995) and Yeh et al. (1994) reported that minority clients seen at ethnically oriented practices had lower dropout rates than those seen in more mainstream practices. Sue et al. (1991) found that matching clients' and therapists' ethnic/cultural background improved retention and outcome for Asian American and Mexican American clients, and length of treatment (but not outcome) for African American clients. Sue (1998) has reported preliminary data indicating that matching therapist–client ethnicity and/or language resulted in better treatment outcomes, and Jerrell (1998) found that this matching improved length of treatment and decreased need for intensive treatment services with children and adolescents. Relatedly, Menapace (1998) found that African American clients treated by European American therapists had better outcomes when the therapists reported multicultural competence in counseling skills and counseling relationships, as well as more social experiences with African Americans. However, Sue (1998) also cautions that clients' degree of acculturation and ethnic identity, and therapist–client belief similarity, may be more important than simply matching therapists to clients on the basis of cultural background alone.

It has been years since the first warning bells were sounded regarding psychology's own ethnocentrism (Guthrie, 1976; Jones, 1983; Ponterotto & Casas, 1987). Despite the formal support of professional organizations such as the APA (1993) and some progress in graduate school training requirements, only small increases have occurred in recruitment of ethnic and other minorities into graduate programs (C. I. Hall, 1997). The ever-increasing pluralism of the U.S. population contrasts glaringly with the underutilization of outpatient psychotherapy services, poor treatment retention among minorities, and paucity of providers who are members of minority groups.

Since there is no likelihood that sufficient numbers of minority therapists will be trained in the near future, there is a huge opportunity for all psychotherapists interested in these underserved populations. Therapists with competence in treating clients from ethnic and other minority groups are in a position to meet an important unmet need. Therapists with ethnic minority group background, experience, and training, and/or who are bilingual or from a sexual minority, will be positioned to offer psychotherapy services that are better attuned to the needs of minority clients, and will benefit from marketing and networking with such clients.

In this niche we will discuss a number of minority groups that differ considerably along different dimensions. Only their unfamiliarity to majority therapists unites them, and this is what our discussion focuses on.

YOUR POTENTIAL SATISFACTIONS

- If you find learning about other cultures and subcultures (or your own) fascinating and enhancing, specializing in this area can be both personally and professionally satisfying. It can add to your professional status as well.

- Because you will be meeting an important need in an area where little competition exists, your services will be very much appreciated.

YOUR SKILL SET

Recycling Your Current Competencies

- Your best assets may be your personal experience, your own cultural background, and your experience in working clinically with a particular group. If you are a member of a minority culture or orientation, you already have invaluable insight and empathy for working with its members, as well as an understanding of the gaps between current practices and those desired. Studies (e.g., Sue & Zane, 1987) indicate that more proximal variables like experience and familiarity predict ethnic counseling competence, whereas more distal variables like knowledge and training do not.
- Brushing up on relevant language skills through coursework and/or tutoring (preferably both) can be an excellent investment in your multicultural competency.
- Expenses may be necessary to make sure that all of your office forms, signs, brochures, and business cards reflect the native language of the group you wish to serve or other cultural variables.
- Although the APA mandates that graduate psychology programs include a multicultural component, there is no special certification required at present in this area. Several states require continuing education in this area, and there are guidelines that can inform and assist you in expanding your knowledge.

NATURE OF THE WORK

Areas of Practice

Ethnically Based Psychotherapies

Although some (e.g., Foulks et al., 1995) would argue that optimal outcomes can be achieved with ethnic minorities utilizing supportive–expressive psychotherapy, and that such therapy is more "effective, feasible, and ethical" than specific ethnic therapies, others maintain that treatment modalities indigenous to a culture can better meet the needs of minority populations. For example, Costantino et al. (1986) make a case for *cuento* therapy, which emphasizes the Puerto Rican cultural context; Reynolds (1989) describes Morita therapy, utilized in Japan. Richeport-Haley (1998) argues for combining ethnic and traditional (structural family therapy) approaches in work with ethnic minority families. Bernal and Scharrón-del-Río (2001) state that any empirically supported treatment that is "actually based on predominantly White, middle-class, English-speaking women is of questionable use for ethnic minorities" (p. 328). They encourage research to determine which treatments are most effective with such groups.

Interventions for Acculturation Stress

Immigrants to North America are a large and growing group. To a greater or lesser degree, all must struggle to adapt to the majority culture, as well as to cope with the loss of their country of origin. In a review of studies of adjustment and acculturation, Moyerman and Forman (1992) concluded that "stress and anxiety may be acute at the very beginning of the acculturation process, and it appears to become less pronounced for Asian-Americans and those with sufficient economic resources" (p. 176). Hovey and King (1996) found that one-quarter of immigrant and second-generation Latino/Latina adolescents reported critical levels of depression and suicidal ideation, and that these were correlated with acculturation stress. Gonsalves (1992) describes the stages of the refugee's adaptation process.

Work with Interethnic or Mixed Couples and Families of Origin

The numbers of ethnically, racially, and religiously mixed marriages and other couple relationships are increasing, and these couples and their families face problems beyond the ones common to all. Barbara Okun (1996) interviewed 187 nontraditional families, some of which were interracial, for her book *Understanding Diverse Families: What Practitioners Need to Know*. She found that the marginalized status of these families, and the lack of support they experienced from the mainstream culture, could accentuate existing problems.

Work with Biracial and Ethnic Minority Children

The increasing numbers of interracial couples (see above) have produced a concomitant rise in the number of biracial individuals (Henriksen, 1997). Winn and Priest (1993) found that biracial children and adolescents feel pulled in two directions, and believe that their parents did not adequately prepare them for a world in which prejudice and bigotry exist. Only a small literature exists on work with this population, but their increasing numbers suggest that this can be a developing area of practice. Herring (1995) provides specific strategies for use with this population, and Brandell (1988) and Gibbs and Moskowitz-Sweet (1991) discuss treatment issues related to biracial children and adolescents. Miller and Miller (1990) discuss parenting issues with a biracial child.

For the interested clinician, there are many guidelines for tailoring treatments to a child's cultural background. McIntyre (1996) identifies seven guidelines for providers of services to ethnic minority children who have emotional and/or behavioral disorders. Vargas and Koss-Chioino (1992) discuss therapy with ethnic minority children and adolescents. Plucker (1996) provides information on counseling gifted Asian American children, and guidance for working with their parents. Robinson-Zanartu (1996) offers guidelines for evaluating and working with Native American children in the school system. Frasier et al. (1995) provide suggestions for improving the identification of giftedness among minority students who are underrepresented in the gifted population. Wright (1995) offers guidance for dealing with minority children with learning disabilities. Groce and Zola (1993) offer information about those with disabilities or chronic illness from culturally and linguistically diverse groups.

Counseling on Transracial Adoption

Several studies suggest that quite successful adjustment occurs in children who are transracially adopted, especially when the adoptions occur during their infancy (see, e.g., Simon et al., 1994; Vroegh, 1997; Bagley, 1993, in England; and Cederblad et al., 1999, in Sweden). Nonetheless, it is clear that these families often face unique challenges and stressors (Silverman & Feigelman, 1990). According to Okun (1996),

> The couple who decides to adopt across racial lines does so with the express knowledge that their decision will forever be a public one. The child's "difference" will be apparent to just about everyone the family encounters. In addition to the stresses that adoption puts on any family, transracial adoption places even further strain on the system. This pressure begins exerting an influence long before the child actually arrives, and forever alters the family system. (p. 237)

In addition to the typical issues raised by adoption, attention may be needed to the parents' assumptions and prejudices, the child's development of a sense of racial identity, the prejudices of others (including other family members), and the effects of these prejudices on the family and its support system. Okun's (1996) book is a good place to start learning more about some of the issues.

Work with Clients of Diverse Sexual Orientation

Although research shows that gays and lesbians seek out psychotherapy in disproportionately greater numbers than those who identify themselves as heterosexual, they tended to report less satisfaction with the services they received, at least until very recently ("Gays, Lesbians Seek . . . ," 1997). Up until perhaps the very recent present (Liddle, 1996), individuals who identify as themselves gay, lesbian, bisexual, or transsexual/transgendered (GLBT) have suffered from our profession's neglect, being rendered invisible by lack of research interest (Buhrke, 1989) and heterocentric theory (McGoldrick et al., 1996). Research has consistently found that a large proportion of individuals identifying themselves as GLBT screen therapists for pro-gay attitudes; that a large proportion of such clients prefer to enter treatment with therapists of a like orientation (Liddle, 1997); and that lesbians overwhelmingly (89%) prefer to see a female therapist. In finding therapists, GLBT-identified individuals have had to endure antitherapeutic, countertransferential, and even iatrogenic barriers engendered by constricted definitions of normality, homophobic attitudes, and "homoignorance" (John T. Patten, MD, cited in McGoldrick, 1996). If you can provide unbiased, sensitive, and knowledgeable services for GLBT-identified clients, you will have an important advantage over most therapists.

The many stressors associated with being part of a marginalized group provide coping challenges. GLBT-identified individuals may experience enormous stress and isolation related to their stigmatized status within a largely heterosexual society (Ritter & Terndrup, 2002). Higher rates of drug and alcohol abuse among those individuals (McKirnan & Peterson, 1989; Skinner, 1994); greater involvement in risky sexual behavior among gay and bisexual men (Lemp et al., 1994), with the attendant increased risk of HIV/AIDS; and higher rates of suicide among this population, particularly among youth (Gibson, 1989, cited in Fontaine et al., 1996) are all areas where our clinical skills can have a significant positive impact.

Cross-References to Related Specializations

Diversity can be cross-referenced with just about every niche presented in this book.

Subspecializations

Here are some examples of subniches related to diversity issues that can be developed:

- Corporate consulting on multicultural issues.
- Interventions for ethnic minority health.
- Counseling on adoptions by same-sex parents (see American Academy of Pediatrics, 2002).

Practice Models

All modalities can be employed. Specific ethnic or multicultural approaches have been utilized, but few outcome data exist on differential efficacy.

Practices with a multicultural focus could consider offering a selection of these services:

- Consultations to public and private sector businesses.
- Culturally relevant and adapted parent groups.
- Bilingual treatment in couple, family, and individual modes.
- Home, as well as office, visits.
- Culturally sensitive psychotherapy.

Financial Considerations

If you are comfortable in a managed care environment, you may be able to obtain a number of referrals by orienting your practice toward minority group members. Managed care organizations have shown eagerness for including such specializations (Zwillich, 1998).

Cautions, Ethical Dilemmas, Culture Clashes, and/or Managed Care Issues

If you work with members of diverse groups, remember that cultural competence is not optional but required by the code of ethics for psychologists, and that it will be expected of others as well (APA, 2002; Dworkin, 1992).

You must have a very clear understanding of your own prejudices, assumptions, and expectancies about families, culture, religion, what is "normal" or "healthy," and so forth to work effectively in this area. For example, according to Rosado and Elias (1993), a number of authors "have asserted that ethical and professional standards are violated when (a) there is a failure to formulate the presenting problems of Hispanics within their 'sociocultural matrix,' and (b) clinicians do not consider innovative or alternative treatment that can be more compatible with the world view, value orientation, or 'sociocentric realities' of Hispanic clients. Because of the diversity within the Hispanic population, Rosado and Elias go on to caution that psychologists must develop "an investigative, non-assumptive, and flexible stance concerning the characteristics of members of the various [Hispanic] groups with whom they work." This recommendation would appear to apply to other diverse minorities as well—for example, "Asians."

Be aware of cultural variations in expectations about your services. Lamenza (1999) discusses some possible culture clashes in working with ethnic minority patients, including negative stereotypes of mental health providers, the likelihood of drop-in patients (sometimes due to different views of time), high expectations of the initial appointment, and lack of awareness of mental health interventions in general. Specifically, for less acculturated clients, you should clarify expectations with regard to keeping appointments, timeliness, and phone calls; your respective roles, obligations, and boundaries; and the general process and goals of treatment (Rosado & Elias, 1993). An article by Garnets et al. (1991) is a resource on these issues for treating GLBT-identified clients.

PROSPECTS AND PROSPECTING

Where Is the Need?

The U.S. Bureau of the Census (2000) found that people of color constitute about one-quarter of the U.S. population. According to the National PTA (2002), the number of students with limited-English proficiency in our schools doubled between 1989 and 2000. Rosado and Elias (1993) point out that the Hispanic community has a growth rate four times that of the black community. These authors predict that, taken together with heightening stress levels in this population, this should lead to greatly increased demand for therapists for this already underserved population.

- Over 200,000 African Americans utilize mental health services each year (Manderscheid & Sonnenschein, 1990).
- According to Stanley Sue, the underutilization of psychotherapy services among Asian Americans is in contrast to their more severe levels of mental disturbances (Meadows, 1997). Not surprisingly, more highly acculturated Asian Americans are more accepting of counseling (Atkinson & Gim, 1989).
- In 2000, about 11.1% of the U.S. population was foreign born (U.S. Bureau of the Census, 2003); those states with the largest numbers of foreign-born persons were California (26.2%), New York (20.4%), New Jersey (17.5%), Florida (16.6%), and Texas (13.9%). But even if you do not live in one of these states, you may be personally aware of a group in your area in need of culturally competent services. For example, I (ELZ) was surprised at the large Spanish-speaking, primarily Puerto Rican population of Erie, Pennsylvania; I (RLL) was surprised to find that my community has a very high rate of cultural intermarriages.
- Native Americans have population concentrations in 34 states, not just in the western United States. You can obtain more information from the Indian Health Services (see "Online Resources," below).

Competition

Given the undersupply of culturally sensitive and informed therapists overall, competition is not a concern.

Reaching Clients/Directions for Marketing

- If you are not already so located, you might situate your practice in a locale with a significantly underserved ethnic population. A large proportion of some minority populations live in the central core of cities, others in specific suburbs, and still others in rural areas (see Niche 5.2).
- It will be important to be involved in the communities and ethnic groups to which you are offering services.
- To lower costs, consider beginning with a sublet or shared office.

INCREASING YOUR FORMAL KNOWLEDGE BASE

Core Readings

Work with Ethnic Minority Clients

Canino, I. A., & Spurlock, J. (2000). *Culturally diverse children and adolescents: Assessment, diagnosis, and treatment* (2nd ed.). New York: Guilford Press.
—Practical information on all aspects of clinical work with economically disadvantaged children and adolescents from ethnic minority groups.
Cuellar, I., & Paniagua, F. A. (Eds.). (2000). *Handbook of multicultural mental health: Assessment and treatment of diverse populations.* San Diego, CA: Academic Press.
—A very comprehensive volume, including chapters on influence of culture on pathology, Asian Americans, African Americans, Latinos/Latinas, American Indians/Alaska Natives, HIV/AIDS in diverse groups, culturally diverse elderly populations, and so on.
Falicov, C. J. (1998). *Latino families in therapy: A guide to multicultural practice.* New York: Guilford Press.
Hays, P. A. (2001). *Addressing cultural complexities in practice: A framework for clinicians and counselors.* Washington, DC: American Psychological Association.
Ivey, A. E., Ivey, M. B., & Simek-Morgan, L. (1997). *Counseling and psychotherapy: A multicultural perspective.* Boston: Allyn & Bacon.
Javier, R. A., & Herron, W. G. (Eds.). (1998). *Personality development and psychotherapy in our diverse society: A source.* Northvale, NJ: Aronson.
—Includes chapters on specific symptomatologies and treatment outcomes.
Lee, E. (Ed.). (1997). *Working with Asian Americans: A guide for clinicians.* New York: Guilford Press.
—Excellent guidance for assessment and treatment.
McGoldrick, M. (Ed.). (1997). *Re-visioning family therapy: Race, culture, and gender in clinical practice.* New York: Guilford Press.

McGoldrick, M., Giordano, J., & Pearce, J. K. (Eds.). (1996). *Ethnicity and family therapy* (2nd ed.). New York: Guilford Press.
— The standard reference on its topic, and very comprehensive.

Okun. B. F. (1996). *Understanding diverse families: What practitioners need to know.* New York: Guilford Press.

Okpaku, S. O. (1998). *Clinical methods in transcultural psychiatry.* Washington, DC: American Psychiatric Press.

Panaigua, F. A. (1998). *Assessing and treating culturally diverse clients: A practical guide* (2nd ed.). Thousand Oaks, CA: Sage.

Panaigua, F. A. (2000). *Diagnosis in a multicultural context.* Thousand Oaks, CA: Sage.

Ponterotto, J. G., Casas, J. M., Suzuki, L., & Alexander, C. M. (Eds.). (2001). *Handbook of multicultural counseling* (2nd ed.). Thousand Oaks, CA: Sage.

Sue, D. W., & Sue, D. (2003). *Counseling the culturally diverse: Theory and practice* (4th ed.). New York: Wiley.
— The latest edition of the book that is widely considered the best introduction to the area.

Suzuki, L. A., Meller, P., & Ponterotto, J. G. (Eds.). (2001). *Handbook of multicultural assessment: Clinical, psychological, and educational applications.* San Francisco: Jossey-Bass.

Work with GLBT-Identified Clients

D'Augelli, A. R., & Patterson, C. J. (Eds.). (2001). *Lesbian, gay, and bisexual identities and youth: Psychological perspectives.* New York: Oxford University Press.

Evosevich, J. M., & Avriette, M. (2000). *The gay and lesbian psychotherapy treatment planner.* New York: Wiley.

Laird, J., & Green, R. J. (Eds.). (1996). *Lesbians and gays in couples and families: A handbook for therapists.* San Francisco: Jossey-Bass Publishers.

Patterson, C. J., & D'Augelli, A. R. (Eds.). (1998). *Lesbian, gay, and bisexual identities in families: Psychological perspectives.* New York: Oxford University Press.

Perez, R. M., DeBord, K. A., & Bieschke, K. J. (Eds.). (2000). *Handbook of counseling and psychotherapy with lesbian, gay, and bisexual clients.* Washington, DC: American Psychological Association.

Ritter, K. Y., & Terndrup, A. I. (Eds.). (2002). *Handbook of affirmative psychotherapy with lesbians and gay men.* New York: Guilford Press.

Ryan, C., & Futterman, D. (1998). *Lesbian and gay youth: Care and counseling.* New York: Columbia University Press.

Journals

Work with Ethnic Minority Clients

Journal of Multicultural Counseling and Development
Psychological Intervention and Cultural Diversity
American Journal of Community Psychology
Journal of Community Psychology

Work with GLBT-Identified Clients

Journal of Homosexuality
Journal of Bisexuality
Journal of Gay and Lesbian Psychotherapy (the official journal of the Association of Gay and Lesbian Psychotherapists; abstracts are online at http://bubl.ac.uk/archive/journals/jgalp)
Journal of Lesbian Studies

Online Resources

The Educational Resources Information Center (ERIC) Clearinghouse provides annotated bibliographies and digests for multicultural issues in education online at http://www.askeric.org/eric/adv_search.shtml.

A list of principles for clinicians working with ethnic minorities is available online (http://www.serve.com/Wellness/culture.html) or by mail from the Bridge to Wellness Partial Hospitalization Program (645 Harrison Street, Suite 100, San Francisco, CA 94107; 415-284-9154; fax 415-284-9157). For health care providers, see another Web site (http://www.stfm.org/corep.html).

American Psychological Association Office of Ethnic Minority Affairs
http://www.apa.org/pi/oema/onlinebr.html
—Click on "Online Brochures" for various relevant online publications.

Bibliography
http://www.whittier.edu/psychology/links/prl.html
—A very well-organized 15-page bibliography on ethnic and other "diverse identities" can be found by clicking on "Academic Resources on the Internet," then "Diverse Identities," then "Diverse Identities Bibliography." Thank you, Chuck Hill, Professor of Psychology at Whittier College, for creating this resource.

Discover with Diversity Rx
http://www.diversityrx.org
—A clearinghouse of information addressing the language and cultural needs of minorities, immigrants, and refugees seeking health care.

Cultural Diversty in Health
http://www.diversityinhealth.com
—This site offers, under "Regions" and its subheadings, about a hundred succinct lists of characteristics and other essential information for understanding and being effective with members of other cultures—invaluable. The fact sheets under "Identity Issues" include "Torture & Trauma," "Refugees," "Gender," "Age," and "Religion" and are similarly informative as are the very helpful items under "General Diversity Tools." The links include sites devoted to Lao families, Romani (Gypsy), and many links to other organizations and resources.

Asian Studies WWW Virtual Library
http://coombs.anu.edu.au/WWWVL-AsianStudies.html

—A very rich source of links and information. An especially good site to start a search for information on any Asian or Pacific country.

Indian Health Service
http://www.ihs.gov
—The federal health program for American Indians and Alaska Natives. Useful for learning about the extensive programs and job openings.

American Civil Liberties Union
http://www.aclu.org/lesbiangayrights/lesbiangaryrightsmain.cfm
—If you want information on legal issues facing GLBT-identified clients, this site has everything.

Professional Organizations

The American Psychological Association has several divisions and sections of relevance. The Web sites for them are all of the same format (http://www.apa.org/divisions/div#, with the division number in place of "#" at the end).

Division 12 (Clinical Psychology) has a section on Clinical Psychology of Ethnic Minorities.

Division 17 (Counseling Psychology) has a section on Racial and Ethnic Diversity, and another on Lesbian, Gay, and Bisexual Awareness.

Division 44 (Society for the Psychological Study of Lesbian, Gay, and Bisexual Issues) publishes *Contemporary Lesbian and Gay Issues in Psychology* and provides *Guidelines for Psychotherapy with Lesbian, Gay, and Bisexual Clients*.

Division 45 (Society for the Psychological Study of Ethnic Minority Issues) publishes a newsletter and a journal, *Cultural Diversity and Ethnic Minority Psychology*.

Division 52 (International Psychology) is concerned with effective assessment and treatment approaches in different cultures as well as the types of psychological problems found in different cultures. Their newsletter, *International Psychology Reporter*, is published three times a year.

ASPIRA Association, Inc.
1444 I Street N.W., Suite 800, Washington, DC 20005; 202-835-3600; fax 202-835-3613
e-mail: info@aspira.org   http://www.aspira.org
—Fact sheets on Hispanic health, education, and violence, and a quarterly newsletter.

International Association for Cross-Cultural Psychology
http://www.fit.edu/CampusLife/clubs-org/iaccp

Association of Black Psychologists
P.O. Box 55999, Washington, DC 20040-5999; 202-722-0808
http://www.abpsi.org
—The Web site offers convention information, searchable directory of psychologists, etc.

Asian American Psychological Association
3003 North Central Avenue, Suite 103-198, Phoenix, AZ 85012; 602-230-4257
http://www.aapaonline.org
—Convention information and contacts are available at the Web site.

Association of Hispanic Mental Health Professionals
P.O. Box 7631, F.D.R. Station, New York, NY 10150-1913; 718-960-0208

Harry Benjamin International Gender Dysphoria Association
1300 South Second Street, Suite 180, Minneapolis, MN 55454; 612-625-1500; fax
     612-626-8311
http://www.hbigda.org
—This group's *Standards of Care for Gender Identity Disorders* has the most current information on the treatment of transgendered individuals, and the whole Web site is of great value.

Sport Psychology, Exercise, and Fitness

OVERVIEW AND OPPORTUNITIES

Sport has so many psychological facets that the combination of sport with psychology is perfectly natural. Whereas professional athletes and performers want to improve their efforts for fame and fortune, many others participate at all levels from semipro to amateur, and they can all benefit from behavioral interventions.

Sport psychology can help some clients improve the benefits of their practice time, reduce and eliminate negative and unhelpful thinking, focus better during performance, and coach and be coached more productively. Others, such as recreational joggers and bikers, want help with maintaining an exercise program. Then there are the millions who don't engage in an active lifestyle at present, but who would like help in doing so. Lastly, the desire for and funds spent on weight loss are extensive, and the outcomes are small and transient. Psychological interventions in this area can be very beneficial in several ways. It is easy to see that sport is an important aspect of life for many people and exercise is of even wider value. Psychologists have many effective ways to help people lead better lives through changes in this area.

The APA Task Force on Envisioning, Identifying, and Accessing New Professional Roles is bullish on sport psychology:

> Sports psychology is an emerging area embedded in a more general approach to enhanced performance (e.g., see Hays, 1995; Petrie & Diehl, 1995). Psychological techniques have been applied to performance of individuals and teams and to the development of team and interteam cohesion and cooperation.

These methods might be applied to community, business, and industrial groups. (Levant et al., 2001, p. 83)

Sophisticated and effective interventions exist to help individuals or teams to rehabilitate painful injuries, raise efficiencies, live healthier lives, pursue their passion for excellence, and continue to achieve their personal best in terms of physical or competitive accomplishments. Sport psychology services can be an extension of your more traditional psychotherapy services (see "Practice Models," below).

YOUR POTENTIAL SATISFACTIONS

- This is an opportunity to combine an interest in exercise or a sport hobby with your clinical skills to benefit those working for athletic achievements.
- Generally, you will be working with mentally healthy clients.
- This is an almost managed-care-free area.
- Due to the pervasiveness of participation in sports, fitness activities, and exercise in today's society, this specialty can be applied to many age groups and locations.

YOUR SKILL SET

Recycling Your Current Competencies

- Techniques with which you are probably already familiar, such as guided imagery, concentration/attentional skills training, and goal setting, are basic components of any sport clinician's approach to enhancing performance. You will only need to learn the specifics of sport psychology applications.
- In addition to your clinical skills and knowledge about the field of sport psychology per se, you should have a solid understanding of the sport each client is involved in, as well as a working knowledge of exercise physiology, biomechanics, and motor learning (Hays, 1995). Knowledge of the psychosocial aspects of sports—such as gender differences; the role of social support, coaching, and mentoring; and team-building principles—is also valuable.
- Interventions for weight control and treating eating disorder issues in athletes (Brownell et al., 1992) are relevant. Experience with eating disorders may open doors to work with athletes and dancers, just as substance abuse training may open other doors on college campuses.
- Techniques developed for the management of chronic or unpredict-

able pain are very useful for injured athletes. Coping methods and concepts of the psychological aspects of pain (Macchi, 1996; Gilbourne & Taylor, 1998) are also relevant to rehabilitation.

- Hypnosis (Morgan, 1993) has been utilized with exercise and sport.
- Substance abuse treatment and relapse prevention techniques are often needed.
- If you have firsthand experience with intensive training for a demanding sport or performance, you will have an advantage.

Retreading for Added Skills

The expansion of clinical practice into the arena of sport psychology has generated a continuing debate about qualifications of practitioners. Petrie and Diehl (1995) found that many psychologists practice in this area without specific training, and that many sports clinicians work in this field with only master's degrees. Nonetheless, those desiring to practice effectively should consider obtaining training and supervision when working in areas unfamiliar to them. See Sachs et al. (2000) or Van Raalte and Williams (1994) for information on graduate programs and training.

Credentialing is an additional option to increase the confidence of your clients and give you further proficiency (Hays, 1995). If you wish to obtain certification as a sport psychologist, you will need to undergo both training and supervision. Considerable time and financial commitment are involved in this undertaking. Coursework may involve one postdoctoral year. Hays (1995) notes that coursework is available online as well as in classrooms.

For psychologists, there are two national certification programs—one run by the Association for the Advancement of Applied Sport Psychology (AAASP), and one by the U.S. Olympic Committee (USOC). The AAASP offers certification as a Consultant in Sport Psychology.

AAASP certification will require education in general psychological principles and knowledge about the biological, cognitive–affective, social, and individual bases of behavior. In addition, you will need supervised practica, training for skills in counseling, knowledge of skills and techniques within sport or exercise, and supervised experience, with a qualified person, in the use of sport psychology principles and techniques. It is also necessary to have knowledge of the biomechanical and/or physiological bases of physical activity. For contact information for the AAASP, see "Professional Organizations," below.

The USOC has established standards for inclusion in its registry as a sport psychologist. You will need to be a member of the APA and have AAASP certification. You can learn more about the certification and the USOC registry by contacting Kirsten Peterson, PhD, Sport Psychology Program, USOC Sport Science and Technology, One Olympic Plaza, Colorado Springs, CO 80909; 719-578-4722

You can also gain skills and knowledge by attending the programs, courses, workshops, and symposia offered at the annual conventions of AAASP and Division 47 of APA (again, see "Professional Organizations," below).

NATURE OF THE WORK

Areas of Practice

Sport and psychology intersect in a surprisingly large number of areas.

Achieving Peak Performance

Depending somewhat on the sport, a great deal of an individual's performance can be accounted for by psychological variables and skills (Ungerleider, 1995). This has led to the development of theories and strategies that use psychological principles for maximizing athletic performance (e.g., Simek & O'Brien, 1981). Techniques include centering to focus one's attention, using imagery to enhance rehearsal and performance, and the assessment and modification of attributional style (Stinson et al., 2000). These techniques can help athletes at an amateur, elite, or professional level, as well as performers such as dancers.

Getting "psyched" is a heterogeneous area that includes the improvement of mental rehearsal effects, attention to an athlete's expectations and beliefs, and enhancing the athlete's coping with the intense emotions that arise during competition (Garza & Feltz, 1998). For example, athletes may lower their performance by self-talk that is either too pessimistic or overly optimistic, or they may cope poorly with a "slump" or "dry spell" in their performance (Grove & Heard, 1997).

Increasing Exercise Adherence

Clinicians are knowledgeable about cognitive, behavioral, social, and environmental factors that affect adherence to training regimens. Psychological concepts such as self-efficacy, focusing on positive outcomes, and locus of control, as well as a functional analysis of an individual's history of exercise success, can improve exercise regularity or intensity. Knowledge about gender differences, stages of change, and maximizing social supports can help athletes overcome barriers to exercise adoption (Hays, 1999).

The Use of Exercise as an Adjunct to Therapy

An easy entry into this area, for those already doing psychotherapy, is using exercise as an adjunct to treatment. Research is showing that regular exercise has positive effects on mood, and some therapists are incorporating it into their treatment to augment the outcomes (Hays, 1993, 1995, 1999). For example, exercising three times a week may be more effective than medication in relieving the symptoms of major depression in elderly people, and may also decrease the chances that the depression will recur over time (Babyak et al., 2000).

Health and Wellness Counseling

Psychologists can work with individuals and apply their methods to help people become healthier through physical activity (Morgan, 1997), improved nutrition, more effective rest and relaxation, and other life management skills. (See Niche 5.5 for more on this topic.) Clinicians can also help identify the early signs of burnout and substance abuse in athletes and institute interventions.

Rehabilitation of Injured Athletes

Clinicians can use their knowledge to assist in recovery from sports injury by raising adherence to rehabilitation procedures and offering pain management (Udry et al., 1997; Brewer, 1998). Dancers, for example, suffer high levels of injury (Kerr et al., 1992), and psychological reactions to injuries can be severely limiting in this group, according to Macchi (1996). Psychologists can use their knowledge of the relationship between stress and psychological factors to help prevent or contain damage (Williams & Andersen, 1998).

Cognitive and behavioral therapy techniques have been useful in coping with injury (Petitpas, 1998) and coping with forced retirement from sports (Grove et al., 1998). Depression is a risk whenever athletes—whether professional or amateur—must stop or decrease their participation in athletics. "Even injured weekend athletes are susceptible to depression, anxiety and other psychological symptoms, including nightmares, flashbacks to the accident, moodiness, irritability, fatigue, insomnia, weight gain and low self-esteem" (Tarkan, 2000, Sect. F, p. 7). Clinicians' skills in treating depression can help athletes who have to restrict their activities either as part of recovery from injury or illness, or when retirement is forced upon them.

Prevention or Treatment of Injuries from Overtraining

Athletes will often continue to train in an injured state (Shuer & Dietrich, 1997), overreach for impossible achievements, or overtrain. The results are often staleness, burnout, and further injury (Raglin, 1993). Clinicians who are knowledgeable about the psychological factors and ramifications can prevent these or treat the consequences.

Coach Effectiveness Training

Training coaches in techniques that enhance team performance, team spirit, and enjoyment of team sports is a developing area. Smith et al. (1979) and Kuchenbecker (1999; Kuchenbecker et al., 1999) found that training coaches to be more positive and less punitive improves the performance and enjoyment of participants.

Cross-References to Related Specializations

Niche 2.4. Competent and Resilient Girls
Niche 2.5. Clinical Interventions for Students and Schools
Niche 3.1. Treating Public Speaking Anxiety (see the "Treating Performance Anxieties" subspecialization)
Niche 5.5. Wellness and Positive Psychology

Subspecializations

Subspecializations can include assessment, referral (as necessary), and interventions for the following:

- Drug use by high school, college, and professional athletes.
- Obesity, weight management, dieting, eating disorders, body dysmorphic disorder, and similar issues.
- Exercise and fitness for those with chronic illness.
- Midlife fitness.
- Aging fitness.

Practice Models

For the present, full-time sport psychology practice is a rarity. If you are interested in becoming a practitioner, your expectation should be for a part-time practice or consultation, at least for the first few years (Hays, 2000).

Work settings can vary enormously. Clinicians in this area may practice in their offices, but they may also accompany athletes to training sessions. Sport medicine clinics, specialty training camps, and briefer programs offer additional opportunities that you might explore. You might work as part of a professional team in a rehabilitation setting, or work with sports teams and team building, and you might employ systems approaches in that work. Consultation on performance and sport psychology can be offered in physical fitness facilities of all kinds. See "Collaboration: Informal Health Club . . ." (2001) for a description of how one practitioner worked as part of a professional team at a health club.

Financial Considerations

Individual and group treatments and consulting fees are about as usual.

Cautions, Ethical Dilemmas, Culture Clashes, and/or Managed Care Issues

- Training and supervision are recommended in this area.
- Confidentiality and boundary issues can be problematic if you are working with coaches and other third parties who are involved with your client (Hays, 1995), so clarifications of boundaries and of who is your "client" are necessary from the start.
- See Sachs (1993) and Whelan et al. (2002) for a fuller description of the ethical issues in sport psychology practice. Petitpas (1998) discusses ethical areas of caution in work with sports medicine clinics.
- Injuries create medical information. HIPAA law is relevant.

PROSPECTS AND PROSPECTING

Where Is the Need?

Despite the evidence and the many areas of application, "only about 2 percent of sports medicine centers have psychologists available to help patients. . . . Although professional and Olympic athletes increasingly turn to sport psychologists, these experts are usually called on to improve the performance of great athletes, not to lift the moods of those on crutches" (Tarkan, 2000, Sect. F, p. 7).

Petrie and Diehl (1995) and Wildenhaus (1997) point to an increasing openness to the use of psychological interventions and sport psychology among athletes and professionals alike. Brewer (1998) predicts increasing opportunities for sport psychologists in clinical sport medicine.

Competition

There is much competition from lesser-trained individuals, especially those who have notable sports achievements. Although these may be inspiring, the techniques of heroes may not generalize to others. We all think that those who can do, can teach.

Reaching Clients

- Volunteering your time to work with local coaches and teams can provide you with credible experience as well as networking opportunities.

- Speaking engagements at camps devoted to specific sports are ways of reaching an already motivated audience.
- Although your sport psychology practice may be distinct from your psychotherapy work, previous and present clients may be interested in this area, because you have already established a relationship of trust.

Directions for Marketing

The consensus seems to be that this is not an area for practitioners who are averse to marketing and networking. A strong business sense and persistence, creativity, and self-direction are required for success in sport psychology practice (Wildenhaus, 1997). Clients frequently will not know how your credentials or skills qualify you to help them achieve their goals. Without using jargon, your educational and marketing efforts must clearly distinguish how you can utilize validated techniques to assist in such areas as adherence, peak performance, burnout prevention, recovery from injury, and improving coping skills.

- Network and explore synergies with college athletics departments, sport medicine clinics, physical rehabilitation clinics, massage therapists, high school athletic coaches, tennis and golf clubs, Little League coaches, and sport camps. Special-interest groups that focus on particular sports can be approached by the usual methods.
- National Physical Fitness and Sports Month (May), or Healthy Weight Week (in January), are some of the many good opportunities for your marketing efforts.

INCREASING YOUR FORMAL KNOWLEDGE BASE
Core Readings

Andersen, M. (Ed.). (2000). *Doing sport psychology*. Champaign, IL: Human Kinetics.
  —Covers all the bases including working with eating disorders, depression and suicidal athletes, injured athletes, and performing artists.
Brownell, K. D., Rodin, J., & Wilmore, J. H. (1992). *Eating, body weight, and performance in athletes: Disorders of modern society*. Philadelphia: Lea & Febiger.
Buckworth, J., & Dishman, R. (2002). *Exercise psychology*. Champaign, IL: Human Kinetics.
  —This book covers the mental health benefits of exercise as well as motivational aspects of exercise.
Hays, K. F. (1995). Putting sport psychology into (your) practice. *Professional Psychology: Research and Practice, 26*(1), 33–40.
Hays, K. F. (1999). *Working it out: Using exercise in psychotherapy*. Washington, DC: American Psychological Association.

Hays, K., & Chan, C. (Eds.). (2001). Sport psychology [Special section]. *Professional Psychology: Research and Practice, 32*(1), 5–39.

—Five high-quality articles explore the current status of work in this area.

Murphy, S. (Ed.). (1995). *Sport psychology interventions.* Champaign, IL: Human Kinetics.

Van Raalte, J. L., & Brewer, B. W. (Eds.). (2002). *Exploring sport and exercise psychology* (2nd ed.). Washington, DC: American Psychological Association.

Weinberg, R., & Gould, D. (1999). *Foundations of sport and exercise psychology* (3rd ed.). Champaign, IL: Human Kinetics.

—This textbook covers a vast array of introductory topics, and so is ideal for those who want a good review of the basics.

Williams, J. M. (Ed.). (2000). *Applied sport psychology: Personal growth to peak performance* (4th ed.). Palo Alto, CA: Mayfield.

Journals

Journal of Applied Sport Psychology
Journal of Sport and Exercise Psychology
The Sport Psychologist

Online Resources

American Kinetics Gateway to Sport Information
http://www.humankinetics.com

—This is the commercial site of a major publisher in the area; it is included here because it gives many links to conferences, associations, events, and careers in sport-psychology-related topics.

Professional Organizations

American College of Sports Medicine
P.O. Box 1440, Indianapolis, IN 46206-1440; 317-637-9200
http://www.acsm.org

—The Web site gives information on meetings, online journals (fee-based), a newsletter (no charge for online access), and products and brochures.

American Fitness Professionals and Associates (AFPA)
P.O. Box 214, Ship Bottom, NJ 08008; 609-978-7583
e-mail: afpa@afpafitness.com   http://www.AFPAfitness.com

—AFPA currently offers a variety of certifications in fitness-related areas. The Web site offers a wide variety of articles on the relationship among fitness, diet, exercise, and health, and a free subscription to the online newsletter.

International Society for Aging and Physical Activity (ISAPA)
Wojtek Chodzko-Zajko, PhD, ISAPA President, Professor and Head, Department of Kinesiology, University of Illinois at Urbana–Champaign, Louise Freer Hall, 906 S. Goodwin Avenue, Urbana, IL 61801; 217-244-0823
e-mail: wojtek@zajko.org   http://www.isapa.org

—According to the Web site, ISAPA is an international not-for-profit society promoting research, clinical practice, and public policy initiatives in the area of aging and physical activity." Browse abstracts from its journal and newsletter online.

Association for the Advancement of Applied Sport Psychology (AAASP)
801 Main Street, Suite 010, Louisville, CO 80027; 303-494-5931
http://www.aaasponline.org
—The *Journal of Applied Sport Psychology* is available online for members, along with a membership directory and newsletter.

The American Psychological Association has a division devoted to sport psychology, as well as two other divisions that are relevant:

Division 47 (Exercise and Sport Psychology)
http://www.psyc.unt.edu/apadiv47

Division 22 (Rehabilitation Psychology)
http://www.apa.org/divisions/div22

Division 38 (Health Psychology)
http://www.health-psych.org

Wellness and Positive Psychology

OVERVIEW AND OPPORTUNITIES

If you are like most practitioners, your professional involvement has focused on the amelioration of problematic behaviors, emotional states, and cognitive pathologies, with little attention to directly promoting positive mental states and actions. Seligman articulates this discrepancy sharply:

> Psychologists rarely think much about what makes people happy. They focus instead on what makes them sad, on what makes them anxious. That is why psychology journals have published 45,000 articles in the last 30 years on depression, but only 400 on joy. Joy is not covered by insurance, nor does it lead to tenure. (quoted in Hall, 1998, p. 9)

Similarly, Fredrickson (1998) comments that "psychologists have inadvertently marginalized the emotions, such as joy, interest, contentment, and love, that share a pleasant subjective feel," but emphasizes that such emotions "are central to human nature and contribute richly to the quality of people's lives" (p. 300). Positive emotions build personal resources by prompting individuals to try new approaches to situations, and they may actually counteract the effect of negative emotions and protect health (Fredrickson & Levenson, 1998). Some researchers are looking into other positive emotional states, such as pride (Fredrickson et al., 2000), elevation (Haidt, 2000), and gratitude (McCullough & Worthington, 1999).

Until recently, psychological growth and wellness were associated almost exclusively with humanistic psychology (Warmoth et al., n.d.) and received little empirical investigation. But the past decade has seen a steady increase in empirically based descriptions of positive emotional states, positive personality characteristics, and positive coping strategies. According to

Seligman and Csikszentmihalyi (2000, p. 12), "As positive psychology finds its way into prevention and therapy, techniques that build the positive traits will become commonplace . . . in therapy and perhaps more importantly in prevention."

Many of the skills and much of the knowledge we already possess can be helpful to clients in promoting positive mental states and emotional resilience. Work in this area can be described as personal development, coaching, or "making well people weller." It has such goals as becoming more creative, finding deeper meaning in work, being more productive in pursuit of personal goals, becoming more spiritual, achieving greater intimacy, and finding greater satisfaction in relationships.

YOUR POTENTIAL SATISFACTIONS

Have you always enjoyed exploring or been curious about this side of the human psyche? Have you believed that professional practice had to be restricted to the scope of the *Diagnostic and Statistical Manual of Mental Disorders*? It no longer is. Health, wellness, prevention, and growth constitute a burgeoning area of practice and need.

- You can be part of an exciting and expanding arena for psychological skills.
- You can apply your clinical skills to upbeat, positive areas with motivated clients.
- You can work outside "mental illness," "medical," and "deficits" models.
- This niche is managed-care-free and likely to remain so, because it is not diagnosis-based. It does not aim to return clients to a previous level of functioning and is not "medically necessary."

YOUR SKILL SET

Recycling Your Current Competencies

Commonly, cognitive and behavioral techniques are refocused for positive goals. Other techniques employed are relationship enrichment, assertiveness training, relaxation training, coaching skills, meditation, expressive interventions (e.g., dance, movement, art, and music), and focused expressive psychotherapy (Daldrup et al., 1988).

The biggest obstacles facing therapists with these skills who wish to work in wellness are their habits of mind: attending only to pathological affects and behaviors, and focusing on deficits and negatives.

NATURE OF THE WORK

Wellness work includes a wonderful variety of efforts.

Clinical work can focus on lifespan issues (e.g., successful transitions, midlife issues, aging well) and can be subniched by cultural group, gender, or sexual orientation.

Prevention, wellness, and growth interventions are also of interest to businesses. Some such interventions might include helping workers achieve career success, increase their workplace creativity, improve their "adversity quotient" (Stoltz, 1997), or raise their "emotional intelligence" or "emotional quotient" (EQ). Leadership training, or augmenting teamwork for optimum performance, are other possibilities.

Preventive interventions with children can include depression-proofing and resiliency-enhancing interventions.

Individual, group, family, and couple modalities can all be utilized.

Areas of Practice

Assessment

Assessment in this specialization focuses on strengths including emotional and other kinds of intelligence, resilience and coping, creativity and talent, intuitiveness, and life satisfaction. Therefore, traditional instruments are often irrelevant. Some commonly used instruments are these:

> Myers–Briggs Type Indicator (Myers et al., 1998).
> Attributional Style Questionnaire (for adults; Seligman, 1990).
> Children's Attributional Style Questionnaire (Seligman et al., 1995).
> Guilford–Zimmerman Temperament Survey (Guilford et al., 1976).
> Oxford Happiness Inventory (Argyle & Lu, 1990).
> Satisfaction with Life Scale (Pavot & Diener, 1993).

Prevention

Preventive interventions, particularly among high-risk groups, have been shown to reduce the frequency, duration, and/or intensity of emotional disorders. For example, Schweinhart and Weikart (1986) have demonstrated this in a school setting, and Dimeff et al. (1999) with screening for drinking behavior among college students. Preventive health interventions can include helping clients develop positive health behaviors related to exercise, dietary choices, sleep hygiene, sexual risk taking, substance use, and stress management.

Because of depression's extreme personal and social costs, the prevention of depression has received much attention (see, e.g., Jaycox et al., 1994; Gillham et al., 1995). In a striking example reported by Moon (2000), standard cognitive therapy methods that created optimism halved the expected rate of depression in both children and adults at as much as a 10-year follow-up. Taking a different approach, Beardslee et al. (1997) developed interventions for fostering resilience among children whose parents had mood disorders and who were thus at high risk for emotional problems.

Therapy

Foci of therapy using a wellness model could include the following:

- Exploring and enhancing subjective well-being, "flow" (Csikszentmihalyi, 1990), happiness (Lykken, 1999), and life satisfaction (with sensitivity to life stage).
- Understanding the behaviors and events that lead to positive emotions in a person's life, as in Fava's (1999) "well-being therapy" for mood disorders.
- Positive parenting, relationship enrichment, optimal family functioning.
- Integrative approaches, such as human–nature, mind–body, and individual–community interaction.
- Spirituality.

Cross-References to Related Specializations

Niche 2.1. Relationship Enrichment Programs
Niche 2.3. Gifted Children
Niche 2.4. Competent and Resilient Girls
Niche 3.3. Improving Work Performance
Niche 5.4. Sports Psychology, Exercise, and Fitness

Practice Models

Practitioners wishing to explore and develop this niche could proceed in a stepwise fashion by offering specialized services within an already existing private or group practice and expanding as opportunities or demands permit.

To launch a full-time practice in psychological growth, prevention, and wellness, you should consider including two or more of areas. You might offer specialty services for specific populations, such as adolescents, married people, singles, "midlifers," "transitioners," or preretirees. Services could be also be tailored for particular subpopulations (e.g., highly creative or high-

IQ persons) or those in a particular field (e.g., lawyers, performers, educators, or health care workers). Such services could be marketed to private individuals, businesses, community organizations, or educational institutions.

Multidisciplinary practice is another option. Working with others interested in growth, prevention, and wellness who have training in such fields as medicine, fitness, athletic coaching, nutrition, spiritual counseling, creativity and talent, substance abuse, human–animal bonding, trauma, coping/resilience, training/development, community development, or business management can augment creative synergies, accelerate your learning curve, and present exciting networking opportunities.

Financial Considerations

As noted earlier, this is a managed-care-free area of practice, so your usual fees and policies can apply.

Cautions, Ethical Dilemmas, Culture Clashes, and/or Managed Care Issues

Seligman (1998b) warns that there is currently a lack of serious science in this area, although much knowledge is available and it is growing. Some of the interventions discussed here have received only minimal empirical testing. It is essential that legitimate providers avoid overpromising, going beyond their data or beyond empirically supported theories, and misrepresenting or distorting what is known.

The APA has given its sanction to a major research consortium on positive psychology, and an APA book series on this topic is also planned. There has been a remarkable growth in PsycINFO abstracts of articles (searched for subject) on topics related to wellness and prevention (from 828 documents in 1990 to 1,849 in 2002). There has also been an increase in the number of persons who value prevention and wellness, auguring well for job growth in this area.

PROSPECTS AND PROSPECTING

Where Is the Need?

Surveys of consumers' use of nontraditional, complementary, and alternative health services indicate that members of the public are willing to pay out of pocket for care that they consider helpful and valid. Eisenberg et al. (1998) found utilization of these services increasing substantially between 1990 and 1997, and expenditures increasing 45.2% over the same period. More than half of these expenditures, some $12.2 billion, were paid for out of pocket.

Competition

See the discussion under "Cautions . . . ," above.

Reaching Clients/Directions for Marketing

We have mentioned "Cultural Creatives" in our introduction to this section. This would be a core group of clients seeking wellness and preventive health services. A *Journal of the American Medical Association* study (Astin, 1998) reported that Cultural Creatives use alternative health approaches and are identifiable by their commitment to environmentalism, feminism, spirituality, and personal growth psychology.

Marketing and networking possibilities include partnering with physicians interested in prevention and wellness and practitioners of alternative or nonmainstream approaches, as well as writing columns or advertising in periodicals that feature information on such approaches.

Publicity for your practice can be associated with such events as World Mental Health Day in October, or National Humor Month (April).

INCREASING YOUR FORMAL KNOWLEDGE BASE

Core Readings

Berger, R., & Hannah, M. T. (Eds.). (1999). *Preventive approaches in couples therapy.* Philadelphia: Brunner/Mazel.

Chang, E. C. (Ed.). (2001). *Optimism and pessimism: Implications for theory, research, and practice.* Washington, DC: American Psychological Association.

Csikszentmihalyi, M. (1990). *Flow: The psychology of optimal experience.* New York: Harper & Row.

Emmons, R. A. (1999). *The psychology of ultimate concerns: Motivation and spirituality in personality.* New York: Guilford Press.

Gillham, J. E. (Ed.). (2000). *The science of optimism and hope: Research essays in honor of Martin E. P. Seligman.* Philadelphia: Templeton Foundation Press.

Glantz, M. D., & Johnson, J. L. (Eds.). (1999). *Resilience and development: Positive life adaptations.* New York: Kluwer Academic/Plenum Press.

Goleman, D. (1998). *Working with emotional intelligence.* New York: Bantam.

Lopez, S., & Snyder, C. R. (Eds.). (2003). *Positive psychological assessment: A handbook of models and measures.* Washington, DC: American Psychological Association.

Lykken, D. (1999). *Happiness: What studies on twins show us about nature, nurture, and the happiness set-point.* New York: Golden Books.

Miller, W. R. (Ed.). (1999). *Integrating spirituality into treatment: Resources for practitioners.* Washington, DC: American Psychological Association.

Seligman, M. E. P., with Revich, K., Jaycox, L., & Gillham, J. (1995). *The optimistic child.* Boston: Houghton Mifflin.

Journals

Prevention and Treatment
American Journal of Preventive Medicine
Applied and Preventive Psychology
The Arts in Psychotherapy
Journal of Creative Behavior
Creativity Research Journal
Journal of Happiness Studies

Online Resources

You may want to explore some of the organizations that reflect Cultural Creatives' world view. Examples include Common Boundary (http://www.commonboundary.org), the Institute of Noetic Sciences (http://www.noetic.org), and the Institute for HeartMath (http://www.heartmath.org). To learn more about Cultural Creatives, try visiting the Cultural Creatives Web ring (http://www.ilovethisplace.com/webring/worldview.htm).

Ed Diener, University of Illinois
http://www.psych.uiuc.edu/~ediener
—Several articles on "subjective emotional well-being" and life satisfaction, as well as a comprehensive bibliography. The Satisfaction with Life Scale is also there.

World Database of Happiness
http://www.eur.nl/fsw/research/happiness
—This site is a "continuous register of scientific research on subjective appreciation of life," directed by Ruut Veenhoven, Erasmus University, Rotterdam, the Netherlands. It includes many readings, list of research, researchers, surveys, and reviews.

David G. Myers, Hope College
http://www.davidmyers.org
—Click on "The Pursuit of Happiness" for several articles and many links.

The Martin Seligman Research Alliance
http://psych.upenn.edu/seligman
—This research group's site lists grants and other resources in the areas of positive psychology, learned helplessness, depression, and optimism–pessimism.

EQ.org
http://www.eq.org
—This is a metasite for EQ/emotional intelligence studies and resources in education, research, assessment tools, and so on.

Professional Organizations

Association for Humanistic Psychology
1516 Oak Street, #320A, Alameda, CA 94501-2947; 510-769-6495; e-mail:
    ahpoffice@aol.com

FRIENDS-OF-PP (Positive Psychology) List
For professionals interested in positive psychology. To request membership in this
listserv, send an e-mail (kashdan@acsu.buffalo.edu).

Patient Education Materials: Online Resources, Printed Resources, and Organizations

Reivich, K., & Shatte, A. (2002). *The resilience factor: 7 essential skills for overcoming life's inevitable obstacles*. New York: Broadway Books.
 —Based largely on the work of Aaron Beck and Martin Seligman, a nuts and bolts approach to traversing the inevitable potholes in the road of life.
Seligman, M. (1990). *Learned optimism: How to change your mind and your life*. New York: Pocket Books.
 —His seminal ideas are here and accessible to the lay reader. A classic.
Seligman, M. (2002). *Authentic happiness: Using the new positive psychology to realize your potential for lasting fulfillment*. New York: Simon and Schuster.
 —Provides research-based advice, rating scales, and directions for a major attitude adjustments for readers. A companion Web site, http://www.authentic-happiness.org, complements the book.

Pet Loss Work and Animal-Assisted Therapy

OVERVIEW AND OPPORTUNITIES

We have placed the two topics of pet loss work and animal-assisted therapy (AAT) together, because they both concern animals. If you become involved with one topic, you can expand into the other. At some places below, we offer information unique to one but most of the information applies to both.

Pet Loss Work

While most people believe that active grieving over the death of a loved one is not only normal but healthy and necessary, many see grieving over the loss of a pet as somewhat childish or overly dramatic. They fail to understand the intensity, qualities, meanings, and history of the bond people often develop with their pets (or, less condescendingly, "companion animals"). Bonas et al. (2000) found similarities between human interrelationships and human–companion animal relationships. In a survey of pet owners (Cain, 1985), most respondents felt that pets were full family members, and almost all agreed on the importance of a pet's role in a family. Using a projective technique, Barker and Barker (1988, 1990) found that one-third of dog owners were emotionally closer to their dogs than they were to any other family member. In one survey, 84% of respondents said that they referred to themselves as their pets' "mom" or "dad"; 72% of married survey respondents greeted their pets first when they returned home; 63% celebrated their pets' birthdays; and 43% gave their pets wrapped gifts ("Survey Says: Owners Taking . . . , " 2000). Wessels (1984) reminds us that the role of the companion animal in a family system is important to consider:

> Numerous studies . . . depict pets in today's society as filling the role of surro-
> gate relatives. . . . In elevating pets in this way, they come to serve as substi-
> tutes for human relationships. Such substitutions run the course from replacing
> extended family members in a nuclear family society to serving as a sibling to
> an only child, to replacing the loss of a human relationship with a pet relation-
> ship. (p. 178)

Although clearly most people cope with the loss of a pet without seeking professional help, a minority exhibit severe grief. Archer and Winchester (1994) found that one-quarter of their survey sample of pet owners reported avoidance or mitigation strategies, and feelings of anger, anxiety, and de-pression following the death of a companion animal. In their social work practice ancillary to the Veterinary Hospital of the University of Pennsylva-nia, Quackenbush and Glickman (1984) reported seeing 14 cases of extreme bereavement reactions to pet loss. Rynearson (1978) discusses types of at-tachment to companion animals that may result in pathological grief reac-tions. Other evidence of the durability of this bond includes the fact that at a pet cemetery in Los Angeles, 60% of the graves receive flowers each week, according to a *Time* magazine article (Levy & Ru, 1993), and 15% of pet owners who have lost a pet say they will not get another one because the loss of a pet is too difficult psychologically (Wilbur, 1976). The proliferation of pet loss hotlines, Web sites, chat lines, and newsgroups is another indica-tor of many people's intense relationship with their pets (see, the "Pet Loss Therapy" section of "Online Resources," below).

Animal-Assisted Therapy

AAT goes beyond such activities as the petting of visiting animals by residents of institutions. AAT should be goal-directed, individualized to the patient, and directed by a therapist who documents progress. When pets are utilized in psychotherapy, they can provide an opportunity for patients to experience the emotions of simpler relationships; to recreate or project feelings; and to give or receive comfort for experiences of loss, loneliness, or closeness. For exam-ple, if you work with children or with difficult-to-reach adult populations, ani-mals can ease their transition from an isolated, nonverbal, alexythymic, de-pressed, or distrusting position to one of greater intimacy and satisfaction.

Despite the fact that animals have been informally employed in the treatment of psychiatric disorders for centuries, the belief that the human–animal bond could provide important psychological benefits has been little more than folklore until very recently. For example, Sigmund Freud kept chows in his office (Coren & Walker, 1997)-. Not only were Lun Yu, JoFi, and Lun dear to Freud's heart, but he sometimes incorporated them into his

interpretations to a patient (taking the potential sting out of a negative interpretation by acting as if the dynamic were between the patient and one of
the dogs). Levinson (1962) was one of the earliest to publish a paper in the
professional literature about the benefit of using pets in psychotherapy.
Findings to date consistently point to benefits of both pet ownership and
AAT—particularly with hard-to-reach populations, such as persons with autism (Law & Scott, 1995), prisoners (Lee, 1983), hospitalized psychiatric patients (Haughie et al., 1992; Barker & Dawson, 1998), patients with Alzheimer's disease (Fritz et al., 1995), and abused and withdrawn children
(Reichert, 1994). Furthermore, AAT has been employed for stress reduction
and for motivational purposes with a variety of populations in acute medical
care facilities (Barba, 1995), hospice care (Chinner & Dalziel, 1991), and
physical rehabilitation[1] for spinal cord injury (Counsell et al., 1997).

Pets appear to be stress buffers for their owners. This buffering may be
particularly important to individuals who have suffered abuse as children.
In a retrospective study, Barker et al. (1997) found that animal companions
during childhood were the only reported support for some sexual abuse survivors. Among another group of abuse survivors, Nebbe (1998) found lower
anger levels and less abuse behavior among those who had a strong bond
with a pet during childhood.

YOUR POTENTIAL SATISFACTIONS

AAT and pet loss work will be attractive to clinicians who would like to combine an interest in human–animal interaction with their psychotherapy
practices.

YOUR SKILL SET

Recycling Your Current Competencies

- Knowledge of and experience with grief therapy is basic for work
  with pet loss.
- You should be familiar with the literature and research on the complex relationships between humans and companion animals.

---

[1]Therapeutic horseback riding has become more popular for patients with various physical disorders, and for those with autism. From my experience (ELZ), I would note that caring for large
animals can be quite therapeutic, and that training such animals requires and stimulates very
high levels of empathy, consistency, and responsibility.

- Using an animal to assist your therapy is an extension of your current treatment methods and skills. There is little empirical literature, but many case examples and vignettes are available to supply ideas about how you might utilize an animal in therapy.

Retreading for Added Skills

Although there is presently no requirement for additional therapists' certification for AAT or pet loss counseling, there are programs that train and certify animals for work in therapeutic settings. State-by-state resources for training animals are listed by the Latham Foundation. Training in AAT is available for you and your animal from organizations such as Therapet or the Delta Society; costs vary. (See "Professional Organizations," below, for more information on these three groups.)

NATURE OF THE WORK

Clinical work with clients who have lost a pet is similar to that with clients who are grieving the loss of a significant person in their life. Because of society's tendency to dismiss the emotional importance of the human–animal bond, however, clinicians will need to be especially sensitive to the client's possible embarrassment, minimizing, or denial of grief feelings (Sharkin & Knox, 2003). Another potential clinical focus is guilt about real or imagined responsibility for the pet's death. Circumstances such as sudden loss, euthanasia, negligence or maltreatment of the pet, or unresolved grief over previous losses will demand special clinical attention.

In AAT animals are partners in helping clinicians help clients. Depending on the specifics of the client, the situation, and the therapy goals, a relationship with a therapy animal can accelerate rapport building, be a catalyst for emotional expression, or serve as a model for more complex human relationships (Fine, 2000). The relationship with a therapy animal might also serve to motivate some clients (particularly children), buffer stressful aspects of psychotherapy, or provide less threatening ways of talking about difficult feelings. If you are considering entering this niche, learn all that you can about its practical aspects, such as selecting and training animals, risk management strategies and the associated costs, and animal maintenance and health.

For those already doing grief counseling, pet loss work represents an opportunity to extend one's services to a related population. Vulnerable children who have lost a pet may represent an important subpopulation.

Cross-References to Related Specializations

Niche 1.2. Supporting Caregivers and Working with Chronic Illnesses
Niche 1.3. Working with Dying and Grieving People
Niche 5.1. Gerontology and Services to Aging Individuals

Subspecialization

Treating Those Who Abuse Animals

Although we are all horrified by reports of abused, neglected, and tortured animals, few perpetrators are prosecuted, fewer receive deterring punishments, and almost none receive mental health treatments designed to prevent recurrence. Currently, perpetrators of three types are commonly seen:

1. "Hoarders," or collectors of too many animals to care for. Most often, hoarders are middle-aged women who become overwhelmed with the burden of caring for the increasing numbers they take in; they are also often repeat offenders.
2. Children harming or killing animals. Animal abuse is very highly correlated with later antisocial behavior, violence, and other kinds of abuse of humans (Felthous & Kellert, 1987). Early intervention in such cases can be very beneficial for all concerned.
3. Adults harming or killing animals as part of family violence, such as child, elder, or spouse/partner abuse (Boat, 1995).

Obviously, each type of perpetrator will require different treatment approaches. Contacting your local animal protection officers or organizations (e.g., the Humane Society, the Society for Prevention of Cruelty to Animals) can result in referrals. Cases are present in every community, and law enforcement and judicial personnel usually do not know where to refer perpetrators.

Training in the treatment of animal abuse perpetrators has been developed and provided in California by Lynn Loar, PhD, LCSW, and Randy Lockwood of the Humane Society of the United States (contact the Mental Health Institute in Palo Alto at 650-321-3055 or http://www.mri.org). The group Psychologists for the Ethical Treatment of Animals (PSYETA) has produced a 90-page practitioner's handbook called *AniCare*, for use with children who abuse animals (this is available in both print and CD-ROM versions from http://www.psyeta.org/anicarechild.html, or from PSYETA at P.O. Box 1297, Washington Grove, MD 20880; 301-963-4751). There is also a version for use with adults, *The AniCare Model of Treatment for Animal Abuse*.

You could develop interventions for animal abuse that veterinarians and shelters can utilize. Ascione (1992) is an example of one such intervention for school children. The Latham Foundation has intervention materials available for use with animal abusers.

Practice Models

Pet Loss Work

Pet loss counseling or other work is usually done in the clinician's office, although arrangements with a veterinarian to be available at specific hours or as a consultant are certainly possible as well.

Animal-Assisted Therapy

AAT is varied in its application. In some programs, clients work intensively with animals, taking responsibility for training, grooming, exercise, and feeding. Other programs (e.g., geriatric) involve a therapy animal's "visiting" with people on a daily or weekly basis. Still other applications could involve inpatient, partial hospital, therapeutic school, and forensic settings. See some of the examples under "Where Is the Need?", below, for ideas and resources.

Financial Considerations

You will be able to charge your usual fees for AAT and for grief counseling involved in pet loss treatment if a client's suffering meets a diagnosis and you provide psychotherapy. Other services could be on contract or *pro bono*.

Cautions, Ethical Dilemmas, Culture Clashes, and/or Managed Care Issues

You will need to obtain liability insurance for any animals you utilize, particularly in order to gain approval to conduct AAT at a facility other than your office. Obtaining liability coverage for an animal may require that the animal be certified by a recognized organization such as the Delta Society. Information on liability coverage is available from those organizations that do training. Also, check with your professional liability insurance provider. Hospital staff members may rightly be concerned about animal-borne diseases, but the data are available to show that these can be easily handled. Again, they may require that the animal be certified by one of the several training programs.

According to an online article by Nolen (2000), additional signs of the increased acceptance of the human–animal bond include the following:

- State regulations barring animals from health care facilities are being lightened, allowing animal-assisted activity and AAT programs for residents and patients in these facilities.
- It is illegal to discriminate against persons requiring assistance from service animals (usually Seeing-Eye Dogs for blind persons, or "assistance dogs" or other animals [e.g., monkeys] for persons who use wheelchairs). Working with other groups, the Delta Society has helped to open hospital doors to therapy animals.
- Federal housing regulations currently allow elderly and disabled individuals living in federally subsidized units to keep their pets, and the American Veterinary Medical Association (AVMA) is lobbying for this to be extended to all residents.

PROSPECTS AND PROSPECTING

Where Is the Need?

Pet Loss Work

There are large numbers of pets, and so there are large numbers of deaths. Fifty million contacts are made with veterinarians each year, and two million involve the death of an animal. An average small-animal vet practice experiences three or four pet deaths a week from illness, accident, or euthanasia. These deaths can be stressful for the veterinarian and owners alike (Stewart, 1999). Budgin (1997) reports that 40% of veterinary clients change veterinarians due to dissatisfaction stemming from the death or euthanasia of their pets, and so veterinarians should be quite interested in your services. For example, Cornell University offers a pet loss hotline (http://www.vet.cornell.edu/public/petloss/).

Animal-Assisted Therapy

The projects described below should give you ideas of where AAT can be applied and there are literally hundreds more programs.

- Mary Jacobs, a school psychologist, does AAT with autistic adults in a sheltered workshop environment according to an article in *Psychotherapy Finances* ("Animals Can Assist . . . ," 1996). Jacobs says that an autistic adult forms a "nonverbal bond" with a therapy animal. She also conducts play therapy with hospitalized children, in which the children get a chance to play "veterinarian" with the therapy dog—an empowering experience for a sick child, says Jacobs.

- The Northeast Rehabilitation Health Network (see "Online Resources," below) in Salem, New Hampshire, uses pets in movement, socialization, and speech therapy for patients undergoing rehabilitation.
- Paws for Health, the Pet Visitation Program of the Children's Medical Center, Medical College of Virginia Hospitals (see "Online Resources," below), utilizes pet-assisted therapy to reduce the traumatic effects of hospitalization for children and to help make their hospital stay a more positive experience.
- At the National Institutes of Health, AAT is utilized for child and adult populations with cancer, HIV, epilepsy and other neurological disorders, heart disorders, schizophrenia and other mental health disorders, and many other conditions. AAT interventions utilized with children focus on lowering anxiety during painful medical procedures, reducing regressive behaviors, and improving compliance with medical procedures (Parker, n.d.).

Competition

- Many veterinarians and humane organizations offer pet loss information, and some offer hotlines and support groups, but very few offer individual or group therapy.
- Recreational and occupational therapists may offer animal-assisted activities in medical and rehabilitation settings, but these are obviously not psychotherapy.
- In mental health, others with lesser degrees and training may also offer these services. Competition with AAT may also involve volunteers who conduct animal-assisted activities, although smaller medical and mental health facilities often are not able to utilize volunteers due to insurance considerations. If you are interested in this area, consider joining with some of the organizations or professionals mentioned in this niche to create a comprehensive AAT program.

Reaching Clients/Directions for Marketing

Pet Loss Work

You can provide a valuable service to veterinarians if you let them know about your practice. Veterinarians who are not comfortable dealing with the strong emotional reactions sometimes seen with the death of a pet may value having the name of someone to whom they can refer their clients. You can send announcements about your specialties to the veterinarians in your locale. Include with your announcement other informative material about grief and how veterinarians can determine when to suggest a referral. Review published materials (see "Core Readings, below) to tailor your materials and approach.

- Offer a presentation or article to your local veterinary organization. Coordinate articles or presentations in your local newspaper with National Pet Week (which is usually in May; dates vary slightly by year). This event is publicized by the AVMA, so you will benefit from its advertising efforts.
- "Vet stress" is not talked about a lot, but vets experience personal stressors related to euthanizing unwanted but healthy pets, reporting suspected pet abuse, giving bad news to families, interacting with some pet owners and office staff, and dealing with business pressures. Writing an article for your local veterinary association on these topics can help get your practice specialty known.
- Many pet adoptions and purchases do not work out well. You could collaborate with vets and animal shelters on maximizing "successful adoptions" of homeless pets. Kidd et al. (1992) showed a significant increase in the rate of successful adoptions after a brief educational intervention that helped potential owners understand what was involved in caring for a pet. This is unlikely to be compensated, but may help you build your practice.
- Disasters such as hurricanes and floods result in pet losses. The AVMA and the American National Red Cross have joined in an official effort to help rescue companion animals injured or threatened by disasters (AVMA, 1998). This is an opportunity for clinicians interested in pet loss issues and disaster response.
- Your local Humane Society can be a referral resource, as can other local animal organizations. You can announce your specialty and provide informative materials, such as articles and fact sheets at their Web sites or offices.
- The Pet Loss Support Web site (see "Online Resources," below) offers a free, camera-ready brochure entitled *Ten Tips on Coping with the Loss of Your Pet* by Moira Anderson Allen, MEd, which you can have personalized and can then utilize in your marketing efforts.
- Periodically running a brief group on pet loss, and letting local veterinarians and others know about it, can also build up a practice specialty.

Animal-Assisted Therapy

- As a provider of new services, you will need to prove their value. Whether you want to work with schools, hospitals, rehabilitation clinics, geriatric facilities, at-risk adolescents, or populations with autism or other psychiatric disorders, you will probably need to give away some services at first in order to build references and referrals, and to develop the experience and expertise of working with your chosen population.
- Develop a brochure describing your services, so that you will have materials to leave with each contact person or at each organization you visit.
- Offer a presentation on the psychological aspects of animals or the human–companion animal bond to local organizations. A few days after a presentation, make a follow-up phone call to express your appreciation, address any other questions or needs, and inquire about any further opportunities.
- A quarterly newsletter describing your activities and some relevant news items will help to remind your contacts of your availability. You can ask your contacts to post the newsletter in their waiting room, note it in their own publications, or offer it to specific potential clients.
- Once you have launched your AAT practice, you might consider creating a video that demonstrates your program, to give to potential referrers and clients.
- Press releases are another inexpensive way of getting information out about your practice.

INCREASING YOUR FORMAL KNOWLEDGE BASE

Core Readings

Pet Loss Work

Kay, W. J., Nieburg, H. A., Kutscher, A. H., & Kutscher, L. G. (Eds.). (1984). *Pet loss and human bereavement*. Ames: Iowa State University Press.
—This volume has articles by the leaders in this area and a section of use to veterinarians.
Nieburg, H. A., & Fischer, A. (1996). *Pet loss: A thoughtful guide for adults and children*. New York: HarperPerennial.
—This book is written from the perspective of psychotherapists.
Ross, C. B., & Baron-Sorensen, J. (1998). *Pet loss and human emotion: Guiding clients through grief*. Philadelphia: Accelerated Development.
—A step-by-step guide for all kinds of professionals to guide the grieving process.

Animal-Assisted Therapy

Abdill, M. N., & Juppe, D. (Eds.). (1997) *Pets in therapy*. Ravensdale, WA: Idyll Arbor.
—A collection of articles on starting a program, sample forms, regulations and policies, stories and program evaluations.

Arkow, P. (1998). *Pet therapy: A study and resource guide for the use of companion animals in selected therapies* (8th ed.). (Available from Phil Arkow, 37 Hillside Rd., Stratford, NJ 08084; for information, e-mail parkow@phlfound.org)
—Arkow is one of the originators of, and leaders in, this area.

Ascione, F. R., & Arkow, P. (Eds.). (1998). *Child abuse, domestic violence, and animal abuse: Linking the circles of compassion for prevention and intervention*. West Lafayette, IN: Purdue University Press.

Bernard, S. (1995). *Animal assisted therapy: A guide for health care professionals and volunteers*. Whitehouse, TX: Therapet.

Davis, K. D. (1992). *Therapy dogs*. New York: Howell Books.
—This handbook for animal-assisted activities and AAT is sponsored by the Delta Society.

Douglas, C. (n.d.). *How to start a people–pet partnership*. (Available from People–Pet Partnership, College of Veterinary Medicine, Pullman, WA 99164-7010; 509-335-1303, 509-335-4569;; e-mail to douglasc@wsuvm1.csc.wsu.edu)

Fine, A. (Ed.). (2000). *Handbook of animal-assisted therapy: Theoretical foundations and guidelines for practice*. San Diego, CA: Academic Press.
—This volume is a very broad and high-quality collection, perfect for an overview and getting started (with assessment tools, guidelines, etc.).

Lebeck, S. L. (1990). *How to set up an animal-assisted therapy program in a psychiatric facility*. Albany, CA: Friendship Foundation.

Levinson, B. M. (rev. by Mallon, G. P.). (1997). *Pet-oriented child psychotherapy* (2nd ed.). Springfield, IL: Thomas.
—A good clinical introduction to the many uses of pets in child and family therapy and in assessment.

Serpell, J. (Ed.). (1996). *The domestic dog: Its evolution, behaviour, and interactions with people*. New York: Cambridge University Press.

Stewart, M. F. (1999). *Companion animal death: A practical and comprehensive guide for veterinary practice*. Boston: Butterworth–Heinemann.
—This book, designed for the veterinarian, provides guidance on how to deal with emotions, actions, and ethics.

Journals

Anthrozoös
Animal Welfare
Animals and Society
Animal Behaviour
The Lantham Letter
Journal of the American Veterinary Medical Association

Online Resources

Pet Loss Work

College of Veterinary Medicine, Michigan State University
http://www.cvm.msu.edu/petloss/index
—Volunteer counselor services and other kinds of support are available, as well as readings and links.

Pet Loss Support Page
http://www.pet-loss.net
—This site provides access to many fine resources and an excellent brochure, *Ten Tips on Coping with the Loss of Your Pet* (see "Reaching Clients/Directions for Marketing," above).

Melanie's Rainbow Bridge
http://www.fortunecity.com/millenium/rainbow/65
—This site includes a fine set of links to resources for pet loss, including rescuing,[2] ceremonies, and grief support.

Ken Pope, PhD
http://kspope.com
—Pope is a psychologist who maintains an extensive list of pet resources, including resources on pet loss, service animals, and pet care.

Animal-Assisted Therapy

Paws for Health: The Pet Visitation Program, Children's Medical Center, Medical College of Virginia Hospitals
http://views.vcu.edu/paws
—Paws for Health is a good example of a pediatric inpatient visitation AAT program. Although it is a volunteer program, there is much information about requirements for participating in the program that you may find helpful.

Northeast Rehabilitation Health Network
http://www.northeastrehab.com/Programs/aft.htm
—This site provides a wealth of information on the use of AAT in medical care and rehabilitation.

---

[2]You may not know of the hundreds of organizations—mostly local and informal, but some widely recognized—that engage in the "rescue" of particular breeds of pets (such as Collie Rescue) or animals in harm's way (such as Farm Animal Rescue) or wounded wild animals (wildlife rehabilitators, with federal licenses). If you wish to adopt a pure-bred (and thus more predictable) pet at little cost, or would like to do some good in this area, investigate these organizations; some have Web sites (try a search at http://www.google.com). Or contact your local shelters (basically for dogs and cats), county humane officers, animal control officers, or veterinarians.

Professional Organizations

Canine Companions for Independence (CCI), National Headquarters
P.O. Box 446, Santa Rosa CA, 95402-0446; 800-572-2275 (V/TDD)
http://www.caninecompanions.org
—CCI is a nonprofit organization that provides highly trained assistance dogs to people with disabilities and to professional caregivers providing AAT.

Delta Society: Pet Partners Programs
289 Perimeter Rd. East, Renton, WA 98055; 800-869-6898; fax 206-235-1076
http://www.deltasociety.org
—The Delta Society provides consultation, continuing education, and many relevant publications. A major resource, it offers a home study course, the *Pet Partners Volunteer Training Manual*, training for human service providers, and other courses.

Latham Foundation
Latham Plaza Building, Clement and Schiller Streets, Alameda, CA 95401; 510-
    521-0920; fax 510-521-9861
e-mail: LATHM@aol.com   http://www.latham.org/
—This group is a superb resource for literature and educational materials focused on the human–companion animal bond and abuse prevention.

Therapet
P.O. Box 1696, Whitehouse, TX 75791
e-mail: Therapet@Juno.com   http://www.therapet.com
—Therapet is involved in education and training of health care professionals, evaluation and training of animals and the establishment of AAT programs. They provide publications, seminars, and professionally developed videos. They have also developed an AAT program with psychiatric inmates.

Patient Education Materials: Online Resources, Printed Resources, and Organizations

All of the following books concern pet loss, and all except the Sife book are intended for children.

Rogers, F. (1988). *Mr. Rogers' first experience: When a pet dies.* New York: Putnam.
Sibbitt, S. (1991). *Oh, where has my pet gone?: A pet loss memory book.* Wayzata,
    MN: B. Libby Press.
Sife, W. (1998). *The loss of a pet* (rev. ed.). New York: Hungry Minds.
Viorst, J. (1971). *The tenth good thing about Barney.* New York: Atheneum.
Wilhelm, H. (1985). *I'll always love you.* New York: Crown.

References

Not all of the works cited in each niche's "Core Readings" are included here.

Aber, J. L. (1999). *Teaching conflict resolution: An effective school-based approach to violence prevention.* New York: National Center for Children in Poverty. (Available from the NCCP Publication Office, 212-304-7195, or at http://www.nccp.org)

Ablard, K. E., & Parker, W. D. (1997). Parents' achievement goals and perfectionism in their academically talented children. *Journal of Youth and Adolescence, 26* (6), 651–667.

Ables, N., & American Psychological Association (APA) Working Group on the Older Adult. (1997). *What practitioners should know about working with older adults.* Washington, DC: American Psychological Association.

Abrams, W. B., Beers, M. H., & Berkow, R. (Eds.). (1995). *Merck geriatric manual* (2nd ed.). Whitehouse Station, NJ: Merck Research Laboratories. (Also available at http://www.merck.com/pubs/mm_geriatrics)

Accordino, M. P., & Guerney, B., Jr. (1998). An evaluation of the Relationship Enhancement® Program with prisoners and their wives. *International Journal of Offender Therapy and Comparative Criminology, 42*(1), 5–15.

Ackley, D. (1997). *Breaking free of managed care: A step-by-step guide to regaining control of your practice.* New York: Guilford Press.

Administration on Aging, U.S. Department of Health and Human Services. (1998). *The National Elder Abuse Incidence Study: Final report* [Online]. Available: http://www.aoa.dhhs.gov/abuse/report

Alabama Associated Resources Corporation. (n.d.). *Shoplifters alternatives* [Online]. Available: http://www.court-referral.com/shoplifting.htm

Albert, M. S., Savage, C. R., Jones, K., Berkman, L., Seeman, T., Blazer, D., & Rowe, J. W. (1995). Predictors of cognitive change in older persons: MacArthur studies of successful aging. *Psychology and Aging, 10*(4), 568–589.

Albert, R. S., & Runco, M. A. (1986). The achievement of eminence: A model based on a longitudinal study of exceptionally gifted boys and their families. In R. J. Sternberg & J. E. Davidson (Eds.), *Conceptions of giftedness* (pp. 332–357). Cambridge, England: Cambridge University Press.

Alday, C. S., Boergers, J., Jelalian, E., & Frank, R. (1999). *Physician survey of attitudes and practices related to pediatric obesity.* Paper presented at the 107th Annual Convention of the American Psychological Association, Boston.

Allen, M., Hunter, J. E., & Donohue, W. A. (1989). Meta-analysis of self-report data on the effectiveness of public speaking anxiety treatment techniques. *Communication Education, 38*(1) 54–76.

Allen, R. F., & Pilnick, S. (1973). Confronting the shadow organization: How to detect and defeat negative norms. *Organizational Dynamics, 1*(4), 2–18.

Alsop, G. (1997). Coping or counseling: Families of intellectually gifted students. *Roeper Review, 20*(1), 28–34.

Altmaier, E. M., Ross, S. L., Leary, M. R., & Thornbrough, M. (1982), Matching stress inoculation's treatment components to client's anxiety mode. *Journal of Counseling Psychology, 29*(3), 331–334.

Alto, W. A. (1995). Prevention in practice. *Primary Care, 22*(4), 543–554.

Ambrosini, P. J., Bianchi, M. D., Rabinovich, H., & Elia, J. (1993). Antidepressant treatments in children and adolescents: I. Affective disorders. *Journal of the American Academy of Child and Adolescent Psychiatry, 32,* 1–6.

American Academy of Child and Adolescent Psychiatry. (1999, November 2). *News release: November marks inaugural National Child Mental Health Month* [Online]. Available: http://www.aacap.org/press_releases/1999/ncmhm.htm

American Academy of Family Physicians. (1995, August). *Position paper on the provision of mental health care services by family physicians* [Online]. Available: http://www.aafp.org/practice/mental_f.html

American Academy of Pediatrics, Committee on Psychosocial Aspects of Child and Family Health. (2001). The new morbidity revisited: A renewed commitment to the psychosocial aspects of pediatric care. *Pediatrics, 108*(5), 1227–1230.

American Academy of Pediatrics, Committee on Psychosocial Aspects of Child and Family Health. (2002, February). Technical report: Coparent or second-parent adoption by same-sex parents. *Pediatrics, 1093,* 339–340. (Also available at http://www.aap.org/policy/020008.html)

American Association of University Women (AAUW). (2001). *Hostile hallways II: Bullying, teasing, and sexual harassment in school.* Washington, DC: Author.

American Council for Drug Education. (1999). *Facts for employers* [Online]. Available: http://www.acde.org/employer

American Family Business Survey [Online]. (2002). Available: http://www.raymondinstitute.org/knowledge/research/AFBSresults_97.pdf

American Psychological Association (APA). (1993). Guidelines for providers of psychological services to ethnic, linguistic, and culturally diverse populations. *American Psychologist, 48,* 45–48. (Also available at http://www.apa.org/pi/oema/guide.html)

American Psychological Association (APA). (2000). *Psychology is a behavioral and mental health profession* [Online]. Available: http://www.apa.org/ppo/issues/ebsprofession.html

American Psychological Association (APA) Practice Directorate. (2001). *Medical cost offset* [Online]. Available: http://www.apa.org/practice/offset3.html

American Psychological Association (APA). (2002). *Ethical principles of psychologists and code of conduct* [Online]. Available: http://www.apa.org/ethics/code2002.html

American Psychological Association (APA) Practice Directorate, with Coopers & Lybrand, LLP. (1996). *Marketing your practice: Creating opportunities for success*. Washington, DC: American Psychological Association.

American Veterinary Medical Association (AVMA). (1998, March 1). *AVMF team with Red Cross to provide disaster relief* [Online]. Available: http://www.prweb.com/releases/1998/prweb3837.php

Ames, G., Grube, J., & Moore, R. (1997). Relationship of drinking and hangovers to workplace problems: An empirical study. *Journal of Studies on Alcohol, 58*(1), 37–47.

Amminger, G. P., Pape, S., Rock, D., Roberts, S. A., Ott,S. L., Squires-Wheeler, E., Kestenbaum, C., & Erlenmeyer-Kimling, L. (1999). Relationship between childhood behavioral disturbance and later schizophrenia in the New York High-Risk Project. *American Journal of Psychiatry, 156*(4), 525–530.

Animals can assist in the therapy process. (1996, November). *Psychotherapy Finances*, pp. 2–3.

Anton, W. D., & Klisch, M. C. (1995). Perspectives on mathematics anxiety and test anxiety. In C. D. Spielberger & P. R. Vagg (Eds.), *Test anxiety: Theory, assessment, and treatment* (pp. 93–106). Philadelphia: Taylor & Francis.

Antonuccio, D. O., Danton, W. G., & DeNelsky, G. Y. (1995). Psychotherapy versus medication for depression: Challenging the conventional wisdom with data. *Professional Psychology: Research and Practice, 26*(6), 574–585.

Arathuzik, D. (1994). Effects of cognitive-behavioral strategies on pain in cancer patients. *Cancer Nursing, 17*(3), 207–214.

Archer, J., & Winchester, G. (1994). Bereavement following death of a pet. *British Journal of Psychology, 85*(Pt. 2), 259–271.

Argyle, M., & Lu, L. (1990). The happiness of extraverts. *Personality and Individual Differences, 11*(10), 1011–1017.

Arnstein, P., Caudill, M., Mandle, C. L., Norris. A., & Beasley, R. (1999). Self efficacy as a mediator of the relationship between pain intensity, disability and depression in chronic pain patients. *Pain, 80*(3), 483–491.

Arthritis Foundation. (2002, December 31). *Delivering on the promise in fibromyalgia* [Online]. Available: http://www.arthritis.org/research/research_ program/fibromyalgia/default.asp

Ascione, F. R. (1992). Enhancing children's attitudes about the humane treatments of animals: Generalization to human directed empathy. *Anthrozoos, 5*(3), 176–191.

Ashcraft, M. H., & Kirk, E. P. (2001). *The relationships among working memory, math anxiety, and performance*. Journal of Experimental Psychology: General, 130(2), 224–237.

Ashley, J. (1997). *Overcoming stage fright in everyday life*. New York: Crown.

Astin, J. A. (1998). Why patients use alternative medicine. *Journal of the American Medical Association, 279*, 548–553.

Atkinson, D. R., & Gim, R. H. (1989). Asian-American cultural identity and attitudes toward mental health services. *Journal of Counseling Psychology, 36*, 209–212.

Azpeitia, L., & Rocamora, M. (1994, November). Misdiagnosis of the gifted. *Mensa Bulletin* [Online]. Available: http://www.rocamora.org/gifted.html

Babyak, M., Blumenthal, J. A., Herman, S., Khatri, P., Doraiswamy, M., Moore, K., Craighead, W. E., Baldewicz, T. T., & Krishnan, K. R. (2000). Exercise treatment for major depression: Maintenance of therapeutic benefit at 10 months. *Psychosomatic Medicine, 62*(5), 633–638.

Bagley, C. (1993). Transracial adoption in Britain: A follow-up study, with policy considerations. *Child Welfare, 72*(3), 285–299.

Ball, K. (1996, August). *Predicting crash risk in older drivers*. Paper presented at the 104th Annual Convention of the American Psychological Association, Toronto.

Banks, R. (1997). *Bullying in schools* [Online]. Available: http://www.ericps.ed.uiuc. edu/eece/pubs/digests/1997/banks97.html

Barba, B. E. (1995). The positive influence of animals: Animal-assisted therapy in acute care. *Clinical Nurse Specialist, 9*(4), 199–202.

Barker, S. B., & Barker, R. T. (1988). The human–canine bond: Closer than family ties? *Journal of Mental Health Counseling, 10,* 46–56.

Barker, S. B., & Barker, R. T. (1990). Investigation of the construct validity of the Family Life Space Diagram. *Journal of Mental Health Counseling, 12,* 506–514.

Barker, S. B., Barker, R. T., Dawson, K. S., & Knisely, J. S. (1997) The use of the Family Life Space Diagram in establishing interconnectedness: A preliminary study of sexual abuse survivors, their significant others and pets. *Individual Psychology, 53*(4), 435–450.

Barker, S. B., & Dawson, K. S. (1998). The effects of animal-assisted therapy on anxiety ratings of hospitalized psychiatric patients. *Psychiatric Services, 49*(6), 797–801.

Bass, A. R., Bharucha-Reid, R., Delaplane-Harris, K., Schork, M. A., Kaufmann, R., McCann, D., Foxman, B., Fraser, W., & Cook, S. (1996). Employee drug use, demographic characteristics, work reactions, and absenteeism. *Journal of Occupational Health Psychology, 1*(1), 92–99.

Batsche, G. M., & Knoff, H. M. (1994). Bullies and their victims: Understanding a pervasive problem in the schools. *School Psychology Review, 23*(2), 165–174.

Baum, S. M. (1988). An enrichment program for gifted learning disabled students. *Gifted Child Quarterly, 32,* 226–230.

Baum, S. M., Olenchak, F. R., & Owen, S. V. (1998). Gifted students with attention deficits: Fact and/or fiction? Or, can we see the forest for the trees? *Gifted Child Quarterly, 42*(2), 96–104.

Baum, S. M., Owen, S. V., & Dixon, J. (1991). *To be gifted and learning disabled: From identification to practical intervention strategies.* Mansfield Center, CT: Creative Learning Press.

Beardslee, W. R., Versage, E. M., Wright, E. J., Salt, P., Rothberg, P. C., Drezner, K., & Gladstone, T. R. G. (1997). Examination of preventive interventions for families with depression: Evidence of change. *Development and Psychopathology, 9,* 109–130.

Beck, E. A., & McIntyre, S. C. (1977). MMPI patterns of shoplifters within a college population. *Psychological Reports, 41*(3, Pt 2), 1035–1040.

Beckwith, H. (1997). *Selling the invisible: A field guide to modern marketing.* New York: Warner Books.

Beery, L. C.., Prigerson, H. G., Bierhals, A. J., Santucci, L. M., Newsom, J. T., Maciejewski, P. K., Rapp, S. R., Fasiczka, A., & Reynolds, C. F., III. (1997). Traumatic grief, depression, and care giving in elderly spouses of the terminally ill. *Omega: Journal of Death and Dying. 35*(3), 261–279.

Beidel, D., & Turner, S. (1997). *Shy children, phobic adults: Nature and treatment of social phobia.* Washington, DC: American Psychological Association.

Bell, I. R., Martino, G. M., Meredith, K. E., Schwartz, G. E., Siani, M. M., & Morrow, F. D. (1993). Vascular disease risk factors, urinary free cortisol, and health histories in older adults: Shyness and gender interactions. *Biological Psychology, 35*(1), 37–49.

Benbow, C. P., & Stanley, J. C. (1996). Inequity in equity: How "equity" can lead to inequity for high-potential students. *Psychology, Public Policy, and Law. 2*(2), 249–292.

Bennis, W. (1994). *On becoming a leader.* Reading, MA: Perseus Books.

Benson, E. (2003, June). Beyond "urbancentrism." *APA Monitor, 34*(6), 54.

Berger, R. (1997). Immigrant stepfamilies. *Contemporary Family Therapy: An International Journal, 19*(3), 361–370.

Bernal, G., & Scharrón-del-Río, M. R. (2001). Are empirically supported treatments valid for ethnic minorities?: Toward an alternative approach for treatment research. *Cultural Diversity and Ethnic Minority Psychology, 7*(4), 328–342.

Beutler, L. E. (2000). David and Goliath: When empirical and clinical standards of practice meet. *American Psychologist, 55*(9), 997–1007.

Blagg, N. (1992). School phobia. In D. A. Lane & A. Miller (Eds.), *Child and adolescent therapy: A handbook.* Buckingham, England: Open University Press.

Blanchard, E. B. (1992). Psychological treatment of benign headache disorders. *Journal of Consulting and Clinical Psychology, 60,* 537–551.

Blanchard, E. B., & Diamond, S. (1996). Psychological treatment of benign headache disorders. *Professional Psychology: Research and Practice, 27*(6), 541–547.

Blanchard, E. B., & Hickling, E. J. (1997). *After the crash: Assessment and treatment of motor vehicle accident survivors.* Washington, DC: American Psychological Association.

Blanchard, E. B., Hickling, E. J., Buckley, T. C., Taylor, A. E., Vollmer, A., & Loos, W. R. (1996). Psychophysiology of posttraumatic stress disorder related to motor vehicle accidents: Replication and extension. *Journal of Consulting and Clinical Psychology, 64,* 742–751.

Blanchard, E. B., Hickling, E. J., Mitnick, N., Taylor, A. E., Loos, W. R., & Buckley, T. C. (1995). The impact of severity of physical injury and perception of life threat in the development of post-traumatic stress disorder in motor vehicle accident victims. *Behaviour Research and Therapy, 33,* 529–534.

Bloom, B. S. (1985). *Developing talent in young people.* New York: Ballantine Books.

Blustein, D. L., Walbridge, M. M., Friedlander, M. L., & Palladino, D. E. (1991). Contributions of psychological separation and parental attachment to the career development process. *Journal of Counseling Psychology, 38,* 39–50.

Boat, B. (1995). The relationship between violence to children and violence to animals. *Journal of Interpersonal Violence, 10*(2), 229–235.

Bodnar, J. C., & Kiecolt-Glaser, J. K. (1994). Caregiver depression after bereavement: Chronic stress isn't over when it's over. *Psychology and Aging, 9*(3), 372–380.

Bonas, S., McNicholas, J., & Collis, G. M. (2000). Pets in the network of family relationships: An empirical study. In A. L. Podberscek & E. S. Paul (Eds.), *Companion animals and us: Exploring the relationships between people and pets* (pp. 209–236). New York: Cambridge University Press.

Bonica, J. J. (Ed.). (1990). *The management of pain.* Philadelphia: Lea & Febiger.

Bork, D., Jaffe, D. T., Lane, S. H., Dashew, L., & Heisler, Q. G. (1996). *Working with family businesses: A guide for professionals.* San Francisco: Jossey-Bass.

Bourne, E. J. (1995). *The anxiety and phobia workbook* (2nd ed.). Oakland, CA: New Harbinger.

Bowman, M., & Garralda, M. E. (1993). Psychiatric morbidity among children who are frequent attenders in general practice. *British Journal of General Practice, 43,* 6–9.

Bradford, J. M., & Balmaceda, R. A. (1983). Shoplifting: Is there a specific psychiatric syndrome? *Canadian Journal of Psychiatry, 28*(4), 248–254.

Bradley, L. A. (1989). Adherence with treatment regimens among adult rheumatoid arthritis patients: Current status and future directions. *Arthritis Care Research, 2*(3), 33–39.

Bramer, J. S. (1996). *Succeeding in college with attention deficit disorders: Issues and strategies for students, counselors and educators.* Plantation, FL: Specialty Press.

Brandell, J. R. (1988). Treatment of the biracial child: Theoretical and clinical issues. *Journal of Multicultural Counseling and Development, 16*(4), 176–187.

Bray, J. H. (1995, 1996). *Interventions that work for stepfamilies* [Online]. Available: http://helping.apa.org/family/step.html

Bray, J. H. (1999). *Therapy for stepfamilies* (Pick 42 Niche Guide Series, Division 42 of the American Psychological Association). Washington, DC: American Psychological Association.

Bray, J. H., & Berger, S. H. (1993). Developmental issues in stepfamilies research project: Family relationships and parent–child interactions. *Journal of Family Psychology, 7,* 76–90.

Bray, J. H., & Harvey, D. M. (1995) Adolescents in stepfamilies: Developmental family interventions. *Psychotherapy, 32*(1), 122–130.

Bray, J. H., & Kelly, J. (1998). *Stepfamilies: Love, marriage, and parenting in the first decade.* New York: Broadway Books.

Bray, J. H., & Rogers, J. G. (1995). Linking psychologists and family phsyicians for collaborative practice. *Professional Psychology: Reasearch and Practice, 26*(2), 132–138.

Brewer, B. W. (1998). Psychological applications in clinical sports medicine: Current status and future directions. *Journal of Clinical Psychology in Medical Settings, 5*(1), 91–102.

Briere, J., & Runtz, M. (1993). Childhood sexual abuse: Long-term sequelae and implications for psychological assessment. *Journal of Interpersonal Violence, 8,* 312–330.

Briere, J., Woo, R., McRae, B., Foltz, J., & Sitzman, R. (1997). Lifetime victimization history, demographics, and clinical status in female psychiatric emergency room patients. *Journal of Nervous and Mental Disease, 185*(2), 95–101.

Britton, B. K., & Tesser, A. (1991). Effects of time-management practices on college grades. *Journal of Educational Psychology, 83*(3), 405–410.

Bronfman, E. T., Campis, L. B., & Koocher, G. P. (1998). Helping children to cope: Clinical issues for acutely injured and medically traumatized children. *Professional Psychology: Research and Practice, 29*(6), 574–581.

Brown, T. L., Henggeler, S. W., Brondino, M. J., & Pickrel, S. G. (1999). Trauma exposure, protective factors and mental health functioning of substance-abusing
and dependent juvenile offenders. *Journal of Emotional and Behavioral Disorders, 7*(2), 94–102.

Brownell, K. D., Rodin, J., & Wilmore, J. H. (1992). *Eating, body weight, and performance in athletes: Disorders of modern society.* Philadelphia: Lea & Febiger.

Bruch, J., Barraclough, B., Nelson, M., & Sainsbury, P. (1971). Suicide following
death of parents. *Social Psychiatry, 6,* 193–199.

Bruyere, S. M., & O'Keeffe, J. (Eds.). (1994). *Implications of the Americans with Disabilities Act for psychology.* Washington, DC: American Psychological Associa-
tion/Springer.

Bryant, R. A., Sackville, T., Dang, S. T., Moulds, M., & Guthrie, R. (1999). Treating
acute stress disorder: An evaluation of cognitive behavior therapy and supporting counseling techniques. *American Journal of Psychiatry, 156*(11), 1780–
1786.

Budgin, J. (1997). Pet loss support hotline established at the College of Veterinary
Medicine. *ISU Veterinarian* [Online]. Available: http://www.vetmed.iastate.
edu/students/current/organizations/isuvet/s97-2.html

Buhrke, R. A. (1989) Incorporating lesbian and gay issues into counselor training: A
resource guide. *Journal of Counseling and Development, 68*(1), 77–80.

Bulman, R. J., & Wortman, C. B. (1977). Attributions of blame and coping in the "real
world": Severe accident victims react to their lot. *Journal of Personality and Social Psychology, 35,* 351–363.

Bunker, K. A. (1997). The power of vulnerability in contemporary leadership. *Consulting Psychology Journal: Practice and Research, 49*(2), 122–136.

Bureau of Labor Statistics, U.S. Department of Labor. (2000). *Occupational outlook handbook, 2000–01 edition* [Online]. Available: http://www.bls.gov/oco/
0c05056.htm

Burgio, K. L. (1990). Behavioral training for stress and urge incontinence in the community. *Gerontology, 36*(Suppl. 2), 27–34.

Business tension can spur consultations. (1999). *Clinical Psychiatry News, 27*(11), 50.

Butler, R. N. (1974). Successful aging and the role of the life review. *Journal of the
American Geriatrics Society, 22*(12), 529–535.

Cain, A. O. (1985). Pets as family members. *Marriage and Family Review, 8*(3–4), 5–
10.

Callan, J. E. (1999). Practice and education issues related to adolescent girls. In N. G.
Johnson, M. C. Roberts, & J. Worell (Eds.), *Beyond appearance: A new look at
adolescent girls* (pp. 355–375). Washington, DC: American Psychological Association.

Camic, P. M., & Brown, F. D. (Eds.). (1989). *Assessing chronic pain: A multidisciplinary clinic.* New York: Springer.

Campbell, P. B. (1999, October). *Bringing girls into SMET in 1999: The state of the
art.* Paper presented at the annual meeting of the principal investigators of the
National Science Foundation, Program for Gender Equity, Washington, DC.

Caplan, R. D., Vinokur, A. D., & Price, R. H. (1997). From job loss to reemployment:
Field experiments in prevention-focused coping. In G. W. Albee & T. Gullota
(Eds.), *Primary prevention works* (pp. 341–379). Thousand Oaks, CA: Sage.

Carducci, B. J. (2000). What shy individuals do to cope with their shyness: A content analysis. In W. R. Crozier (Ed.), *Shyness: Development, consolidation and change* (pp. 171–185). New York: Routledge Falmer

Carlson, C. I., Tharinger, D. J., Bricklin, P. M., DeMers, S. T., & Paavola, J. C. (1996). Health care reform and psychological practice in schools. *Professional Psychology: Research and Practice, 27*(1), 14–23.

Caroll, R. (1988). Siblings and the family business. In M. D. Kahn & K. G. Lewis (Eds.), *Siblings in therapy: Life span and clinical issues.* New York: Norton.

Carson, J. F., Warren, B. L., & Doty, L. (1994–1995). An investigation of the grief counseling services available in the middle schools and high schools in the state of Mississippi. *Omega: Journal of Death and Dying, 30*(3), 191–204.

Caudill, M., Schnable, R., Zuttermeister, P., Benson, H., & Friedman, R. (1991). Decreased clinic utilization by chronic pain patients: Response to behavioral medicine intervention. *Clinical Journal of Pain, 7,* 305–310.

Cederblad, M.. Hoeoek, B., Irhammar, M., & Mercke, A. (1999). Mental health in international adoptees as teenagers and young adults: An epidemiological study. *Journal of Child Psychology and Psychiatry, 40*(8), 1239–1248.

Cellucci, T., & Vik, P. (2001). Training for substance abuse treatment among psychologists in a rural state. *Professional Psychology: Research and Practice, 32*(3), 248–252.

Center for the Advancement of Health. (n.d.). *Skills not pills: Caring for pain.* (Available from Center for the Advancement of Health, 2000 Florida Avenue, NW, Suite 210, Washington, DC 20009-1231)

Chamberlin, J. (2003, June). At home on the range: Rural texas offers opportunities aplenty to psychologists. *APA Monitor, 34*(6), 69.

Chandy, J. M., Blum, R. W., & Resnick, M. D. (1996). Female adolescents with a history of sexual abuse: Risk outcome and protective factors. *Journal of Interpersonal Violence, 11*(4), 503–518 .

Cheng, G.-S. (2000). Cognitive behavior treatment for chronic pain. *Clinical Psychiatry News, 28*(2), 23.

Chiles, J. A., Lambert, M. J., & Hatch, A. L. (1999). The impact of psychological interventions on medical cost offset: A meta-analytic review. *Clinical Psychology: Science and Practice, 6*(2), 204–224.

Chinner, T. L., & Dalziel, F. R. (1991). An exploratory study on the viability and efficacy of a pet-facilitated therapy project within a hospice. *Journal of Palliative Care, 7*(4), 13–20.

Classen, C., Koopman, C., Angell, K., & Spiegel, D. (1996). Coping styles associated with psychological adjustment to advanced breast cancer. *Health Psychology, 15*(6), 434–437.

Clement, P. W. (1999). *Outcomes and incomes: How to evaluate, improve, and market your psychotherapy practice by measuring outcomes.* New York: Guilford Press.

Clevenger, T., Jr., Halvorson, S. K., & Bledsoe, D. L. (1992). *Identification and validation of independent factors in the speech anxiety state.* Paper presented at the annual convention of the Speech Communication Association, Atlanta, GA.

Colangelo, N. (1988). Families of gifted children: The next ten years. *Roeper Review, 11*(1), 16–18.

Cole, J. D. (1998). Psychotherapy with chronic pain patients. *Independent Practitioner, 18*(1), 29–30.

Collaboration: Informal health club links bolster strong referrals. (2001, December). *Practice Strategies, 7*(12), 1, 8.

Comprehensive study focuses on conflict, education, and cultural issues. (n.d.). *Family Business Quarterly* [Online]. Available: http://www.fambiz.com/template.cfm?Article=Conflicts/NECFB-2131-dup.html&Keywords=&Button=fambiz

Consulting to family businesses. (1998). *Psychotherapy Finances, 24*(3), 1–2.

Cooke, B. E. M. (1995). Health promotion, health protection, and preventive services. *Primary Care, 22,* 555–565.

Cooper, S., & Wagenfeld, M. O. (n.d.). *Delivering mental health services to children and adolescents with serious mental illness in frontier areas: Parent and provider views* (Letter to the Field No. 17) [Online]. Available: http://www.wiche.edu/MentalHealth/Frontier

Corcoran, K. J., & Fischer, J. (2000). *Measures for clinical practice: A sourcebook* (3rd ed.). New York: Free Press.

Cordova, J. V., & Gee, C. B. (2001). Couples therapy for depression: Using healthy relationships to treat depression. In S. R. H. Beach (Ed.), *Marital and family processes in depression: A scientific foundation for clinical practice* (pp. 185–204). Washington, DC: American Psychological Association.

Coren, S., & Walker, J. (1997). *What do dogs know?* New York: Simon and Schuster.

Costantino, G., Malgady, R. G., & Rogler, D. (1986). *Cuento* therapy: A culturally-sensitive modality for Puerto Rican children. *Journal of Consulting and Clinical Psychology, 54,* 639–645.

Costas, M., & Landreth, G. (1999). Filial therapy with non-offending parents of children who have been sexually abused. *International Journal of Play Therapy, 8*(1), 43–66.

Counsell, C. M., Abram, J., & Gilbert, M. (1997). Animal assisted therapy and the individual with spinal cord injury. *SCI Nursing, 14*(2), 52–55.

Covey, S. R. (1990). *The seven habits of highly effective people: Restoring the character ethic.* New York: Fireside.

Cowen, E. (1994). The enhancement of psychological wellness: Challenges and opportunities. *American Journal of Community Psychology, 22*(2), 149–179.

Coyle, B. R. (1999). Practical tools for rural psychiatric practice. *Bulletin of the Menninger Clinic, 63*(2), 202–222.

Coyne, J. C., Fechner-Bates, S., & Schwenk, T. L. (1995) Nondetection of depression by primary care physicians reconsidered. *General Hospital Psychiatry, 16,* 267–276.

Cradock, C., Cotler, S., & Jason, L. A. (1978). Primary prevention: Immunization of children for speech anxiety. *Cognitive Therapy and Research, 2*(4), 389–396.

Crandall, R. (1998). *1001 ways to market your services: Even if you hate to sell.* Lincolnwood, IL: Contemporary Books.

Crespi, T. D., & Fieldman, J. P. (2001). Post-doctoral re-specialization experience: Lessons from the field. *School Psychologist, 55*(3), 68–70.

Crespi, T. D., & Nissen, K. S. (1998, February). Privatization of mental health services: Considerations, concerns and credentialing. *Communique* [Online]. Available: http://www.nasponline.org/publications/cq265privat.html

Cryer, B. A. (1996, June 12). *Neutralizing workplace stress: The physiology of human performance and organizational effectiveness.* Paper presented at Psychological Disabilities in the Workplace, Centre for Professional Learning, Toronto.

Csikszentmihalyi, M. (1990). *Flow: The psychology of optimal experience.* New York: Harper & Row.

Csikszentmihalyi, M., Rathunde, K. R., Whalen, S., & Wong, M. (1993). *Talented teenagers: The roots of success and failure.* New York: Cambridge University Press.

Culbertson, J. L. (1993). Clinical child psychology in the 1990's: Broadening our scope. *Journal of Clinical Child Psychology, 22,* 116–122.

Cummings, N. (1992). Psychologists in the medical surgical setting: Some reflections. *Professional Psychology: Research and Practice, 20,* 390–394.

Cummings, N. A., Dorken, H., Pallack, M. S., & Henke, C. J. (1993). Managed mental health care, Medicaid, and cost-offset: The impact of psychological services in the Hawaii HCFA Medicaid project. In N. A. Cummings, H. Dorken, M. S. Pallack, & C. Henke (Eds.), *Medicaid, managed behavioral health and implications for public policy: Vol. 2. Healthcare and utilization cost series* (pp. 323–333). San Francisco: Foundation for Behavioral Health.

Cupchik, W. (n.d.). *Shoplifting and other thefts by usually honest adults* [Online]. Available: http://members.aol.com/wcupchik

Cupchik, W. (1997). *Why honest people shoplift or commit other acts of theft: Assessment and treatment of atypical theft offenders.* Toronto: Tagami Communications.

Cupchik, W., & Atcheson, J. D. (1983). Shoplifting: An occasional crime of the moral majority. *Bulletin of the American Academy of Psychiatry and the Law, 11*(4), 343–354.

Curran, J. (1992). *JOBS: A manual for teaching people successful job search strategies.* Ann Arbor: Michigan Prevention Research Center, Institute for Social Research.

Dabrowski, K., & Piechowski, M. M. (1977). *Theory of levels of emotional development* (2 vols.). Oceanside, NY: Dabor Science.

Daldrup, R. J., Beutler, L. E., Engle, D., & Greenberg, L. S. (1988). *Focused expressive psychotherapy: Freeing the overcontrolled patient.* New York: Guilford Press.

Daly, J. A., Vangelisti, A. L., & Weber, D. J. (1995). Speech anxiety affects how people prepare speeches: A protocol analysis of the preparation process of speakers. *Communication Monographs, 62*(4), 383–397.

Davidson, J. R., Hughes, D. C., George, L. K., & Blazer, D. G. (1996). The association of sexual assault and attempted suicide within the community. *Archives of General Psychiatry, 53*(6), 550–555.

Dean, B. (1999). Marketing a virtual coaching practice on a national scale. *Independent Practitioner, 19*(4), 195–198.

Deardorff, W. W. (2002, January 3). *New codes, many issues* [Online]. Available from Division 42 newsgroup: News://Division 42.

A dearth of school counselors. (1999, November–December). *Family Therapy Networker,* pp. 19–20.

Deffenbacher, J. L., Lynch, R. S., Oetting, E. R., & Kemper, C. C. (1996). Anger reduction in early adolescents. *Journal of Counseling Psychology, 43*(2), 149–157.

Delahanty, D. L., Herberman, H. B., Craig, K. J., Hayward, M. C., Fullerton, C. S., Ursano, R. J., et al. (1997). Acute and chronic distress and posttraumatic stress disorder as a function of responsibility for serious motor vehicle accidents. *Journal of Consulting and Clinical Psychology, 65*(4), 560–567.

Desberg, P., & Marsh, G. D. (1999). *Controlling stagefright with audiences from one to one thousand.* Oakland, CA: New Harbinger.

de Vries, A. P., Kassam-Adams, N., Canaan, A., Sherman-Slate, E., Gallagher, P. R., & Winston, F. K. (1999). Looking beyond the physical injury: Posttraumatic stress disorder in children and parents after pediatric traffic injury. *Pediatrics, 104*(6), 1293–1299.

Diamond, M. A. (1996). Innovation and diffusion of technology: A human process. *Consulting Psychology Journal: Practice and Research, 48*(4), 221–229.

Dimeff, L. A., Baer, J. S., Kivlahan, D. R., & Marlatt, G. A. (1999). *Brief alcohol screening and intervention for college students (BASICS): A harm reduction approach.* New York: Guilford Press.

Directions. (1998, June). *Practice Strategies,* p. 10.

Dobratz, M. C. (1995). Analysis of variables that impact psychological adaptation in home hospice patients. *Hospice Journal, 10*(1), 75–88.

Doghramji, K. (2000). *Sleepless in America: Diagnosing and treating insomnia* [Online]. Available: http://www.medscape.com/viewprogram/347

Dougherty, D. M. (1999). Health care for adolescent girls. In N. G. Johnson, M. C. Roberts, & J. P. Worell (Eds.), *Beyond appearance: A new look at adolescent girls* (pp. 301–325). Washington, DC: American Psychological Association.

Dubow, E. F., Lovko, K. R., Jr., & Kausch, D. F. (1990). Demographic differences in adolescents' health concerns and perceptions of helping agents. *Journal of Clinical Child Psychology, 19,* 44–54.

Durant, R. H., Pendergrast, R. A., & Cadenhead, C. (1994). Exposure to violence and victimization and fighting behavior by urban black adolescents. *Journal of Adolescent Health, 15,* 311–318.

Dworkin, S. (1992). Some ethical considerations when counseling gay, lesbian, and bisexual clients. In S. Dworkin & F. Gutierrez (Eds.), *Counseling gay men and lesbians: Journey to the end of the rainbow* (pp. 325–334). Alexandria, VA: Counseling Association.

Edens, J. F. (1998). School-based consultation services for children with externalizing behavior problems. In L. VandeCreek, S. Knapp, & T. L. Jackson (Eds.), *Innovations in clinical practice: A source book* (Vol. 16, pp. 337–353). Sarasota, FL: Professional Resource Press.

Edwards, L. C., Lim, B. R. K. B., McMinn, M. R., & Dominguez, A. W. (1999). Examples of collaboration between psychologists and clergy. *Professional Psychology: Research and Practice, 30,* 547–551.

Eisenberg, D. M., Davis, R. B., Ettner, S. L., Appel, S., Wilkey, S., Van Rompay, M., & Kessler, R. C. (1998). Trends in alternative medicine use in the United States, 1990–1997: Results of a follow-up national survey. *Journal of the American Medical Association, 280*(18), 1569–1575.

Eisenberg, L. (1992). Treating depression and anxiety in primary care: Closing the gap between knowledge and practice. *New England Journal of Medicine, 326,* 1080–1083.

Ejime, P. (1996, August 26). NASP: America will need 3,000 more school psychologists by 2006. *US Newswire.*

Embry, D. D., Flannery, D. J., Vazsoni, A. T., Powell, K. E., & Atha, H. (1996). Peace Builders: A theoretically driven, school-based model for early violence prevention. *American Journal of Preventive Medicine, 12,* 91–100.

Emmelkamp, P. M., & van Oppen, P. (1993). Cognitive interventions in behavioral medicine. *Psychotherapy and Psychosomatics, 59*(3–4), 116–130.

Epstein, E. E., & McCrady, B. S. (1998). Behavioral couples treatment of alcohol and drug use disorders: Current status and innovations. *Clinical Psychology Review, 18*(6), 689–711.

Equal Employment Opportunity Commission. (1992). *Americans with Disabilities Act: Technical assistance manual on the employment provisions* (Title I). Washington, DC: Author. (Also available at http://www.eeoc.gov)

Ermer, D. J. (1999). Experience with a rural telepsychiatry clinic for children and adolescents. *Psychiatric Services, 50*(2), 260–261.

Espleage, D., Bosworth, K., Karageorge, K., & Daytner, G. (1996). *Family environment and bullying behaviors: Interrelationships and treatment implications.* Paper presented at the 104th Annual Convention of the American Psychological Association, Toronto.

Evers-Szostak, M. (1998). Psychological practice in pediatric primary care settings. In L. VandeCreek, S. Knapp, & T. Jackson (Eds.), *Innovations in clinical practice: A source book* (Vol. 16, pp. 325–335). Sarasota, FL: Professional Resource Press.

Family therapy transfers to corporate setting. (1999). *Practice Strategies, 5*(9), 3.

Farrell, P. A. (1996). Psychological disorders and medical illness in the elderly: A double-edged sword. In L. VandeCreek, S. Knapp,, & T. L. Jackson (Eds.), *Innovations in clinical practice: A source book* (Vol. 15, pp. 283–309). Sarasota, FL: Professional Resource Press.

Fava, G. A. (1999). Well-being therapy: Conceptual and technical issues. *Psychotherapy and Psychosomatics, 68*(4), 171–179.

Federal Communications Commission (FCC). (2002, September 25). *The FCC's universal service program for rural health care providers* [Online]. Available: http://ftp.fcc.gov/cgb/consumerfacts/usp_RuralHealthcare.html

Felthous, A. R., & Kellert, S. R. (1987). Childhood cruelty to animals and later aggression against people: A review. *American Journal of Psychiatry, 144*(6), 710–717.

Felton, B. J., Revenson, T. A., & Hinrichsen, G. A. (1984). Stress and coping in the explanation of psychological adjustment among chronically ill adults. *Social Science and Medicine, 8*(10), 889–898.

Fergusson, D. M.., Horwood, L. J., &. Lynskey, M. T. (1996). Child sexual abuse and psychiatric disorder in young adulthood: II. Psychiatric outcomes of childhood sexual abuse. *Journal of the American Academy of Child and Adolescent Psychiatry, 35*(10), 1365–1374.

Ferrari, J. R., Johnson, J. L., & McCown, W. G. (1995). *Procrastination and task avoidance: Theory, research, and treatment.* New York: Plenum Press.

Fine, A. H. (2000). Animals and therapists: Incorporating animals in outpatient psychotherapy. In A. H. Fine (Ed.), *Handbook of animal-assisted therapy: Theoretical foundations and guidelines for practice.* San Diego, CA: Academic Press.

Fine, M. A., & Kurdek, L. A. (1995). Relation between marital quality and (step)parent/child relationship quality for parents and stepparents in stepfamilies. *Journal of Family Psychology, 9*(2), 216–223.

Fink, P., Sorensen, L., Engberg, M., Holm, M., & Munk-Jorgensen, P. (1999). Somatization in primary care: Prevalence, health care utilization, and general practitioner recognition. *Psychosomatics, 40*(4), 330–338.

Fiore, J., Becker, J., & Coppel, D. (1983). Social network interactions: A buffer or a stress? *American Journal of Community Psychology, 11*, 423–439.

Fischetti, M. (1999). *Building strong family teams*. Philadelphia: Family Business.

Fisher, A. (1999, May 17). Ask Annie: Real world career advice. *Fortune* [Online]. Available: http://www.fortune.com/fortune/askannie

Flemons, D. G., & Cole, P. M. (1994). Playing with contextual complexity: Relational consultation to family businesses. In C. H. Huber (Ed.), *Transitioning from individual to family counseling* (pp.). Alexandria, VA: American Counseling Association.

Flor, H., Kerns, R. D., & Turk, D. C. (1987). The role of spouse reinforcement, perceived pain, and activity levels of chronic pain patients. *Journal of Psychosomatic Research, 31*(2), 251–259.

Fontaine, J. H., & Hammond, N. L. (1996, December 1). Counseling issues with gay and lesbian adolescents. *Adolescence, 31*(124), 817–830.

Foote, W. E. (2000). A model for psychological consultation in cases involving the Americans with Disabilities Act. *Professional Psychology: Research and Practice, 31*, 190–196.

Foulks, E. F., Bland, I. J., & Shervington, D. (1995). Psychotherapy across cultures. *American Psychiatric Press Review of Psychiatry, 14*, 511–528.

Fox, R. (1999). Clinical psychologists as executive coaches. *Independent Practitioner, 19*(3), 121–123.

Foxhall, K. (2000, November). New CPT codes will recognize psychologists' work with physical health problems. *APA Monitor* [Online], 31(10). Available: http://www.apa.org/monitor/nov00/codes.html

Foxhall, K. (2001, July–August). A spark to the business–psychology connection. *APA Monitor* [Online], 32(7). Available: http://www.apa.org/monitor/julaug01/spark.html

Foy, S. S., & Mitchell, M. M. (1990). Factors contributing to learned helplessness in the institutionalized aged: A literature review. *Physical and Occupational Therapy in Geriatrics, 9*(2), 1–23.

Frasier, M. M., García, J. H., & Passow, A. H. (1995). *A review of assessment issues in gifted education and their implications for identifying gifted minority students* (Report No. RM95204). Storrs: University of Connecticut, National Research Center on the Gifted and Talented.

Frederickson, R. H. (1979). Career development and the gifted. In N. Colangelo & R. Zaffrann (Eds.), *New voices in counseling the gifted* (pp. 264–276). Dubuque, IA: Kendall-Hunt.

Fredrickson, B. L. (1998). What good are positive emotions? *Review of General Psychology, 2*(3), 300–319.

Fredrickson, B. L., & Levenson, R. W. (1998). Positive emotions speed recovery from the cardiovascular sequelae of negative emotions. *Cognition and Emotion, 12*, 191–220.

Fredrickson, B. L., Mancuso, R. A., Branigan, C., & Tugade, M. M. (2000). The undoing effect of positive emotions. *Motivation and Emotion, 24*(4), 237–258.

Freeman, J. (1994). Some emotional aspects of being gifted. *Journal for the Education of the Gifted, 17*(2), 180–197.

Freeman, J. (1995). Recent studies of giftedness in children. *Journal of Child Psychology and Psychiatry, 36*(4), 531–547.

Freudenberger, H. J., Freedheim, D. K., & Kurtz, T. S. (1989). Treatment of individuals in family business. *Psychotherapy, 26*(1), 47–53.

Frey, C. P. (1998). Struggling with identity: Working with seventh- and eighth-grade gifted girls to air issues of concern. *Journal for the Education of the Gifted, 21*(4), 437–451.

Friedan, B. (1993). *The fountain of age.* New York: Simon & Schuster.

Friedman, R., Sobel, D., Myers, P., Caudill, M., & Benson, H. (1995). Behavioral medicine, clinical health psychology, and cost offset. *Health Psychology, 14*(6), 509–518.

Fritz, C. L., Farver, T. B., Kass, P. H., & Hart, L. A. (1995). Association with companion animals and the expression of noncognitive symptoms in Alzheimer's patients. *Journal of Nervous and Mental Disease, 183*(7), 459–463.

Gagliese, L., & Melzack, R. (1997). Chronic pain in elderly people. *Pain, 70*(1), 3–14.

Galagan, P. (1985). Between family and firm. *Training and Development Journal, 39*(4), 68–71.

Ganong, L. H., & Coleman, M. (1993). A meta-analytic comparison of the self-esteem and behavior problems of stepchildren to children in other family structures. *Journal of Divorce and Remarriage, 19*(3–4), 143–163.

Gardner, H. (1983). *Frames of mind: The theory of multiple intelligences.* New York: Basic Books.

Garnets, L., Hancock, K. A., Cochran, S. D., Goodchilds, J., & Peplau, L. A. (1991). Issues in psychotherapy with lesbians and gay men. *American Psychologist, 46,* 964–972.

Garza, D. L., & Feltz, D. L. (1998). Effects of selected mental practice on performance, self-efficacy, and competition confidence of figure skaters. *Sport Psychologist, 12*(1), 1–15.

Gauthier, J., & Pellerin, D. (1982). Management of compulsive shoplifting through covert sensitization. *Journal of Behavior Therapy and Experimental Psychiatry, 13*(1), 73–75.

Gays, lesbians seek out MH care disproportionately but report dissatisfaction. (1997, April 18). *Psychiatric Times.*

Gendreau, P. Goggin, C., & Cullen, F. T. (1999). *The effects of prison sentences on recidivism.* Ottawa: Solicitor General Canada.

Gendreau, P., Goggin, C., & Paparozzi, M. (1996). Principles of effective assessment for community corrections. *Federal Probation, 60*(3), 64–70.

Gersick, K. E., Davis, J. A., Hampton, M. M., & Landsberg, I. (1997). *Generation to generation: Life cycles of the family business.* Boston: Harvard Business School Press.

Gevirtz, R. N., Hubbard, D. R., & Harpin, R. E. (1996). Psychophysiologic treatment of chronic lower back pain. *Professional Psychology: Research and Practice, 27*(6), 561–566.

Gibbs, J. T., & Moskowitz-Sweet, G. (1991). Clinical and cultural issues in the treatment of biracial and bicultural adolescents. *Families in Society, 72*(10), 579–592.

Gilbourne, D., & Taylor, A. H. (1998). From theory to practice: The integration of goal perspective theory and life development approaches within an injury-specific goal-setting program. *Journal of Applied Sport Psychology, 10*(1), 124–139.

Gillham, J., Reivich, K., Jaycox, L., & Seligman, M. E. P. (1995). Prevention of depressive symptoms in school children: Two year follow up. *Psychological Science, 6*(6), 343–351.

Ginsberg, B. (1997). *Relationship Enhancement family therapy.* New York: Wiley.

Glover, J. H. (1985). A case of kleptomania treated by covert sensitization. *British Journal of Clinical Psychology, 24*(3), 213–214.

Goleman, D. (1993, December 15). Use of antidepressants in children at issue. *The New York Times,* p. C17.

Goleman, D. (1998). *Working with emotional intelligence.* New York: Bantam.

Gonsalves, C. (1992). Psychological stages of the refugee process: A model for therapeutic interventions. *Professional Psychology: Research and Practice, 23*(5), 382–389.

Gonzalez, H. P. (1995). Systematic desensitization, study skills counseling, and anxiety-coping training in the treatment of test anxiety. In C. D. Spielberger & P. R. Vagg (Eds.), *Test anxiety: Theory, assessment, and treatment* (pp. 117–132). Washington, DC: Taylor & Francis.

Goswami, M., Pollak, C. P., Cohen, F. L., Thorpy, M. J., Kavey, N. B., & Kutscher, A. H. (Eds.). (1996). *Psychosocial aspects of narcolepsy.* New York: Haworth Press.

Gottfredson, L. S., & Lapan, R. T. (1997). Assessing gender-based circumscription of occupational aspirations. *Journal of Career Assessment, 5*(4), 419–441.

Gottman, J., with Silver, N. (1994). *Why marriages succeed or fail: What you can learn from the breakthrough research to make your marriage last.* New York: Simon & Schuster.

Gottman, J. M. (1994). *What predicts divorce?: The relationship between marital processes and marital outcomes.* Hillsdale, NJ: Erlbaum.

Greenberg, L. S., & Johnson, S. M. (1988). *Emotionally focused therapy for couples.* New York: Guilford Press.

Groce, N. E., & Zola, I. K. (1993). Multiculturalism, chronic illness, and disability. *Pediatrics, 91,* 1048–1055.

Grodzki, L. (1999). *Building your ideal private practice: A guide for therapists and other healing professionals.* New York: Norton.

Grossman, D. C., Neckerman, H. J., Koepsell, T. D., Liu, P. Y., Asher, K. N., Beland, K., Frey, K., & Rivara, F. P. (1997). Effectiveness of a violence prevention curriculum among children in elementary school. *Journal of the American Medical Association, 277,* 1605–1611.

Grove, J. R., & Heard, N. P. (1997). Optimism and sport confidence as correlates of slump-related coping among athletes. *Sport Psychologist, 11*(4), 400–410.

Grove, J. R., Lavallee, D., Gordon, S., & Harvey, J. H. (1998). Account-making: A model for understanding and resolving distressful reactions to retirement from sport. *Sport Psychologist, 12*(1), 52–67.

Guerney, B. G. (1977). *Relationship Enhancement: Skill-training programs for therapy, problem prevention, and enrichment.* San Francisco: Jossey-Bass.

Guglielmo, W. J. (2001, July 23). Organized medicine's new turf: e-services. *Medi-*

cal Economics [Online]. Available: http://www.medem.com/corporate/news/ corporate_medeminthenews_new041.cfm

Guilford, J. S., Zimmerman, W. S., & Guilford, J. P. (1976). *The Guilford–Zimmerman Temperament Survey handbook*. San Diego, CA: Educational and Industrial Testing Service.

Guthrie, R. (1976). *Even the rat was white*. New York: Harper & Row.

Haber, S., Rodino, E., & Lipner, I. (2000). *Saying good-bye to managed care: Building your independent psychotherapy practice*. New York: Springer.

Haberstroh, C., Hayslip, B., Jr., & Essandoh, P. (1998). The relationship between stepdaughters' self-esteem and perceived parenting behavior. *Journal of Divorce and Remarriage, 29*(3–4), 161–175.

Hadjistavropoulos, T. (1996). The systematic application of ethical codes in the counseling of persons who are considering euthanasia. *Journal of Social Issues, 53*(2), 169–188.

Haidt, J. (2000). The positive emotion of elevation. *Prevention and Treatment, 3*, n.p.

Hall, C. I. (1997). Cultural malpractice: The growing obsolescence of psychology with the changing U.S. population. *American Psychologist, 52*(6), 642–651.

Hall, D. T., Otazo, K. L., & Hollenbeck, G. P. (1999). Behind closed doors: What really happens in executive coaching. *Organizational Dynamics, 27*(3), 39–53.

Hall, L. L. (1997). Making the ADA work for people with psychiatric disabilities.In R. J. Bonnie & J. Monohan (Eds.), *Mental disorder, work disability, and the law* (pp. 241–280). Chicago: University of Chicago Press.

Hall, T. (1998, May 4). A call for psychology to celebrate virtues. *International Herald Tribune*, Section FE, p. 9.

Halpain, M. C., Harris, M. J., McClure, F. S., & Jeste, D. V. (1999). Training in geriatric mental health: Needs and strategies. *Psychiatric Services, 50*(9), 1205–1208.

Hamer, R. J., & Bruch, M. A. (1997). Personality factors and inhibited career development: Testing the unique contribution of shyness. *Journal of Vocational Behavior, 50*(3), 382–400.

Hansson, R. O., DeKoekkoek, P. D., Neece, W. M., & Patterson, D. W. (1997). Successful aging at work: Annual review, 1992–1996. The older worker and transitions to retirement. *Journal of Vocational Behavior, 51*(2), 202–233.

Harris, L., Blum, R. W., & Resnick, M. (1991). Teen females in Minnesota: A portrait of quiet disturbance. In C. Gilligan, A. G. Roger, & D. L. Tolman (Eds.), *Women, girls, and psychotherapy: Reframing resistance* (119–135). New York: Haworth Press.

Harris, Z. L., & Landreth, G. L. (1997). Filial therapy with incarcerated mothers: A five week model. *International Journal of Play Therapy, 6*(2), 53–73.

Haughie, E., Milne, D., & Elliot, V. (1992). An evaluation of comparison pets with elderly psychiatric patients. *Behavioural Psychotherapy, 20*, 367–372.

Hauri, P. J. (1997). Can we mix behavioral therapy with hypnotics when treating insomniacs? *Sleep: Journal of Sleep Research and Sleep Medicine, 20*(12), 1111–1118.

Hawk, K. (1997). Personal reflections on a career in correctional psychology. *Professional Psychology: Research and Practice, 28*(4), 335–337.

Hays, K. F. (1993). The use of exercise in therapy. In L. VandeCreek, S. Knapp, & T. L. Jackson (Eds.), *Innovations in clinical practice: A source book* (Vol. 12, pp. 155–168). Sarasota, FL: Professional Resource Press.

Hays, K. F. (1995). Putting sport psychology into (your) practice. *Professional Psychology: Research and Practice, 26*(1), 33–40.

Hays, K. F. (1999). *Working it out: Using exercise in psychotherapy.* Washington, DC: American Psychological Association.

Hays, K. F. (2000). Sport psychology. *The Register Report, 26,* 17–19.

Heckman, T. G., Kalichman, S. C., Roffman, R. R., Sikkema, K. J., Heckman, B., Davantes, E., Somlai, A. M., & Walker, J. (1999). A telephone-delivered coping improvement intervention for persons living with HIV/AIDS in rural areas. *Social Work with Groups, 21*(4), 49–62.

Heimberg, R. G., Becker, R. E., Goldfinger, K., & Vermilyea, J. A. (1985). Treatment of social phobia by exposure, cognitive restructuring and homework assignments. *Journal of Nervous and Mental Disease, 173*(4), 236–245.

Heimberg, R. G., Liebowitz, M. R., Hope, D. A., & Schneier, F. R. (Eds.). (1995). *Social phobia: Diagnosis, assessment, and treatment.* New York: Guilford Press.

Hekmat, H., Deal, R., & Lubitz, R. (1985). Instructional desensitization: A semantic behavior treatment of anxiety disorder. *Psychotherapy, 22*(2), 273–280.

Heller, K. M. (1997). *Strategic marketing: How to achieve independence and prosperity in your mental health practice.* Sarasota, FL: Professional Resource Press.

Henderson, L. (1992). Shyness groups. In M. McKay & K. Paleg (Eds.), *Focal psychotherapy groups.* Oakland, CA: New Harbinger.

Henderson, L., & Zimbardo, P. (1998). Shyness. In H. S. Friedman (Ed.), *Encyclopedia of mental health.* San Diego, CA: Academic Press. (Also available at http://www.shyness.com/encyclopedia.html)

Henderson, L., Zimbardo, P., & Rodino, E. (2001). *Painful shyness in children and adults* [Online]. Available: http://www.division42.org/PublicArea/Brochures/shyness.html

Henriksen, R. C. (1997). Counseling mixed parentage individuals: A dilemma. *Texas Classics in Action (TCA) Journal, 25*(2), 68–74.

Henry, J. D., Henry, V. M., & Krug, S. E. (1984). *GROW: Relationship counseling.* Champaign, IL: MetriTech.

Herring, R. D. (1995). Developing biracial ethnic identity: A review of the increasing dilemma. *Journal of Multicultural Counseling and Development, 23*(1), 29–38.

Hetherington, E. M. (1989). Coping with family transitions: Winners, losers, and survivors. *Child Development, 60,* 1–14.

Hiebert, B., Kirby, B., & Jaknavorian, A. (1989). School-based relaxation: Attempting primary prevention. *Canadian Journal of Counselling, 23*(3), 273–287.

Hilburt-Davis, J. (1996, Spring). Consultation to the work place: Thoughts for family therapists. *American Family Therapy Academy Newsletter* [Online]. Available: http://www.familybusinessconsulting.com/resources/therapists.shtml

Hilburt-Davis, J. (1997, Summer). Consulting to family businesses: New opportunity for family therapists. *American Family Therapy Academy Newsletter,* pp. 33–35.

Hilburt-Davis, J., & Senturia, P. (1995). Using the process/content framework: Guidelines for the content expert. *Family Business Review, 8*(3), 189–199.

Hillman, J. L. (2000). *Clinical perspectives on elderly sexuality.* New York: Kluwer Academic/Plenum Press.

Hodges, E. V., & Perry, D. G. (1996). Victimization is never just child's play. *School Safety* [published by the National School Safety Center, Research Triangle Park, NC], p. 4.

Hoffman, C., Rice, D., & Sung, H.-Y. (1996). Persons with chronic conditions: Their prevalence and costs. *Journal of the American Medical Association, 276,* 1473–1479.

Hogarty, G. E., Anderson, C. M., Reiss, D. J., Kornblith, S. J., Greenwald, D. P., Ulrich, R. F., & Carter, M. (1991). Family psychoeducation, social skills training, and maintenance chemotherapy in the aftercare treatment of schizophrenia. *Archives of General Psychiatry, 48,* 340–347.

Holliday, G. A., Koller, J. R., & Thomas, C. D. (1999). Post-high school outcomes of high IQ adults with learning disabilities. *Journal for the Education of the Gifted, 22*(2), 266–281.

Hope, D. A., Heimberg, R. G., Juster, H. R., & Turk, C. L. (2000). *Managing social anxiety: A cognitive-behavioral therapy approach.* San Diego, CA: Academic Press.

Hopf, T., Ayres, J., & Colby, N. (1994). Using visualization to reduce communication apprehension in initial interaction: A brief report. *Communication Reports, 7*(1), 57–60.

Horowitz, A., & Shindelman, L. (1983). Reciprocity and affection: Past influences on current caregiving. *Journal of Gerontological Social Work, 5,* 5–20.

Hotopf, M., Mayou, R., Wadsworth, M., & Wessely, S. (1999). Psychosocial and developmental antecedents of chest pain in young adults. *Psychosomatic Medicine, 61*(6), 861–867.

Houlihan, J. P., & Reynolds, M. D. (2001). Assessment of employees with mental health disabilities for workplace accommodations: Case reports. *Professional Psychology: Research and Practice, 32*(4), 380–385.

Hovey, J. D., & King, C. A. (1996). Acculturative stress, depression, and suicidal ideation among immigrant and second-generation Latino adolescents. *Journal of the American Academy of Child & Adolescent Psychiatry, 35*(9), 1183–1192.

How one provider revitalized his practice by moving. (1995, November). *Psychotherapy Finances, 21*(11), 6–7.

Hultsch, D. F., Hertzog, C., Small, B. J., & Dixon, R. A. (1999). Use it or lose it: Engaged lifestyle as a buffer of cognitive decline in aging. *Psychology and Aging, 14*(2), 245–263.

Human J., & Wasem, C. (1991). Rural mental health in America. *American Psychologist, 46*(3), 232–239.

Humphrey, L. L. (1988). Comparison of bulimic-anorexic and nondistressed families using structural analysis of social behavior. *Journal of the American Academy of Child and Adolescent Psychiatry, 26,* 248–255.

International Coach Federation. (1998, September 15). *ICF survey of coaching clients: Survey reveals emerging profession of coaching having measurable impact on clients* [Online]. Available: http://www.coachfederation.org/nmember.htm# Client

International Labor Organization. (2000, November). ILO examines mental health in the workplace. *ILO News* [Online]. Available: http://us.ilo.org/news/ilowatch/0011.html

Intrieri, R. C., & Rapp, S. R. (1994). Self-control skillfulness and caregiver burden among help-seeking elders. *Journal of Gerontology, 49*(1), 19–23.

Israel, Y., Hollander, O., Sanchez-Craig, M., Booker, S., Miller, V., Gingrich, R., & Rankin, J. G. (1996). Screening for problem drinking and counseling by the primary care physician–nurse team. *Alcoholism: Clinical and Experimental Research, 20*(8), 1443–1450.

Jacobs, G. D. (1999) *Say goodnight to insomnia.* New York: Holt.

Jacobs, G. D., Benson, H., & Friedman, R. (1996). Perceived benefits in a behavioral medicine insomnia program: A clinical report. *American Journal of Medicine, 100,* 212–216.

Jacobs, R. H. (1997). *Be an outrageous older woman.* New York: HarperCollins.

Jacobs, S., & Kim, K. (1990). Psychiatric complications of bereavement. *Psychiatric Annals, 20,* 314–317.

Jaffe, D. T., Scott, C. D., & Tobe, G. R. (1994). *Rekindling commitment: How to revitalize yourself, your work, and your organization.* San Francisco: Jossey-Bass.

James, M. (1994). Child abuse prevention: A perspective on parent enhancement programs from the United States. *Issues in Child Abuse Prevention* http://www.aifs.org.au/external/nch/issues3.html#con

Jaremko, M. E. (1980). The use of stress inoculation training in the reduction of public speaking anxiety. *Journal of Clinical Psychology, 36*(3), 735–738.

Jay, S., C. H., Fitzgibbons, I., & Woody, P. (1995). A comparative study of cognitive behavior therapy versus general anesthesia for painful medical procedures in children. *Pain, 62*(1), 3–9.

Jaycox, L., Reivich, K., Gillham, J., & Seligman, M. E. P. (1994). Prevention of depressive symptoms in school children. *Behaviour Research and Therapy, 32,* 801–816.

Jerrell, J. M. (1998). Effect of ethnic matching of young clients and mental health staff. *Cultural Diversity and Ethnic Minority Psychology, 4*(4), 297–302.

Johnson, S. (1997). *Taking the anxiety out of taking tests: A step-by-step guide.* Oakland, CA: New Harbinger.

Johnson, S. M. (1996). *The practice of emotionally focused marital therapy: Creating connection.* New York: Brunner/Mazel.

Johnson, S. M., & Greenberg, L. S. (1994). *The heart of the matter: Emotion in marital therapy.* New York: Brunner/Mazel.

Jones, B. C. (1997, March 3). Brown University poll finds no more loyalty in workplace. *Knight-Ridder/Tribune Business News.*

Jones, J. (1983). The concept of race in social psychology. In L. Wheeler & P. Shaver (Eds.) *Review of personality and social psychology* (Vol. 4, pp. 117–150). Beverly Hills, CA: Sage.

Jones, L. R., Badger, L. W., Ficken, R. P., Leeper, J. D., & Anderson, R. L. (1987). Inside the hidden mental health network: Examining mental health care delivery of primary care physicians. *General Hospital Psychiatry, 9,* 287–293.

Joseph, L. M., & Greenberg, M. A. (2001). The effects of a career transition program on reemployment success in laid-off professionals. *Consulting Psychology Journal: Practice and Research, 53*(3), 169–181.

Judd, L. L. (1994). Social phobia: A clinical overview. *Journal of Clinical Psychiatry, 55*(Suppl.), 5–9.

Kainz, K. (2002, April). Barriers and enhancements to physician–psychologist collaboration. *Professional Psychology: Research and Practice, 33*(2), 169–175.

Kanter, R. M. (1985). Managing the human side of change. *Management Review, 74*(4), 52–56.

Kaslow, F. W. (1993). The lore and lure of family business. *American Journal of Family Therapy, 21*(1), 3–16.

Katon, W. (1995). Collaborative care: Patient satisfaction, outcomes, and medical cost-offset. *Family Systems Medicine, 13*(3–4), 351–365.

Katon, W., Von Korff, M., Lin, E., Simon, G., Walker, E., Bush, T., & Ludman, E. (1997). Collaborative management to achieve depression treatment guidelines. *Journal of Clinical Psychiatry, 58*(Suppl. 1), 20–23.

Katz, J. H., & Miller, F. A. (1996). Coaching leaders through culture change. *Consulting Psychology Journal: Practice and Research, 48*(2), 104–114.

Katzelnick, D. J., Kobak, K. A., DeLeire, T., Henk, H. J., Greist, J. H., Davidson, J. R. T., Schneider, F. R., Stein, M. B., & Helstad, C. P. (2001). Impact of generalized social anxiety disorder in managed care. *American Journal of Psychiatry, 158*, 1999–2007.

Kavanagh, D. J. (1992). Recent developments in expressed emotion and schizophrenia. *British Journal of Psychiatry, 160*, 601–620.

Kazdin, A. E., & Weisz, J. R. (1998). Identifying and developing empirically supported child and adolescent treatments. *Journal of Consulting and Clinical Psychology, 66*(1), 19–36.

Kearney, C. A. (2001). *School refusal behavior in youth: A functional approach to assessment and treatment.* Washington, DC: American Psychological Association.

Kearney, C. A., & Silverman, W. K. (1995). Family environment of youngsters with school refusal behavior: A synopsis with implications for assessment and treatment. *American Journal of Family Therapy, 23*(1), 59–72.

Keefe, F. J., Dunsmore, J., & Burnett, R. (1992). Behavioral and cognitive-behavioral approaches to chronic pain: Recent advances and future directions. *Journal of Consulting and Clinical Psychology. 60*(4), 528–536.

Kelley, P. (1996). Family-centered practice with stepfamilies. *Families in Society, 77*(9), 535–544.

Kerr, B. A. (1997). *Smart girls: A new psychology of girls, women, and giftedness.* Scottsdale, AZ: Gifted Psychology Press.

Kerr, B. A., & Erb, C. (1991). Career counseling with academically talented students: Effects of a value-based intervention. *Journal of Counseling Psychology, 38*(3), 309–314.

Kerr, G., Krasnow, D., & Mainwaring, L. (1992). The nature of dance injuries. *Medical Problems of Performing Artists, 7*(1), 25–29.

Kets de Vries, M. F. R. (1996). *Family business: Human dilemmas in the family firm: Text and cases.* Boston: International Thomson Business Press.

Key issues as viewed by family business owners. (1999, July). *Relatively Speaking* [Online]. Available: http://www.regeneration-partners.com/NL_articles/nl_july_99_art02.html

Khehgi-Genovese, Z., & Genovese, T. A. (1997). Developing the spousal relationship within stepfamilies. *Families in Society, 78*(3), 255–264.

Kibby, M. Y., Tyc, V. L., & Mulhern, R. K. (1998). Effectiveness of psychological intervention for children and adolescents with chronic medical illness: A meta-analysis. *Clinical Psychology Review, 18*(1), 103–117.

Kidd, A. H., Kidd, R. M., & George, C. C. (1992). Veterinarians and successful pet adoptions. *Psychological Reports, 71*(2), 551–557.

Kilpatrick, D. G., Edmunds, C., & Seymour, A. (1992). *Rape in America: A report to the nation*. Arlington, VA: National Center for Victims of Crime.

King, N. J., Ollendick, T. H., & Tonge, B. J. (1995). *School refusal: Assessment and treatment*. Boston: Allyn & Bacon.

Klein, A. G., & Zehms, D. (1996). Self-concept and gifted girls: A cross sectional study of intellectually gifted females in grades 3, 5, 8. *Roeper Review, 19*(1), 30–34.

Klerman, G. L., & Weissman, M. M. (1989). Increasing rates of depression. *Journal of the American Medical Association, 261*(15), 2229–2235.

Knight, B. G., & McCallum, T. J. (1998). Adapting psychotherapeutic practice for older clients: Implications of the contextual, cohort-based, maturity, specific challenge model. *Professional Psychology: Research and Practice, 29*(1), 15–22.

Koch, W. J., & Taylor, S. (1995). Assessment and treatment of motor vehicle accident victims. *Cognitive and Behavioral Practice, 2*(2), 327–342.

Koder, D.-A. (1998). Treatment of anxiety in the cognitively impaired elderly: Can cognitive-behavior therapy help? *International Psychogeriatrics, 10*(2), 173–182.

Kojlak, J., Keenan, S. P., Plotkin, D., Giles-Fysh, N., & Sibbald, W. J. (1998). Determining the potential need for a bereavement follow-up program: How well are family and health care workers' needs currently being met? *Official Journal of the Canadian Association of Critical Care Nurses, 9*(1), 12–16.

Kolt, L. (1999). *How to build a thriving fee-for-service practice*. San Diego, CA: Academic Press.

Kravets, M., & Wax, I. F. (2000). *K&W guide to colleges for the learning disabled* (5th ed.). New York: Random House.

Kroenke, K., & Mangelsdorff, A. D. (1989) Common symptoms in ambulatory care: Incidence, evaluation, therapy, and outcome. *American Journal of Medicine, 86*(3), 262–266.

Krugman, M., Kirsch, I., Wickless, C., Milling, L., Golicz, H., & Toth, A. (1985). Neuro-linguistic programming treatment for anxiety: Magic or myth? *Journal of Consulting and Clinical Psychology, 53*(4), 526–530.

Kubeck, J. E., Delp, N. D., Haslett, T. K., & McDaniel, M. A. (1996). Does job-related training performance decline with age? *Psychology and Aging, 11*(1), 92–107.

Kuchenbecker, S. (1999, August). *Positive coaching through formative feedback*. Poster presented at the 107th Annual Convention of the American Psychological Association, Boston.

Kuchenbecker, S., Rigg, C. M., Weglarz, C. M., Alvarez, E. E., Fleming, S. R., Robera, S., et al. (1999, August). *Who's a winner?: Coaches' views of winning young athletes*. Paper presented at the 107th Annual Convention of the American Psychological Association, Boston.

Kurlychek, R. T., & Morganstern, K. P. (1978). The use of self-control procedures in the treatment of chronic shoplifting. *Corrective and Social Psychiatry and Journal of Behavior Technology, Methods and Therapy, 24*(2), 86–87.

Kushnir, T., Malkinson, R., & Kasan, R. (1996). Reducing work/home conflicts in employed couples: A proposed program to balance job and family demands. *Contemporary Family Therapy: An International Journal, 18*(1), 147–159.

Lacks, P., & Morin, C. M. (1992). Recent advances in the assessment and treatment of insomnia. *Journal of Consulting and Clinical Psychology, 60*(4), 586–594.

LaCroix, R. P. (1998, May 11). Questions and answers—Marketing your practice. *Selfhelp Magazine* [Online]. Available: http://www.shpm.com/ppc/mar/qamktyp.html

Lam, D. H. (1991). Psychosocial family intervention in schizophrenia: A review of empirical studies. *Psychological Medicine, 21*(2), 423–441.

Lamenza, L. (1999). A newcomer practicing in an inner city community. *Independent Practitioner, 19,* (3), 153–155.

Larson, J. D. (1992). Anger and aggression management techniques through the Think First curriculum. *Journal of Offender Rehabilitation, 18,* 101–117.

Larson, J. D. (1994). Violence prevention in the schools: A review of selected programs and procedures. *School Psychology Review, 23*(2), 151–164.

Larsson, B., & Carlsson, J. (1966). School-based, nurse-administered relaxation training for children with chronic tension type headaches. *Journal of Pediatric Psychology, 21,* 603–614.

Last, C. G., & Strauss, C. C. (1990). School refusal in anxiety disordered children and adolescents. *Journal of the American Academy of Child and Adolescent Psychiatry, 29,* 31–35.

Law, S., & Scott, S. (1995). Tips for practitioners: Pet care: A vehicle for learning. *Focus on Autistic Behavior, 10*(2), 17–18.

Lawless, L. L. (1997). *Therapy, Inc: A hands-on guide to developing, positioning, and marketing your mental health practice in the 1990's.* New York: Wiley.

Lawton, J. M., & Sanders, M. R. (1994). Designing effective behavioral family interventions for stepfamilies. *Clinical Psychology Review, 141*(5), 463–496.

Learning Commons, University of Guelph [Guelph, Ontario, Canada]. (2002). Controlling procrastination [Online]. Available: http://www.learningcommons.uoguelph.ca/learning/fastfax/procrastination.htm

Lechnyr, R. (1992). Cost savings and effectiveness of mental health services. *Journal of the Oregon Psychological Association, 38,* 8–12.

Lee, D. R. (1983). Pet therapy: Helping patients through troubled times. *California Veterinarian, 5,* 24–40.

Leitman, R., Binns, K., & Duffett, A. (1995). *Between hope and fear: Teens speak out on crime and the community.* New York: Louis Harris & Associates.

Lemp, G. F., Hirozawa, A. M., Givertz, D., Nieri, G. N., Anderson, L., Lindegren, M. L., Janssen, R. S., & Katz, M. (1994). Seroprevalence of HIV and risk behaviors among young homosexual and bisexual men. *Journal of the American Medical Association, 272,* 449–454.

Leukefeld, C. G., Godlaski, T. M., Hays, L. R., & Clark, J. (1999). Developing a rural therapy with big city approaches. *Substance Use and Misuse, 34*(4–5), 747–762.

Levant, R., Reed, G., Ragusea, S., Stout, C., DiCowden, M., Murphy, M., Sullivan, F., & Craig, P. (2001). Envisioning and accessing new professional roles. *Professional Psychology: Research and Practice, 32*(1), 79–87.

Levering, R., & Moskowitz, M. (1994). *The 100 best companies to work for in America.* New York: Plume Books.

Levinson, B. (1962). The dog as "co-therapist." *Mental Hygiene, 46,* 59–65.

Levinson, H. (1996). Executive coaching. *Consulting Psychology Journal: Practice and Research, 48*(2), 115–123.

Levy, D. S., & Ru, E. (1993, August 16). Society: Reigning cats and dogs: For Americans and their pets . . . er, companion animals . . . it's the best—and worst—that money can buy. *Time*, p. 50.

Lewin, M. R., McNeil, D. R., & Lipson, J. M. (1996). Enduring without avoiding: Pauses and verbal dysfluencies in public speaking fear. *Journal of Psychopathology and Behavioral Assessment, 18*(4), 387–402.

Lewis, B. L. (2001). Health psychology specialty practice opportunities in a rural community hospital: Practicing local clinical science. *Professional Psychology: Research and Practice, 32,*(1), 59–64.

Li, G. (1995). The interaction effect of bereavement and sex on the risk of suicide in the elderly: An historical cohort study. *Social Science and Medicine, 40*(6), 825–828.

Lidbeck, J. (1997). Group therapy for somatization disorders in general practice: Effectiveness of a short cognitive-behavioural treatment model. *Acta Psychiatrica Scandanavica, 96*(1), 14–24.

Liddle, B. J. (1996). Therapist sexual orientation, gender, and counseling practices as they relate to ratings on helpfulness by gay and lesbian clients. *Journal of Counseling Psychology, 43*(4), 394–401.

Liddle, B. J. (1997). Gay and lesbian clients' selection of therapists and utilization of therapy. *Psychotherapy, 34*(1), 11–18.

Liebowitz, B, (1998). *Resolving conflict in the family owned business* [Online]. Available: http://www.liebowitzassoc.com/art11.htm

Lin, E. H., Katon, W. J., Simon, G. E., Von Korff, M., Bush, T. M., Rutter, C. M., Saunders, K. W., & Walker, E. A. (1997). Achieving guidelines for the treatment of depression in primary care: Is physician education enough? *Medical Care, 35*(8), 831–842.

Linn, M., Linn, B., & Harris, R. (1982). Effects of counseling for late-stage cancer patients. *Cancer, 49,* 1048–1055.

Lipsitt, D. R. (1996). Primary care of the somatizing patient: A collaborative model. *Hospital Practice, 31*(6), 77–80.

Logan, J. M., Sanders, A. L., Snyder, A. Z., Morris, J. C., & Buckner, R. L. (2002). Under-recruitment and nonselective recruitment: Dissociable neural mechanisms associated with aging. *Neuron, 33,* 827–840.

Longlett, S., & Kruse, J. (1992). Behavioral science education in family medicine: A survey of behavioral science educators and family physicians. *Family Medicine, 24*(1), 28–35.

Lowenstein, L. F. (1997). Research into causes and manifestations of aggression in car driving. *Police Journal, 70*(3), 263–270.

Luquet, W. (1996). *Short-term couples therapy: The Imago model in action.* New York: Brunner/Mazel.

Luquet, W., & Hannah, M. T. (1998). *Healing in the relationship paradigm: The Imago Relationship Therapy casebook.* New York: Brunner/Mazel.

Lykken, D. (1999). *Happiness: What studies on twins show us about nature, nurture, and the happiness set-point.* New York: Golden Books.

Lynch, J. (2000). *The broken heart.* Baltimore: Bancroft Press.

Lynch, T. (1997). *The undertaking: Life studies from the dismal trade.* New York: Norton.

Lyster, R. F., Russell, M. N., & Hiebert, J. (1995). Preparation for remarriage: Consumers' views. *Journal of Divorce and Remarriage, 24*(3–4), 143–157.

Maas, J. B. (1999). *Power sleep: The revolutionary program that prepares your mind for peak performance.* New York: HarperCollins.

Macchi, R. (1996). After the fall: Reflections of injured classical ballet dancers. *Journal of Sport Behavior, 19*(3), 221–235.

Maccoby, M. (1995). *Why work?: Motivating the new workforce* (2nd ed.). Alexandria, VA: Miles River Press.

MacDevitt, J. W., & Kedzierzawski, G. D. (1990). A structured group format for first offense shoplifters. *International Journal of Offender Therapy and Comparative Criminology, 34*(2), 155–164.

Maddi, S. R. (1997). Strengths and weaknesses of organizational consulting from a clinical psychology background. *Consulting Psychology Journal: Practice and Research, 49,* 207—219.

Mahoney, A. S. (1998). In search of the gifted identity: From abstract concept to workable counseling constructs. *Roeper Review, 20*(3), 222–226.

Malone, R. P., Luebbert, J. F., Delaney, M. A., Biesecker, K. A., Blaney, B. L., Rowan, A. B., & Campbell, M. (1997). Nonpharmacological response in hospitalized children with conduct disorder. *Journal of the American Academy of Child and Adolescent Psychiatry, 36*(2), 242–247.

Malta, L. S., Blanchard, E. B., Taylor, A. E., Hickling, E. J., & Freidenberg, B. M. (2002). Personality disorders and posttraumatic stress disorder in motor vehicle accident survivors. *Journal of Nervous and Mental Disease, 190*(11), 767–774.

Maly, R. C. (1993). Early recognition of chemical dependence. *Primary Care, 20*(1), 33–50.

Mancino, M., Cunningham, M. R., Davidson, P., & Fulton, R. L. (1996). Identification of the motor vehicle accident victim who abuses alcohol: An opportunity to reduce trauma. *Journal of Studies on Alcohol, 57,* 652–658.

Manderscheid, R. W., & Sonnenschein, M. A. (Eds.). (1990). *Mental health, United States, 1990* (DHHS Publication No. ADM 90-1708). Washington, DC: U.S. Government Printing Office.

Mangione, T. W., Howland, J., Amick, B., Cote, J., Lee, M., Bell, N., & Levine, S. (1999). Employee drinking practices and work performance. *Journal of Studies on Alcohol, 60*(2), 261–270.

Mantyselka, P., Kumpusalo, E., Ahonen, R., & Takala, J. (2001, December). Patients' versus general practitioners' assessments of pain intensity in primary care patients with non-cancer pain. *British Journal of General Practice, 51*(473), 995–997.

Mari, J. J., & Streiner, D. (1996). The effects of family intervention for those with schizophrenia. *Cochrane Database of Systematic Reviews* [Online], Issue 3. Available: http://www.update_software.com/abstracts/ab000088.htm

Marita, A., & Mermelstein-Lopez, R. J. (1995). A cognitive-behavioral program to improve geriatric rehabilitation outcome. *The Gerontologist, 35*(5), 696–701.

Markman, H., Stanley, S., Blumberg, S. L., & Edell, D. S. (1996). *Fighting for your marriage: Positive steps for preventing divorce and preserving a lasting love.* San Francisco: Jossey-Bass.

Marsh, D. T., & Johnson, D. L. (1997). The family experience of mental illness: Implications for intervention. *Professional Psychology: Research and Practice, 28*(3), 229–237.

Marshall, W. L., Parker, L., & Hayes, B. J. (1982). Treating public speaking problems:

A study using flooding and the elements of skills training. *Behavior Modification, 6*(2), 147–170.

Martin, I. (1996). *From couch to corporation.* New York: Wiley.

Marshall, W. L., Presse, L., & Andrews, W. R. (1976). A self-administered program for public speaking anxiety. *Behaviour Research and Therapy, 14*(1), 33–39.

Marwit, S. J. (1997). Professional psychology's role in hospice care. *Professional Psychology: Research and Practice, 28*(5), 457–463.

Massachusetts Mutual Life Insurance Company. (1994). *1994 research findings of American family businesses.* Springfield, MA: Author.

Maurer, M. (1997). *Americans behind bars: U.S. and international use of incarceration, 1995.* Washington, DC: The Sentencing Project.

Mawson, D., Marks, I. M., Ramm, E., & Stern, R. (1981). Guided mourning for morbid grief: A controlled study. *British Journal of Psychiatry, 138,* 185–193.

Mayfield, D., McLeod, G., & Hall, P. (1974). The CAGE questionnaire: Validation of a new alcoholism instrument. *American Journal of Psychiatry, 131,* 1121–1123.

McAleer, D. (1997). Psychology and medicine: A partnership for the future. *Independent Practitioner, 17*(4), 204–206.

McCroskey, J. C., Beatty, M. J., Kearney, P., & Plax, T. G. (1985). The content validity of the PRCA-24 as a measure of communication apprehension across communication contexts. *Communication Quarterly, 33,* 165–173.

McCullough M. E., & Worthington E. L., Jr. (1999). Religion and the forgiving personality. *Journal of Personality, 67*(6), 1141–1164.

McDaniel, S. H. (1995). Collaboration between psychologists and family physicians: Implementing the biopsychosocial model. *Professional Psychology: Research and Practice, 26*(2), 117–122.

McIntyre, T. (1996). Guidelines for providing appropriate services to culturally diverse students with emotional and/or behavioral disorders. *Behavioral Disorders, 21*(2), 137–144.

McKimmy, S. (1996, Winter). Survey: An inventory of family business experiences. *Succeeding Generations* [published by the University of Toledo Center for Family Business]. Available: http://www.msu.edu/course/prr/473/oldstuff/familybusiness.htm

McKirnan, D. J., & Peterson, P. L. (1989). Alcohol and drug use among homosexual men and women: Epidemiology and population characteristics. *Addictive Behaviors, 14,* 1307–1310.

McLeod, C. C., Budd, M. A., & McClelland, D. C. (1997). Treatment of somatization in primary care. *General Hospital Psychiatry, 19*(4), 251–258.

McMinn, M. R., Meek, K. R., Canning, S. S., & Pozzi, C. F. (2001). Training psychologists to work with religious organizations: The center for church-psychology collaboration. *Professional Psychology: Research & Practice, 32*(3), 324–328.

McNees, M. P., Schnelle, J. F., Kirchner, R. E., & Thomas, M. M. (1980). An experimental analysis of a program to reduce retail theft. *American Journal of Community Psychology, 8*(3), 379–385.

Meadows, M. (1997, September). Cultural considerations in treating Asians. *Newsletter of the Office of Minority Health* [Online]. Available: http://www.omhrc.gov/ctg/full-mhm.htm#mhm-01

Meeks, S. (1996). Psychological consultation to nursing homes: Description of a six-year practice. *Psychotherapy, 33*(1), 19–29.

Megargee, E. I. (1995). Assessment research in correctional settings: Methodological issues and practical problems. *Psychological Assessment, 7*(3), 359–366.

Meichenbaum, D., & Biemiller, A. (2000). *Nurturing independent learning: Helping students take charge of their learning.* Cambridge, MA: Brookline Books.

Melamed, B. G., et al. (1978). Effects of film modeling on the reduction of anxiety-related behaviors in individuals varying in level of previous experience in the stress situation. *Journal of Consulting and Clinical Psychology, 46*(6), 1357–1367.

Melchior, L. A., & Cheek, J. M. (1990). Shyness and anxious self-preoccupation during a social interaction. *Journal of Social Behavior and Personality, 5*(2), 117–130.

Menapace, B. (1998). *Correlates of effectiveness for white psychotherapists working with African-American clients.* Paper presented at the 106th Annual Convention of the American Psychological Association, San Francisco.

Mendaglio, S. (1993). Counseling gifted learning disabled: Individual and group counseling techniques. In L. K. Silverman (Ed.), *Counseling the gifted and talented* (pp. 131–149). Denver, CO: Love.

Mental disabilities no barrier to smooth and efficient work: Employers may have exaggerated fears about the costs of employing people with psychiatric disabilities, psychologists find. (1998, July). *APA Monitor* [Online], *29*(7). Available: http://www.apa.org/monitor/jul98/integrate.html

Michigan Adult Foster Care. (n.d.). Impact of schizophrenia on caregiver underestimated; family caregivers may be at personal mental health risk, based on national survey [Online] Available: http://www.miafc.com/Public/MentHlth/3000/ImpOfSz..html

Mikulincer, M., & Florian, V. (1996). Coping and adaptation to trauma and loss. In M. Zeidner & N. S. Endler (Eds.), *Handbook of coping: Theory, research, applications.* New York: Wiley.

Milhorn, H. T. J. (1988). The diagnosis of alcoholism. *American Family Physician, 37*, 175–183.

Miller, B. (1998). *Families matter: A research synthesis of family influences on adolescent pregnancy.* Washington DC: National Campaign to Prevent Teen Pregnancy.

Miller, R. L., & Miller, B. (1990). Mothering the biracial child: Bridging the gaps between African-American and white parenting styles. *Women and Therapy, 10*(1–2), 169–179.

Mintz, S. (1996). "Caregiver disorder": An unacknowledged illness. *Take Care* [Online], *5*(4). Available: http://www.seniorconnections-va.org/caregivers/disorder.htm

Mlynarek, L. S., & Mondoux, L. C. (1996, September). Pulling together for restraint reduction. *Nursing Homes, 45*(8), 12.

Moak, G. S., Zimmer, B., & Stein, E. M. (1988). Clinical perspectives on elderly first-offender shoplifters. *Hospital and Community Psychiatry, 39*(6), 648–651.

Moon, M. A. (2000). Positive psychology halved depression in kids. *Clinical Psychiatry News, 28*(5), 29.

Moon, S. M., & Hall, A. S. (1998). Family therapy with intellectually and creatively gifted children. *Journal of Marital and Family Therapy, 24*(1), 59–80.

Moon, S. M., Kelly, K. R., & Feldhusen, J. F. (1997). Specialized counseling services for gifted youth and their families: A needs assessment. *Gifted Child Quarterly, 41*(1), 16–25.

Moore, R. H. (1983). College shoplifters: Rebuttal of Beck and McIntyre. *Psychological Reports, 53*(3, Pt. 2), 1111–1116.

More clinical psychologists move into organizational consulting realm: Meet three clinical psychologists who have expanded their practices to the world of work. (1998, July). *APA Monitor* [Online], *29*(7). Available: http://www.apa.org/monitor/jul98/consult.html

Morgan, R. D., Winterowd, C. L., & Ferrell, S. W. (1999). A national survey of group psychotherapy services in correctional facilities. *Professional Psychology: Research and Practice, 30*(6), 600–606.

Morgan, W. P. (1993). Hypnosis and sport psychology. In J. W. Rhue, S. J. Lynn, & I. Kirsch (Eds.), *Handbook of clinical hypnosis* (pp. 649–670). Washington, DC: American Psychological Association.

Morgan, W. P. (Ed.). (1997). *Physical activity and mental health.* Washington, DC: Taylor & Francis.

Mori, D. L., LoCastro, J. S., Grace, M., & Costello, T. (1999). Implementing the direct contact model to increase referrals for psychological services in primary care settings. *Professional Psychology: Research and Practice, 30*(2), 143–146.

Morin, C. M. (1993). *Insomnia: Psychological assessment and management.* New York: Guilford Press.

Morin, C. M., & Colecchi, C. A. (1994). Clinical guidelines for the treatment of insomnia. In L. Vandecreek, S. Knapp, & T. L. Jackson (Eds.), *Innovations in clinical practice: A source book* (Vol. 12, pp. 179–195). Sarasota, FL: Professional Resource Press.

Morin, C. M., Kowatch, R. A., Barry, T., & Walton, E. (1993). Cognitive-behavior therapy for late-life insomnia. *Journal of Consulting and Clinical Psychology, 61*(1), 137–146.

Morin, C. M., & Wooten, V. (1996). Psychological and pharmacological approaches to treating insomnia: Critical issues in assessing their separate and combined effects. *Clinical Psychology Review, 16*(6), 521–542.

Morris, J. A. (Ed.). (1997). *Practicing psychology in rural settings: Hospital privileges and collaborative care.* Washington, DC: American Psychological Association.

Morrison, G. M., Storino, M. H., Robertson, L. M., Weissglass, T., & Dondero, A. (2000). The protective function of after-school programming and parent education and support for students at risk for substance abuse. *Evaluation and Program Planning, 23*(3), 365–371.

Morse, D. S., Suchman, A. L., & Frankel, R. M. (1997). The meaning of symptoms in 10 women with somatization disorder and a history of childhood abuse. *Archives of Family Medicine, 6*(5), 468–476.

Mossman, D. (1995). Violence prediction, workplace violence, and the mental health expert. *Consulting Psychology Journal: Practice and Research, 47*(4), 223–233.

Motley, M. T., & Molloy, J. L. (1994). An efficacy test of a new therapy ("communication-orientation motivation") for public speaking anxiety. *Journal of Applied Communication Research, 22*(1), 48–58.

Moye, J., & Brown, E. (1995). Postdoctoral training in geropsychology: Guidelines for formal programs and continuing education. *Professional Psychology: Research and Practice, 26*(6), 591–597.

Moyerman, D. R., & Forman, B. D. (1992). Acculturation and adjustment: A meta-analytic study. *Hispanic Journal of Behavioral Sciences, 14,* 163–200.

Mulder, P. L., & Chang, A. F. (1997). Domestic violence in rural communities: A literature review and discussion. *Journal of Rural Community Psychology [Online], E*(1). Available: http://www.marshall.edu/jrcp/VolE1/Vol_E1_1/Mulder_Chang.html

Multi-disciplinary business team creates the California Family Business Institute. (1997, April 18). *Business Wire.*

Murphy, S. A., Johnson, C., Cain, K., Gupta, A. D., Dimond, M., Lohan, J., & Baugher, R (1998). Broad-spectrum group treatment for parents bereaved by the violent deaths of their 12- to 28-year-old children: A randomized controlled trial. *Death Studies, 22*(3), 209–235

Murray, B. (1997, September). School phobias hold many children back: It takes a team effort to help children overcome fear of school. *APA Monitor,* p. 1.

Murray, J. D., & Keller, P. A. (1991). Psychology and rural America. *American Psychologist, 46*(3), 220–231.

Murtagh, D. R. R., & Greenwood, K. M. (1995). Identifying effective psychological treatments for insomnia: A meta-analysis. *Journal of Consulting and Clinical Psychology, 63*(1), 79–89.

Muszynski, S. Y., & Akamatsu, T. J. (1991). Delay in completion of doctoral dissertations in clinical psychology. *Professional Psychology: Research and Practice, 22*(2), 119–123.

Myers, I. B., McCaulley, M. H., Quenk, N. L., & Hammer, A. L. (1998). *Manual: A guide to the development and use of the Myers–Briggs Type Indicator.* Palo Alto, CA: Consulting Psychologists Press.

Nagy, S., Adcock, A. G., & Nagy M. C. (1994). A comparison of risky health behaviors of sexually active, sexually abused, and abstaining adolescents. *Pediatrics, 93,* 570–575.

Nansel, T. R., Overpeck, M., Pilla, R. S., Ruan, W. J., Simons-Morton, B., & Scheidt, P. (2001). Bullying behaviors among US youth: Prevalence and association with psychosocial adjustment. *Journal of the American Medical Association, 285,* 2094–2100.

Naseef, R. (1997). *Special children, challenged parents: The struggles and rewards of raising a child with a disability.* Secaucus, NJ: Carol.

National Association for Home Care. *Basic statistics about home care* [Online]. Available: http://www.paragonventures.com/home_care_stats.htm

National Association of Psychiatric Health Systems. (2000, May 19). *Behavioral health is an integral part of overall health* [Online]. Available: http://www.naphs.org/news/benefits.html

National Center for Education Statistics. (1996, November). *1996 digest of education statistics* [Online]. Available: http://nces.ed.gov/pubs/D96/d96t053.html

National Center for Education Statistics. (1998). *The condition of education* (NCES Document No. 98-013). Jessup, MD: ED Publications. (Also available at http://www.nces.ed.gov/pubs98/condition98/c9847a01.html)

National Center for Health Statistics. (1999, June 10). *New report documents improvement in American's health: Best rating in two decades for Annual Progress Review.* Washington, DC: U.S. Department of Health and Human Services.

National Commission on Sleep Disorders Research. (1993, January). *Wake up America: A national sleep alert, executive summary and executive report* (Vol. 1) [Online]. Available: http://www.stanford.edu/~dement/overview-ncsdr.html

National Institute on Drug Abuse. (1998). *The economic costs of alcohol and drug abuse in the United States—1992* [Online]. Available: http://www.nida.nih.gov/EconomicCosts

National Institutes of Health. (1995, October). *Integration of behavioral and relaxation approaches into the treatment of chronic pain and insomnia: NIH Technology Assessment Conference statement.* Bethesda, MD: Author.

National Mental Health Association. (1988). *Report of the National Action Commission on the Mental Health of Rural Americans.* Alexandria, VA: Author.

National PTA. (2002). *Bilingual education* [Online]. Available: http://www.pta.org/ptawashington/issues/bilingual.asp

National Sleep Foundation. (1997a). *Omnibus sleep in America poll* [conducted by Louis Harris & Associates]. Washington, DC: Author.

National Sleep Foundation. (1997b, March). *Sleeplessness, pain and the workplace* [poll conducted by Louis Harris & Associates]. Washington, DC: Author.

National Sleep Foundation. (1998). *Omnibus sleep in America poll* [conducted by Louis Harris & Associates]. Washington, DC: Author.

National Sleep Foundation. (1999). *Omnibus sleep in America poll* [conducted by Louis Harris & Associates]. Washington, DC: Author.

National Transportation Safety Board. (1990). *Safety study: Fatigue, alcohol, other drugs, and medical factors in fatal-to-the-driver heavy truck crashes.* Washington, DC: Author.

Nebbe, L. (1998). *The human–animal bond's role with the abused child.* Paper presented at the 17th Annual Conference of the Delta Society, Seattle, WA.

Newman, E. (1996). *No more test anxiety: Effective steps for taking tests and achieving better grades.* Los Angeles: Learning Skills.

Newman, R. (1995). Psychologist–physician collaboration helps fill primary care gap: Protecting the mind and body of rural America. *Rural Health Bulletin* [Online], 2(1). Available: http://www.apa.org/rural/rbullet2

Nicholson, J. M., & Sanders, M. R. (1999). Randomized controlled trial of behavioral family intervention for the treatment of child behavior problems in stepfamilies. *Journal of Divorce and Remarriage, 30*(3–4), 1–23.

Noer, D. M. (1993). *Healing the wounds: Overcoming the trauma of layoffs and revitalizing downsized organizations.* San Francisco: Jossey-Bass.

Noer, D. M. (1997). *Breaking free.* San Francisco: Jossey-Bass.

Nolen, R. S. (2000, January 1). "Animals helping people; people helping animals": Delta Society to explore influence of animals on human health. *Journal of the American Veterinary Medical Association* [Online]. Available: http://www.avma.org/onlnews/javma/jan00/s010100b.asp

Notarius, C. I., & Markman, H. (Eds.). (1994). *We can work it out: How to solve conflicts, save your marriage, and strengthen your love for each other.* Los Angeles: Perigee.

Novack, D. H., Suchman, A. L., Clark, W., Epstein, R. M., Najberg, E., & Kaplan, C. (1997). Calibrating the physician: Personal awareness and effective patient care. *Journal of the American Medical Association, 278,* 502–509.

Novaco, R. W. (1977). A stress inoculation approach to anger management in the training of law enforcement officers. *American Journal of Community Psychology, 5*(3), 327–346

Novaco, R. W. (1980). Training of probation counselors for anger problems. *Journal of Counseling Psychology, 27*(4), 385–390.

O'Farrell, T. J., Choquette, K. A., & Cutter, H. S. G. (1998). Couples relapse prevention sessions after behavioral marital therapy for male alcoholics: Outcomes during the three years after starting treatment. *Journal of Studies on Alcohol, 59*(4), 357–370.

Okun, B. F. (1996). *Understanding diverse families: What practitioners need to know.* New York: Guilford Press.

Olfson, M. W., Broadhead, E., Weissman, M. M, Leon, A. C., Farber, L., Hoven, C., & Kathol, R. (1996). Subthreshold psychiatric symptoms in a primary care group practice. *Archives of General Psychiatry, 53,* 880–886.

Olfson, M., Shea, S., Feder, A., Milton, P., Fuentes, M., Nomura, Y., Gameroff, M., & Weisman, M. M. (2000). Prevalence of anxiety, depression, and substance use disorders in an urban general medicine practice. *Archives of Primary Care, 9*(9), 876–883.

Oliver, R., Hoover, J. H., & Hazler, R. (1994). The perceived roles of bullying in small-town Midwestern schools. *Journal of Counseling and Development, 72*(4), 416–419.

Olivero, G. M., Bane, K. D., & Kopelman, R. E. (1997). Executive coaching as a transfer of training tool: Effects on productivity in a public agency. *Public Personnel Management, 26*(4), 461–469.

Orange, C. (1997). Gifted students and perfectionism. *Roeper Review, 20*(1), 39–41.

Pace, T. M., Chaney, J. M., Mullins, L. L., & Olson, R. A. (1995). Psychological consultation with primary care physicians: Obstacles and opportunities in the medical setting. *Professional Psychology: Research and Practice, 26*(2), 123–131.

Paige, L. Z. (1993). *The identification and treatment of school phobia.* Silver Spring, MD: National Association of School Psychologists.

Pallak, M. S., Cummings, N. A., Dorken, H., & Henke, C. J. (1995). Effect of mental health treatment on medical costs. *Mind/Body Medicine, 1,* 7–12.

Papas, R. K., Robinson, M. E., & Riley, J. (2001, October). Perceived spouse responsiveness to chronic pain: Three empirical subgroups. *Journal of Pain, 2*(5), 262–269.

Parente, S., Dorosh, L., & Mueller, C. (1998). *Has managed care arrived in rural physician practices?* Bethesda, MD: Project HOPE, Walsh Center for Rural Health Analysis.

Parker, H. (n.d.). *Animal-facilitated therapy at the NIH: Use of animals to ease anxiety and facilitate treatment in children with cancer, AIDS, and other chronic diseases* [Online]. Available: http://www.tufts.edu/vet/cfa/parker.html

Pasley, K., Rhoden, L., Visher, E. B., & Visher, J. S. (1996). Successful stepfamily therapy: Clients' perspectives. *Journal of Marital and Family Therapy, 22*(3), 343–357.

Patterson, G. R., DeGarmo, D. S., & Knutson, N. (2000). Hyperactive and antisocial behaviors: Comorbid or two points in the same process? *Development and Psychopathology, 12,* 91–106.

Paul, G. L. (1966). *Insight versus desensitization in psychotherapy.* Stanford, CA: Stanford University Press.

Pavot, W., & Diener, E. (1993). Review of the Satisfaction with Life Scale. *Psychological Assessment, 5,* 164–172.

Paz, J. (1998). The drug free workplace in rural Arizona. *Alcoholism Treatment Quarterly, 16*(1–2), 133–145.

Pear, R. (2002, March 31). In shift, Medicare has begun funding Alzheimer's care. *New York Times News Service* [Online]. Available: http://www.eldercare.uniontrib.com/news/news_medicalz.cfm

Pedro-Carroll, J. (1998, April 29). Promoting healthy child development: Successful prevention programs for children and families. *APA Congressional Briefing* [Online]. Available: http://www.apa.org/ppo/old/carohl.html

Pelletier, K. R. (1977). *Mind as healer, mind as slayer.* New York: Delacorte Press/Seymour Lawrence.

Perrott, L. A. (1998). When will it be coming to the large discount chain stores?: Psychotherapy as commodity. *Professional Psychology: Research and Practice, 29*(2), 168–173.

Perrott, L. A. (1999). *Reinventing your practice as a business psychologist: A step-by-step guide.* San Francisco: Jossey-Bass.

Peterson, C., Seligman, M. E., & Vaillant, G. E. (1988). Pessimistic explanatory style is a risk factor for physical illness: A thirty-five-year longitudinal study. *Journal of Personality and Social Psychology, 55*(1), 23–27.

Peterson, L., & Shigetomi, C. (1981). The use of coping techniques to minimize anxiety in hospitalized children. *Behavior Therapy, 12*(1), 1–14.

Petitpas, A. J. (1998). Practical considerations in providing psychological services to sports medicine clinic patients. *Journal of Applied Sport Psychology, 10*(1), 157–167.

Petrie, T. A., & Diehl, N. S. (1995). Sport psychology in the profession of psychology. *Professional Psychology: Research and Practice, 26*(3), 288–291.

Pfeiffer, S. I. (2001). Professional psychology and the gifted: Emerging practice opportunities. *Professional Psychology: Research and Practice, 32*(2), 175–180.

Phillips, G. C., Jones, G. E., Rieger, E. J., & Snell, J. B. (1997). Normative data for the Personal Report of Confidence as a Speaker. *Journal of Anxiety Disorders, 11*(2), 215–220.

A physician-centered approach keeps this group's waiting room full. (1997). *Managed Care Strategies, 5*(2), 2–3.

Piechowski, M. M. (1991). Emotional development and emotional giftedness. In N. Colangelo & G. A. Davis (Eds.), *Handbook of gifted education* (pp. 285–306). Boston, MA: Allyn & Bacon.

Plucker, J. A. (1996). Gifted Asian-American students: Identification, curricular, and counseling concerns. *Journal for the Education of the Gifted, 19*(3), 315–343.

Ponterotto, J., & Casas, J. (1987). In search of multicultural competence within counselor education programs. *Journal of Counseling and Development, 65,* 430–434.

Practice building: Six steps to increase your physician referrals. (1995). *Psychotherapy Finances, 21*(3), 1–2.

Pratt, C. A., Nosiri, U. I., & Pratt, C. B. (1997). Michigan physicians' perceptions of their role in managing obesity. *Perceptual and Motor Skills, 84,* 848–850.

Pressman, M. R., & Orr, W. C. (Eds.). (1997). *Understanding sleep: The evaluation and treatment of sleep disorders.* Washington, DC: American Psychological Association.

Price, R. H., & Vinokur, A. D. (1995). Supporting career transitions in a time of organizational downsizing: The Michigan JOBS Program. In M. London (Ed.), *Employees, careers and job creation: Developing growth-oriented human resource strategies and programs* (pp. 191–209). San Francisco: Jossey-Bass.

Primary care docs report poor access to quality mental health care. (1997, November 7). *Psychiatric News* [Online]. Available: http://www.psych.019/pnews/97-11-07/primary.html

Psychological treatments for insomnia: Is there a sleeper effect? (1995). *Clinician's Research Digest: Briefings in Behavioral Science, 13*(12), 5.

Pursch, J. A. (1978). Physicians' attitudinal changes in alcoholism. *Alcoholism: Clinical and Experimental Research, 2*(4), 358–361.

Quackenbush, J. E., & Glickman, L. (1984). Helping people adjust to the death of a pet. *Health and Social Work, 9*(1), 42–48.

Qualls, S. H. (1998). Training in geropsychology: Preparing to meet demand. *Professional Psychology: Research and Practice, 29*(1), 23–28.

Quick, J. C. (1999). Occupational health psychology: The convergence of health and clinical psychology with public health and preventive medicine in an organizational context. *Professional Psychology: Research and Practice, 30,* 123–128.

Raglin, J. S. (1993). Overtraining and staleness: Psychometric monitoring of endurance athletes. In R. N. Singer, M. Murphey, & L. K. Tennant (Eds.), *Handbook of research on sport psychology* (pp. 840–850). New York: Macmillan.

Rainer, J. P. (1998). A family systems approach to grief. In L. VandeCreek, S. Knapp, & T. L. Jackson (Eds.), *Innovations in clinical practice: A source book* (Vol. 16, pp. 179–190).Sarasota, FL: Professional Resource Press.

Rainer, J. P. (2000). Compassion fatigue: When caregiving begins to hurt. In L. VandeCreek & T. L. Jackson (Eds.), *Innovations in clinical practice: A source book* (Vol. 18, pp. 441–453). Sarasota, FL: Professional Resource Press.

Rainey, L. M., & Borders, L. D. (1997). Influential factors in career orientation and career aspiration of early adolescent girls. *Journal of Counseling Psychology, 44*(2), 160–172.

Rando, T. (Ed.). (1986). *Parental loss of a child.* Champaign, IL: Research Press.

Rando, T. (1992). The increasing prevalence of complicated mourning: The onslaught is just beginning. *Omega: Journal of Death and Dying, 26,* 43–59.

Rapee, R. M., & Sanderson, W. C. (1998). *Social phobia: Clinical application of evidence-based psychotherapy.* Northvale, NJ: Aronson.

Raphael, B., Middleton, W., Martinek, N., & Misso, V. (1993). Counseling and therapy of the bereaved. In M. S. Stroebe, W. Stroebe, & R. O. Hansson (Eds.), *Handbook of bereavement : Theory, research, and intervention* (pp. 427–453). New York: Cambridge University Press.

Ray, P. H. (1997, February). The emerging culture. *American Demographics Magazine* [Online]. Available: http://www.demographics.com

Ray, P. H., & Anderson, S. R. (2000). *The cultural creatives: How 50 million people are changing the world.* New York: Harmony Books.

Redinbaugh, E. M., MacCallum, R. C., & Kiecolt-Glaser, J. K. (1995). Recurrent syndromal depression in caregivers. *Psychology and Aging, 10*(3), 358–368.

Regier, D. A., Narrow, W. E., Rae, D. S., Manderscheid, R. W., Locke, B. Z., & Goodwin, F. K. (1993). The de facto U.S. mental and addictive disorders service system: Epidemiologic Catchment Area prospective 1–year prevalence rates of disorders and services. *Archives of General Psychiatry, 50,* 85–94.

Reichert, E. (1994). Play and animal-assisted therapy: A group-treatment model for sexually abused girls ages 9–23. *Family Therapy, 21*(1), 55–62.

Reinecke, M. A., Ryan, N. E., & DuBois, D. L. (1998). Cognitive-behavioral therapy of depression and depressive symptoms during adolescence: A review and meta-analysis. *Journal of the American Academy of Child and Adolescent Psychiatry, 37*(1), 26–34.

Reis, S. M., & McCoach, D. B, (2000). The underachievement of gifted students: What do we know and where do we go? *Gifted Child Quarterly, 44*(3), 152–170.

Reis, S. M., Westberg, K. L., Kulikowich, J. M., & Purcell, J. H. (1998). Curriculum compacting and achievement test scores: What does the research say? *Gifted Child Quarterly, 42*(2), 123–129.

Resnick, P. J., & Kausch, O. (1995). Violence in the workplace: Role of the consultant. *Consulting Psychology Journal: Practice and Research, 47,* 213–222.

Reynolds, D. K. (1990). *Flowing bridges, quiet waters.* Albany: State University of New York Press.

Richardson, V. E. (1993). *Retirement counseling: A handbook for gerontology practitioners.* New York: Springer.

Richeport-Haley, M. (1998). Ethnicity in family therapy: A comparison of brief strategic therapy and culture-focused therapy. *American Journal of Family Therapy, 26*(1), 77–90.

Richmonds, V. P., & McCroskey, J. C. (1998). *Communication: Apprehension, avoidance, and effectiveness* (5th ed.). Boston, MA: Allyn & Bacon.

Rigaud, M.-C., & Flynn, C. F. (1995). Fitness for duty (FFD) evaluation in industrial and military workers. *Psychiatric Annals, 25,* 246–250.

Ritter, K. Y., & Terndrup, A. I. (Eds.). (2002). *Handbook of affirmative psychotherapy with lesbians and gay men.* New York: Guilford Press.

Robert Wood Johnson Foundation. (1996). *Chronic care in America: A 21st century challenge* [Online]. Available: http://www.rwjf.org/main

Robinson, C. R. (1991). *Women, girls, and psychotherapy: Reframing resistance.* Binghamton, NY: Harrington Park Press.

Robinson, T. E., II. (1997). Communication apprehension and the basic public speaking course: A national survey of in-class treatment techniques. *Communication Education, 46*(3), 188–197.

Robinson-Zanartu, C. (1996). Serving Native American children and families: considering cultural variables. *Language, Speech, and Hearing Services in Schools, 27*(4), 373–384.

Roedell, W. C. (1984). Vulnerabilities of highly gifted children. *Roeper Review, 6*(3), 1–5.

Rokke, P. D., & Klenow, D. J. (1999). Prevalence of depressive symptoms among rural elderly: Examining the need for mental health services. *Psychotherapy, 35*(4), 545–558.

Romano, J. M., Turner, J. A., Friedman, L. S., Bulcroft, R. A., Jensen, M. P., & Hops, H. (1991). Observational assessment of chronic pain patient–spouse behavioral interactions. *Behavior Therapy, 22*(4), 549–567.

Rosado, J. W., & Elias, M. J. (1993). Ecological and psychocultural mediators in the delivery of services for urban, culturally diverse Hispanic clients. *Professional Psychology: Research and Practice, 24*(4), 450–459.

Rosen, J, C., Gross, J., & Vara, L. (1987). Psychological adjustment of adolescents attempting to lose or gain weight. *Journal of Consulting and Clinical Psychology, 55*(5), 742–747.

Rosen, R. C., Rosekind, M., Rosevear, C., Cole, W. E., & Dement, W. C. (1993). Physician education in sleep and sleep disorders: A national survey of U.S. medical schools. *Sleep, 16,* 249–254.

Rosenblatt, P. C., de Mik, L., Anderson, R. M., & Johnson, P. A. (1985). *The family in business.* San Francisco: Jossey-Bass.

Ross, P. O. (1993). *National excellence: A case for developing America's talent.* Washington, DC: Office of Educational Research and Improvement, Programs for the Improvement of Practice.

Rowe, J. W., & Kahn, R. L. (1998). *Successful aging.* New York: Pantheon.

Rowell, L. L., McBride, M. C., & Nelson-Leaf, J. (1996). The role of the school counselor in confronting peer sexual harassment. *School Counselor, 43*(3), 196–197.

Royse, D., & Buck, S. A. (1991). Evaluating a diversion program for first-time shoplifters. *Journal of Offender Rehabilitation, 17*(1–2), 147–158.

Rural mental health: Familiar problems in a changing world. (1998, Spring). *Rural Health News* [Online], *4*(3). Available: http://www.muskie.usm.maine.edu/research/ruralheal/ruralnews/ruralMH.html

Rynearson, E. K. (1978). Humans and pets and attachment. *British Journal of Psychiatry, 133,* 550–555.

Sachs, M. L. (1993). Professional ethics in sport psychology. In R. N. Singer, M. Murphey, & L. K. Tennant (Eds.), *Handbook of research on sport psychology* (pp. 921–932). New York: Macmillan.

Sachs, M. L., Burke, K. L., & Schrader, D. C. (Eds.). (2000). *Directory of graduate programs in applied sport psychology* (6th ed.). Morgantown, WV: Fitness Information Technology.

Sadker, D., & Sadker, M. (1994). *Failing at fairness: How America's schools cheat girls.* New York: Scribner.

Salganicoff, M. (1990). Women in family business: Challenges and opportunities. *Family Business Review, 3*(2), 125–137.

Sapadin, L. (1999). *Beat procrastination and make the grade: The six styles of procrastination and how students can overcome them.* New York: Penguin.

Saporito, T. J. (1996). Business-linked executive development: Coaching senior executives. *Consulting Psychology Journal: Practice and Research, 48,* 96–103.

Sarasalo, E., Bergman, B., & Toth, J. (1997). Kleptomania-like behaviour and psychosocial characteristics among shoplifters. *Legal and Criminological Psychology, 2*(Pt. 1), 1–10.

Sartorius, T. B., Ustun, J. A., Costa e Silva, J. A., Goldberg, D., Lecrubier, Y., Ormel, H., & Von Korff, M. (1993). *An international study of psychological problems in primary care* (Preliminary report from the WHO Collaborative Project on Psychological Problems in General Health Care). Geneva: World Health Organization.

Saunders, T., Driskell, J. E., Johnston, J. H., & Salas, E. (1996). The effect of stress inoculation training on anxiety and performance. *Journal of Occupational Health Psychology, 1*(2), 170–186.

Schaie, K. W. (1994). The course of adult intellectual development. *American Psychologist, 49*(4), 304–313.

Schaie, K. W. (1996). *Intellectual development in adulthood: The Seattle Longitudinal Study.* New York: Cambridge University Press.

Schank, J. A. (1998). Ethical issues in rural counselling practice. *Canadian Journal of Counselling, 32*(4), 270–283.

Schank, J. A., & Skovholt, T. M. (1997). Dual-relationship dilemmas of rural and small-community psychologists. *Professional Psychology: Research and Practice, 28*(1), 44–49.

Schneier, F., & Welkowitz, L. (1996). *The hidden face of shyness: Understanding and overcoming social anxiety.* New York: Avon Books.

Schoen, C., Davis, K. S., Collins, L., Greenberg, C., Des Roches, C., & Abrams, M. (1997). *The Commonwealth Fund survey of the health of adolescent girls.* New York: Commonwealth Fund.

Schoenberger, N. E., Kirsch, I., Gearan, P., Montgomery, G., & Pastyrnak, S. L. (1997). Hypnotic enhancement of a cognitive behavioral treatment for public speaking anxiety. *Behavior Therapy, 28*(1), 127–140.

Schonert-Reichl, K. A., & Muller, J. R. (1996). Correlates of help-seeking in adolescence. *Journal of Youth and Adolescence, 25*(6), 705–731.

Schroeder, C. S. (1997). Psychologists and pediatricians in collaborative practice. In R. Resnick & R. H. Rozensky (Eds.), *Health psychology through the life span: Practice and research opportunities* (pp. 109–131). Washington, DC: American Psychological Association.

Schulz, M. S., & Masek, B. J. (1996, April). Medical crisis intervention with children and adolescents with chronic pain. *Professional Psychology: Research and Practice, 27*(2), 121–129.

Schwartz, L., Slater, M. A., & Birchler, G. R. (1994). Interpersonal stress and pain behaviors in patients with chronic pain. *Journal of Consulting and Clinical Psychology, 62*(4), 861–864.

Schwartz, S., & Wood, H. V. (1991). Clinical assessment and intervention with shoplifters. *Social Work, 36*(3), 234–238.

Schweinhart, L., & Weikart, D. (1986). Consequences of three preschool curriculum models through age 15. *Early Childhood Research Quarterly, 1*(1), 15–45.

Scogin, F., & McElreath, L. (1994). Efficacy of psychosocial treatments for geriatric depression: A quantitative review. *Journal of Consulting and Clinical Psychology, 62*(1), 69–73.

Scogin, F., Jamison, C., & Gochneaur, K. (1989).Comparative efficacy of cognitive and behavioral bibliotherapy for mildly and moderately depressed older adults. *Journal of Consulting and Clinical Psychology, 57*(3), 403–407.

Seligman, M. E. P. (1990). *Learned optimism.* New York: Knopf.

Seligman, M. E. P. (1998a, April 29). Opening remarks of Martin Seligman, PhD. *APA Congressional Briefing* [Online]. Available: http://www.apa.org/ppo/marty.html

Seligman, M. E. P. (1998b). *Positive psychology network concept paper* [Online]. Available: http://www.positivepsychology.org/ppgrant.htm

Seligman, M. E. P., & Csikszentmihalyi, M. (2000). Positive psychology: An introduction. *American Psychologist, 55*(1), 5–14.

Seligman, M. E. P., with Reivich, K., Jaycox, L., & Gillham, J. (1995). *The optimistic child.* Boston: Houghton Mifflin.

Sharkin, B. S., & Knox, D. (2003). Pet loss: Issues and implications for the psychologist. *Professional Psychology: Research and Practice, 34*(4), 414–421.

Shaywitz, S. E., Shaywitz, B. A., Fletcher, J. M., & Escobar, M. D. (1990). Prevalence of reading disability in boys and girls: Results of the Connecticut Longitudinal Study. *Journal of the American Medical Association, 264*(8), 998–1002.

Sheehan, N., & Nuttall, P. (1988). Conflict, emotion, and personal strain among family caregivers. *Family Relations, 37,* 92–98.

Shell Oil Company. (1999). *News release: America's teens speak out: Pressures many, but future looks bright. Shell Survey, 1999.* (Available from Shell's media line: 713-241-4544)

Shipherd, J. C., Beck, J. G., Hamblen, J. L., & Freeman, J. B. (2000). Assessment and treatment of PTSD in motor vehicle accident survivors. In L. VandeCreek & T. L. Jackson (Eds.), *Innovations in clinical practice: A source book* (Vol. 18, pp. 132–135). Sarasota, FL: Professional Resource Press.

Shneidman, E. S., Farberow, N. L., & Litman, R. E. (Eds.). (1995). *The psychology of suicide.* New York: Science House.

Shuer, M. L., & Dietrich, M. S. (1997). Psychological effects of chronic injury in elite athletes. *Western Journal of Medicine, 166,* 104–109.

Silverman, A. R., & Feigelman, W. (1990). Adjustment in interracial adoptees: An overview. In D. M. Brodzinsky & M. D. Schechter (Eds.), *The psychology of adoption* (pp. 187–200). New York: Oxford University Press.

Silverman, E., Range, L., & Overholser, J. C. (1994–1995). Bereavement from suicide as compared to other forms of bereavement. *Omega: Journal of Death and Dying, 30*(1), 41–51.

Silverman, L. K. (1983). Personality development: The pursuit of excellence. *Journal for the Education of the Gifted, 6*(1), 5–19.

Silverman, L. K. (1986). Parenting young gifted children. In J. R. Whitmore (Ed.), *Intellectual giftedness in young children* (pp. 73–87). New York: Haworth Press.

Silvia, E. S., & Thorne, J. (1997). *School-based drug prevention programs: A longitudinal study in selected school districts.* (Available from Research Triangle Institute, 3040 Cornwallis Road, Research Triangle Park, NC 27709; 919-541-6000)

Simantov, E., Schoen, C., & Klein J. D. (2000). Health-compromising behaviors: Why do adolescents smoke or drink? Identifying underlying risk and protective factors. *Archives of Pediatric Adolescent Medicine, 154,* 1025–1033.

Simek, T. C., & O'Brien, R. M. (1981). *Total golf: A behavioral approach to lowering your score and getting more out of your game.* New York: Doubleday.

Simmons, J. W., Avant, W. S., Demski, J., & Parisher, D. (1988). Determining successful pain clinic treatment through validation of cost effectiveness. *Spine, 13,* 342–344.

Simon, E. P., & Folen, R. A. (2001). The role of the psychologist on the multidisciplinary pain management team. *Professional Psychology: Research and Practice, 32*(2), 125–134.

Simon, R. J., Altstein, H., & Melli, M. S. (1994). *The case for transracial adoption.* Washington, DC: American University Press.

Sirkin, M. I. (1996, May–June). Consulting to family businesses: The dollars and sense of family values. *Networker*, pp. 71–78.

Skinner, W. F. (1994). The prevalence and demographic predictors of illicit and licit drug use among lesbians and gay men. *American Journal of Public Health, 84,* 1307–1310.

Slomski, A. J. (2000, June 5). What a behavioral specialist could add to your practice. *Medical Economics, 77*(11), 149–150.

Smith, D. (2001, September). Sleep psychologists in demand: The success of cognitive behavioral therapy has made behavioral sleep medicine a fast-growing field. *APA Monitor*, pp. 36–39.

Smith, R. E., Smoll, F. L., & Curtis, B. (1979). Coach effectiveness training: A cognitive behavioral approach to enhancing relationship skills in youth sport coaches. *Journal of Sports Psychology, 1,* 59–75.

Snook, P., Hyman, I., Brown, R., Waren, L., DuCette, J., & Savage, S. (1999). *Do dangerous schools produce dangerous students?: Conceptualizing and measuring Student Alienation Syndrome.* Paper presented at the 107th Annual Convention of the American Psychological Association, Boston.

Snowdon, D. A., Kemper, S. J., Mortimer, J. A., Greiner, L. H., Wekstein, D. R., & Markesbery, W. R. (1996). Linguistic ability in early life and cognitive function and Alzheimer's disease in late life: Findings from the Nun Study. *Journal of the American Medical Association, 275*(7), 528–532.

Sobel, D. S. (1995). Rethinking medicine: Improving health outcomes with cost-effective psychosocial interventions. *Psychosomatic Medicine, 57,* 234–244.

Solomon, C. R. (1995). The importance of mother–child relations in studying stepfamilies. *Journal of Divorce and Remarriage, 24*(1–2), 89–98.

Solomon, G. S., & Ray, J. B. (1984). Irrational beliefs of shoplifters. *Journal of Clinical Psychology, 40*(4), 1075–1077.

Somerville, K. (1998). Where is the business of business psychology headed? *Consulting Psychology Journal: Practice and Research, 50,* 237–241.

Sommers, C. (1999, October 17). By the way; working wonders. *New York Times,* Sect. 14NJ, p. 3.

Sperry, L. (1993). Working with executives: Consulting, counseling, and coaching. *Individual Psychology: Journal of Adlerian Theory, Research and Practice, 49*(2), 257–266.

Spiegel, D. (1996). Cancer and depression. *British Journal of Psychiatry*, Suppl.(30) 109–116.

Spiegel, D., & Classen, C. (2000). *Group therapy for cancer patients: A research-based handbook of psychosocial care.* New York: Basic Books.

Spiegel, D., & Sands, S. H. (1988). Pain management in the cancer patient. *Journal of Psychosocial Oncology, 6*(3–4), 205–216.

Spitzer, R. L., Kroenke, K., Linzer, M., Hahn, S. R., Williams, J. B., deGruy, F. V., III, Brody, D., & Davies, M. (1995). Health-related quality of life in primary care patients with mental disorders: Results from the PRIME-MD 1000 Study. *Journal of the American Medical Association, 274*(19), 1511–1517.

Spitzer, R. L., Kroenke, K., & Williams, J. B. (1999). Validation and utility of a self-report version of PRIME-MD: The PHQ primary care study. Primary Care Evaluation of Mental Disorders. Patient Health Questionnaire. *Journal of the American Medical Association, 282*(18), 1737–1744.

Sprang, G. (1997). Victim impact panels: An examination of the effectiveness of this program on lowering recidivism and changing offenders' attitudes about drinking and driving. *Journal of Social Service Research, 22*(3), 73–84.

Stacks, D. W., & Stone, J. D. (1984). An examination of the effect of basic speech courses, self-concept, and self-disclosure on communication apprehension. *Communication Education, 33,* 317–331.

Stanley, S., Trathen, D. W., & Bryan, B. M. (1998). *A lasting promise: A Christian guide to fighting for your marriage.* San Francisco: Jossey-Bass.

Statistical Assessment Service. (1997, August 1). *Interracial marriage* [Online]. Available: http://www.stats.org/record.jsp?type=news&ID=22

Stefan, S. (2000). Unequal rights: Discrimination against people with mental disabilities and the Americans with Disabilities Act. Washington, DC: American Psychological Association.

Stein, M. B., Walker, J. R., & Forde, D. R. (1996). Public speaking fears in a community sample: Prevalence, impact on functioning, and diagnostic classification. *Archives of General Psychiatry, 53*(2), 169–174.

Stepfamilies. (1998, December). *Psychotherapy Finances,* p. 8.

Sternberg, R. J. (1996a). Equal protection under the law: What is missing in education. *Psychology, Public Policy, and Law, 2*(3–4), 575–583.

Sternberg, R. J. (1996b). The sound of silence: A nation responds to its gifted. *Roeper Review, 18*(3), 168–172.

Sternberg, R. J. (1997). *Thinking styles.* New York: Cambridge University Press.

Sternberg, R. J., & Lubart, T. I. (1996). Investing in creativity. *American Psychologist, 51*(7), 677–688.

Stewart, M. F. (1999). *Companion animal death: A practical and comprehensive guide for veterinary practice.* Boston: Butterworth-Heinemann.

Stiles, P. G., & McGarrahan, J. F. (1998). The Geriatric Depression Scale: A comprehensive review. *Journal of Clinical Geropsychology, 4*(2), 89–110.

Stinson, B. L., II, Friedberg, R. D., Page, R. A., & Cusak, M. J. (2000). Improving athletic performance and motivating athletes. In L. VandeCreek & T. L. Jackson (Eds.), *Innovations in clinical practice: A source book* (Vol. 18, pp. 349–367). Sarasota, FL: Professional Resource Press.

Stipek, D. J., & Gralinski, J. H. (1991). Gender differences in children's achievement-related beliefs and emotional responses to success and failure in mathematics. *Journal of Educational Psychology, 83*(3), 361–371.

Stitt-Gohdes, W. L. (1997). *Career development: Issues of gender, race, and class* (Information Series No. 371). Columbus, OH: ERIC Clearinghouse on Adult, Career, and Vocational Education. (ERIC Document Reproduction Service No. ED413533)

Stoltz, P. (1997). *Adversity quotient: Turning obstacles into opportunities.* New York: Wiley.

Straatmeyer, A. J., & Watkins, J. T. (1974). Rational-emotive therapy and the reduction of speech anxiety. *Rational Living, 9*(1), 33–37.

Strawbridge, W., & Wallhagen, M. (1991). Impact of family conflict on adult–child caregivers. *The Gerontologist, 31,* 770–777.

Striegel-Moore, R. H., & Cachelin, F. M. (1999). Body image concerns and disordered eating in adolescent girls: Risk and protective factors. In N. G. Johnson,

M. C. Roberts, & J. Worell (Eds.), *Beyond appearance: A new look at adolescent girls* (pp. 85–108). Washington, DC: American Psychological Association.

Study: Exercise treats elderly depression [Online]. (2000). Available: http://www.abcnews.go.com/sections/living/DailyNews/depression_elderly000921.html

Sue, S. (1977). Community mental health services to minority groups: Some optimism, some pessimism. *American Psychologist, 32*, 616–624.

Sue, S. (1998). In search of cultural competence in psychotherapy and counseling. *American Psychologist, 53*(4), 440–448.

Sue, S., Fujino, D., Hu, L., Takeuchi, D., & Zane, N. (1991). Community mental health services for ethnic minority groups: A test of the cultural responsiveness hypothesis. *Journal of Consulting and Clinical Psychology, 59*, 533–540.

Sue, S., & Zane, N. (1987). The role of culture and cultural techniques in psychotherapy: A critique and reformulation. *American Psychologist, 42*, 37–45.

Suinn, R. M. (1997). Working with cancer patients: Expanding your practice. *Independent Practitioner, 17*(2), 82–85.

Survey says: Owners taking good care of their pets. (2000, February 1). *Journal of the American Veterinary Medical Association* [Online]. Available: http://www.avma.org/onlnews/javma/feb00/s020100d.asp

Takeuchi, D. T., Sue, S., & Yeh, M. (1995). Return rates and outcomes from ethnicity-specific mental health programs in Los Angeles. *American Journal of Public Health, 85*, 638–643.

Tamblyn, R., Berkson, L., Dauphinee, W. D., Gayton, D., Grad, R., Huang, A., Isaac, L., McLeod, P., & Snell, L. (1997). Unnecessary prescribing of NSAIDs and the management of NSAID-related gastropathy in medical practice. *Annals of Internal Medicine, 127*, 429–438.

Tarkan, L. (2000, September 26). Athletes' injuries go beyond the physical. *The New York Times,* Sect. F, p. 7.

Taylor, A. W. (1992). Ageing: A normal degenerative process—with or without regular exercise. *Canadian Journal of Sport Sciences, 17*(3), 163–167.

Tebbutt, J., Swanston, H., Oates, R. Kim, A., & O'Toole, B. I. (1997). Five years after child sexual abuse: Persisting dysfunction and problems of prediction. *Journal of the American Academy of Child and Adolescent Psychiatry, 36*(3), 330–340.

Technology: 9 steps for building a cheap and easy Web site. (2002, October). *Psychotherapy Finances* [Online], *28*(10). Available: http://www.psyfin.com/articles/021002.htm

Teno, J. M., Weitzen, S., Wetle, T., & Mor, V. (2001). Persistent pain in nursing home residents. *Journal of the American Medical Association, 285*(16), 2081.

Tharinger, D. J., Lambert, N. M., Bricklin, P. M., Feshbach, N., Johnson, N. F., Oakland, T. D., Paster, V. S., & Sanchez, W. (1996, February). Education reform: Challenges for psychology and psychologists. *Professional Psychology: Research and Practice, 27*(1), 24–33

Thompson, L. W., Gallagher, D., & Breckenridge, J. S. (1987). Comparative effectiveness of psychotherapies for depressed elders. *Journal of Consulting and Clinical Psychology, 55*(3), 385–390.

Thorpe, G. L., Amatu, H. I., Blakey, R. S., & Burns, L. E. (1976). Contribution of overt instructional rehearsal and specific insight to the effectiveness of self-instructional training: A preliminary study. *Behavior Therapy, 4*, 504–511.

Tiemens, B. G., Ormel, J., & Simon, G. E. (1996). Occurrence, recognition, and outcome of psychological disorders in primary care. *American Journal of Psychiatry, 153*(4), 636–644.

Tobin, T. J., & Sugai, G. M. (1999). Using sixth grade school reports to predict violence, chronic discipline problems, and high school outcomes. *Journal of Emotional and Behavioral Disorders, 7*(1), 40–53.

Tong, C. (1998). *Are you an architect of trust?* [Online]. Available: http://www.feel. org/article/trust.html

Trent, J. T. (1998, July/August). Forensic psychology: Rewarding the risks? *National Psychologist*, p. 8.

Turk, D. C., & Melzack, R. (Eds.). (2001). *Handbook of pain assessment* (2nd ed.). New York: Guilford Press.

Uchino, B., Kiecolt-Glaser, J., & Cacioppo, J. (1994). Construals of pre-illness relationship quality predict cardiovascular response in family caregivers of Alzheimer's disease victims. *Psychology and Aging, 9*, 113–120.

Udry, E., Gould, D., Bridges, D., & Tuffey, S. (1997). People helping people?: Examining the social ties of athletes coping with burnout and injury stress. *Journal of Sport and Exercise Psychology, 19*(4), 368–395.

Underwood, M. (1992). The older driver: Clinical assessment and injury prevention. *Archives of Internal Medicine, 152*(4), 735–740.

Ungerleider, S. (1995). *Mental training for peak performance.* Emmaus, PA: Rodale Press.

U.S. Bureau of the Census. (1995). *Statistical abstract of the United States* (115th ed.). Washington, DC: U.S. Government Printing Office.

U.S. Bureau of the Census. (1997). *Disabilities affect one-fifth of all americans proportion could increase in coming decades* [Online]. Available: http://www.census.gov/prod/3/97pubs/cenbr975.pdf

U.S. Bureau of the Census. (2000). *Census 2000 summary file 1: 1990 census of population, general population, characteristics, United States* (1990 CP-1–1). Washington, DC: U.S. Government Printing Office.

U.S. Bureau of the Census. (2001). *Population by race and hispanic or latino origin for the United States: 1990 and 2000* [Online]. Available: http://www.census.gov/population/cen2000/phc-t1/tab01.pdf

U.S. Bureau of the Census. (2003). *State and county QuickFacts* [Online]. Available: http://quickfacts.census.gov/qfd/states/00000.html

U.S. Bureau of Prisons. (2003). *Employment* [Online]. Available: http://www.bop.gov

Vagg, P. R., & Papsdorf, J. D. (1995). Cognitive therapy, study skills training, and biofeedback in the treatment of test anxiety. In C. D. Spielberger & P. R. Vagg (Eds.), *Test anxiety: Theory, assessment, and treatment* (pp. 183–194). Washington, DC: Taylor & Francis.

Van der Hart, O. (1988). An imaginary leave-taking ritual in mourning therapy: A brief communication. *International Journal of Clinical and Experimental Hypnosis, 36*(2), 63–69.

VanFleet, R. (1994). *Filial therapy: Strengthening parent–child relationships through play.* Sarasota, FL: Professional Resource Press.

VanFleet, R. (2000). Short-term play therapy for families with chronic illness. In H. G. Kaduson & C. E. Schaefer (Eds.), *Short-term play therapy for children* (pp. 175–193). New York: Guilford Press.

Van Raalte, J. L., & Williams, J. M. (1994). *Graduate training and career possibilities in exercise and sport psychology* [Online]. Available: http://www.psyc.unt.edu/apadiv47/careers

Vargas, L. A., & Koss-Chioino, J. D. (Eds.). (1992). *Working with culture: Psychotherapeutic interventions with ethnic minority children and adolescents.* San Francisco: Jossey-Bass.

Vinturella, J., Elstrott, J. B., & Galiano, A. (1994, July 28–30). *University programs for family businesses: Survey and projections.* Paper presented at Strategies for Growth: Inaugural Conference of the International Family Business Program Association, Portsmouth, NH.

Violence in the workplace: Employers' concerns on the rise. (1997, March 24). *Business Wire.*

Vroegh, K. S. (1997). Transracial adoptees: Developmental status after 17 years. *American Journal of Orthopsychiatry, 67*(4), 568–575.

Vuchinich, S., Vuchinich, R. A., Hetherington, E. M., & Clingempeel, W. G. (1991). Parent–child interaction and gender differences in early adolescents' adaptation to stepfamilies. *Developmental Psychology, 27,* 618–626.

Wachelka, D., & Katz, R. C. (1999). Reducing test anxiety and improving academic self-esteem in high school and college students with learning disabilities. *Journal of Behavior Therapy and Experimental Psychiatry, 30*(3), 191–198.

Wagner, A. (2000, October 16). *Suicide rate in rural areas soars* [Online]. Available: http://www.saljournal.com/stories/101500/lif_ap_suicide.html

Waldren, T., Bell, N. J., Peek, C. W., & Sorell, G. (1990). Cohesion and adaptability in post-divorce remarried and first married families: Relationships with family stress and coping styles. *Journal of Divorce and Remarriage, 14,* 13–27.

Walfish, S. (2001, August). *Clinical practice strategies outside the realm of managed care.* Paper presented at the 109th Annual Convention of the American Psychological Association, San Francisco.

Walker, A., Martin, S., & Jones, L. (1992). The benefits and costs of caregiving and care receiving for daughters and mothers. *Journal of Gerontology: Social Sciences, 47,* 130–139.

Warmoth, A., Resnick, S., & Serlin, I. (n.d.). *Contributions of humanistic psychology to positive psychology* [Online]. Available: http://www.westga.edu/~psydept/os2/papers/serlin2.htm

Weaver, A. J., Samford, J. A., Kline, A. E., Lucas, L. A., Larson, D. B., & Koenig, H. G. (1997). What do psychologists know about working with the clergy?: An analysis of eight APA journals, 1991–1994. *Professional Psychology: Research and Practice, 28*(5), 471–474.

Weinberger, L. E., & Sreenivasan, S. (1994). Ethical and professional conflicts in correctional psychology. *Professional Psychology: Research and Practice, 25*(2), 161–167.

Weisinger, H. D., & Williams, S. (Eds.). (1997). *Emotional intelligence at work: The untapped edge for success.* San Francisco: Jossey-Bass.

Weiss, A. (1992). *Million dollar consulting: The professional's guide to growing a practice.* New York: McGraw-Hill.

Weisz, J. R., Weiss, B., Han, S. S., Granger, D. A., & Morton, T. (1995). Effects of psychotherapy with children revisited: A meta-analysis of treatment outcome studies. *Psychological Bulletin, 117*(3), 450–468.

Wells, M. (1998). *Dog presence effects on children's stress responses during medical procedures*. Paper presented at the 17th Annual Conference of the Delta Society, Seattle, WA.

Wessels, D. T. (1984). Family psychotherapy methodology: A model for veterinarians and clinicians. In W. J. Kay, H. A. Nieburg, A. H. Kutscher, & L. G. Kutscher (Eds.), *Pet loss and human bereavement* (pp. 175–184). Ames: Iowa State University Press.

Whelan, J. P., Meyers, A. W., & Elkins, T. D. (2002). Ethics in sport and exercise psychology. In J. L. Van Raalte & B. W. Brewer (Eds.), *Exploring sport and exercise psychology* (2nd ed., pp. 503–523). Washington, DC: American Psychological Association.

Whitmore, J., & Maker, J. (1985). *Intellectual giftedness among disabled persons*. Rockville, MD: Aspen Press.

Whitworth, R. H., & Cochran, C. (1996). Evaluation of integrated versus unitary treatments for reducing public speaking anxiety. *Communication Education, 45*, 306–314.

Wiesendanger, B. (1995). Shrink rap. *Journal of Business Strategy, 16*(1), 22–29.

Wilbur, R. H. (1976). Pets, pet ownership, and animal control: Social and psychological attitudes. In *Proceedings of the National Conference on Dog and Cat Control* (pp. 21–34). Chicago: American Veterinary Medicine Association.

Wildenhaus, K. J. (1997). Sport psychology services in a clinical practice. In L. VandeCreek, S. Knapp, & T. L. Jackson (Eds.), *Innovations in clinical practice* (Vol. 15, pp. 365–383). Sarasota, FL: Professional Resource Press.

Williams, J. M., & Andersen, M. B. (1998). Psychosocial antecedents of sport injury: Review and critique of the stress and injury model. *Journal of Applied Sport Psychology, 10*(1), 5–25.

Williams, R. A., Pruitt, S. D., Doctor, J. N., Epping-Jordan, J. E., Wahlgren, D. R., Grant, I., & Patterson, T. L. (1998). The contribution of job satisfaction to the transition from acute to chronic low back pain. *Archives of Physical Medicine and Rehabilitation, 79*(4), 366–374.

Winn, N. N., & Priest, R. (1993) . Counseling biracial children: A forgotten component of muticultural counseling. *Family Therapy. 20*(1) 29–36.

Winner, E. (1996). *Gifted children: Myths and realities*. New York: Basic Books.

Winner, E. (2000). The origins and ends of giftedness. *American Psychologist, 55*(1) 159–169.

Wolfson, A. R., & Carskadon, M. A. (1998, August). Sleep schedules and daytime functioning in adolescents. *Child Development, 69*(4),875–887.

Woody, S. R., Chambless, D. L., & Glass, C. R. (1997). Self-focused attention in the treatment of social phobia. *Behaviour Research and Therapy, 35*(2), 117–129.

Worden, J. W., & Silverman, P. R. (1996). Parental death and the adjustment of school-age children. *Omega: Journal of Death and Dying, 33*(2), 91–102.

Workers comp: Tapping underdeveloped markets: Managing pain with group therapy. (1997). *Managed Care Strategies, 5*(6), 1–3.

Worthington, E. L., Tipton, R. M., Cromley, J. S., Richards, T., & Janke, R. H. (1984). Speech and coping skills training and paradox as treatment for college students anxious about public speaking. *Perceptual and Motor Skills, 59*(2), 394.

Wright, J. V. (1995). Multicultural issues and attention deficit disorders. *Learning Disabilities: Research and Practice, 10*(3), 153–159.

Yeh, M., Takeuchi, D. T., & Sue, S. (1994). Asian American children in the mental health system: A comparison of parallel and mainstream outpatient service centers. *Journal of Clinical Child Psychology, 23,* 5–12.

Young, L. D., Bradley, L. A., & Turner, R. A. (1995). Decreases in health care resource utilization in patients with rheumatoid arthritis following a cognitive behavioral intervention. *Biofeedback and Self-Regulation, 20*(3), 259–268.

Young, T., Blustein, J., Finn, L. I., & Palta, M. (1997). Sleep-disordered breathing and motor vehicle accidents in a population-based sample of employed adults. *Sleep, 20*(8), 608–613.

Zarit, S. H., & Knight, B. G. (1996). *A guide to psychotherapy and aging.* Washington, DC: American Psychological Association.

Zarit, S. H., & Zarit, J. M. (1998). *Mental disorders in older adults: Fundamentals of assessment and treatment.* New York: Guilford Press.

Zaubler, T. S., & Katon, W. (1996). Panic disorder and medical comorbidity: A review of the medical and psychiatric literature. *Bulletin of the Menninger Clinic, 60*(2, Suppl. A), A12–A38.

Zeidner, M. (1998). *Test anxiety: The state of the art.* New York: Plenum Press.

Zeilinski, J. J. (1999). Discovering Imago relationship therapy. *Psychotherapy, 36*(1), 91–101.

Zeiss, A. M., Lewinsohn, P. M., Rohde, P., & Seeley, J. R. (1996). Relationship of physical disease and functional impairment to depression in older people. *Psychology and Aging, 11*(4), 572–581.

Zemore, R. (1975). Systematic desensitization as a method of teaching a general anxiety-reducing skill. *Journal of Consulting and Clinical Psychology, 43*(2), 157–161.

Zimbardo, P. (1990). *Shyness: What it is, what to do about it.* Reading, MA: Addison-Wesley.

Zimmerman, B. J., Greenberg, D., & Weinstein, C. E. (1994). Self-regulating academic study time: A strategy approach. In D. H. Schunk & B. J. Zimmerman (Eds.), *Self-regulation of learning and performance: Issues and educational applications* (pp. 181–199). Hillsdale, NJ: Erlbaum.

Zimmerman, M. A., & Wienckowski, L. A. (1991). Revisiting health and mental health linkages: A policy whose time has come . . . again. *Journal of Public Health Policy, 12,* 510–524.

Zur, O. (2000). Marketing 101. *Independent Practitioner, 20*(1), 28–31.

Zwillich, T. (1998). Small fish swims in managed care sea. *Clinical Psychiatry News, 26*(1), 1.

Index

READER FEEDBACK REQUEST LETTER

Dear Reader,

We hope this book has helped you, and we ask you to tell us about what you found valuable, or not, so that we might make it even more useful. Please take the time to tell us; we promise to listen carefully, get back to you if we have questions, and use your comments to improve the next edition of this book.

1. What are your current *major* professional activities?

_____

_____

2. What has caused you to consider diversifying into a other practice areas?

_____

_____

3. Which practice specializations in this book appeal most to you?

_____

_____

4. Which practice specializations do you wish we had explored for you?

_____

_____

_____

5. We know we have missed materials about each niche. Please help us by telling us of additional materials you found valuable which should be added for the next edition of this book.

Specialization: Resource(s) to be added:

_____   _____

_____   _____

_____   _____

6. If you have additional experiences with a specialization not covered, won't you please tell us about the specialization and of your preparation, difficulties, successes, tricks you learned, satisfactions, or whatever will help our colleagues? Please note the area here and tell us more by mail or e-mail.

_____

_____

Here is how to reach us: Rona LoPresti or Edward L. Zuckerman, P. O. Box 222, Armbrust, PA 15616; or e-mail: mail@nichesforclinicians.

Thank you, and best wishes for a satisfying and prosperous professional life.

Rona and Ed

Visit our Web site (http://www.nichesforclinicians.com) for more information on these and other niche opportunities, and for updated information that we have collected or that people like you have sent to us. All of the URLs from this book can be copied and pasted from the site, so you do not have to type them in.